ADVANCED SURGICAL RECALL
2nd edition

"'SCUT'. . . . . Forgive me for this; I HATE this word. Ward work is patient care. It's the work of Angels and Saints. It is a privilege to do. It's fun. It is necessary to the care of patients. If you call this patient care scut, you (and your protégés) won't do it. If you call an admission a 'hit,' you won't take care of them. Your language defines your feelings. Your feelings determine what you have energy for. I get energy from getting a patient a cup of coffee, drawing their blood well, and closing their skin in a nice manner. . . . . as much energy as I get from transplanting their hearts and lungs, and bypassing their vessels. I can't do what I don't have energy for."

—Curt Tribble, M.D.

2nd Edition

ADVANCED SURGICAL RECALL
2nd edition

RECALL SERIES EDITOR AND SENIOR EDITOR:

LORNE H. BLACKBOURNE, M.D.
Fellow, Trauma/Critical Care
Department of Surgery
University of Miami
Jackson Memorial Hospital
Miami, Florida

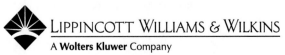
LIPPINCOTT WILLIAMS & WILKINS
A **Wolters Kluwer** Company
Philadelphia · Baltimore · New York · London
Buenos Aires · Hong Kong · Sydney · Tokyo

Editor: Neil Marquardt
Managing Editor: Emilie Linkins
Marketing Manager: Scott Lavine
Production Editor: Christina Remsberg
Compositor: Peirce Graphic Services
Printer: Malloy

Printed in the United States of America

First Edition, 1997

Library of Congress Cataloging-in-Publication Data

The publishers have made every effort to trace the copyright holders for borrowed material. If they have inadvertently overlooked any, they will be pleased to make the necessary arrangements at the first opportunity.

To purchase additional copies of this book, call our customer service department at **(800) 638–3030** or fax orders to **(301) 824–7390**. International customers should call **(301) 714-2324**.

Visit Lippincott Williams & Wilkins on the Internet: http://www.LWW.com. Lippincott Williams & Wilkins customer service representatives are available from 8:30 am to 6:00 pm, EST.

03 04 05 06 07
1 2 3 4 5 6 7 8 9 10

EDITORS:

DAMLE SAGAR
Medical Student
University of Virginia School of Medicine
Charlottesville, Virginia

ANIKAR CHHABRA, MD
Resident in Orthopedic Surgery
University of Virginia School of Medicine
Charlottesville, Virginia

ADVISOR:

CURTIS G. TRIBBLE, MD
Professor and Vice Chairman
Department of Surgery
University of Virginia School of Medicine
Charlottesville, Virginia

ARTIST:

HOLLY FISCHER, MFA

FIRST EDITION EDITORS:

KIRK J. FLEISCHER, M.D.
OLIVER A.R. BINNS, M.D.
TANANCHAI A. LUCKTONG, M.D.
JOSEPH WELLS, M.D.

ASSOCIATE EDITORS, Second Edition

Fellows in Trauma and Critical Care at Ryder Trauma Center, University Of Miami School of Medicine, Miami, Florida:

Fahim Habib, M.D.
Dror Soffer, M.D.
Carl Schulman, M.D.
Teofilo Lama, M.D.
Bruce Crookes, M.D.
Robert Benjamin, M.D.
Jana Macleod, M.D.

Residents in General Surgery, University of Miami School of Medicine, Jackson Memorial Hospital, Miami, Florida:

Tekin Akin, M.D.
Moises Salama, M.D.
Tobi Greene, M.D.

Billy Johnson
Medical Student
University of Hawaii
Hawaii

ASSOCIATE EDITORS, First Edition

Fouad M. Abbas, M.D.
Kyle D. Bickel, M.D.
Duke E. Cameron, M.D.
H. Ballantine Carter, M.D.
Martin A. Goins, III, M.D.
David D. Graham, M.D.
Richard F. Heitmiller, M.D.
David Holt, M.D.
Brian Jones, M.D.
Scott Langenburg, M.D.
John Minasi, M.D.
Stanley L. Minken, M.D.
Michael A. Mont, M.D.
Marcia Moore, M.D.
Paul J. Mosca, M.D., Ph.D.
Charles N. Paidas, M.D.
John Pilcher, M.D.
Donald Schmit, M.D.
R. Scott Stuart, M.D.
Rafael Tamargo, M.D.
Curtis G. Tribble, M.D.

Contributors

The following contributed to the second edition of this book:

Joshua B. Alley, M.D.
General Surgery Resident
Wilford Hall Medical Center
The University of Texas
San Antonio, Texas

Robert Benjamin, M.D.
Fellow-Trauma/Critical Care
Ryder Trauma Center
General Surgery
University of Miami
Miami, Florida

Kyrie Bernstein
Medical Student
University of Virginia School of
    Medicine
Charlottesville, Virginia

Shawn A. Birchenough
Medical Student
University of Virginia School of
    Medicine
Charlottesville, Virginia

Vernon L. Christenson
Medical Student
University of Virginia School of
    Medicine
Charlottesville, Virginia

Sagar Damle
Medical Student
University of Virginia School of
    Medicine
Charlottesville, Virginia

Soffer Dror, M.D.
Trauma/Critical Care
General Surgery
University of Miami
Miami, Florida

Charity Forstmann
Medical Student
University of Virginia School of
    Medicine
Charlottesville, Virginia

Penelope A. Goode
Medical Student
University of Virginia School of
    Medicine
Charlottesville, Virginia

Sharon Goyal, M.D.
Medical Student
University of Virginia School of
    Medicine
Charlottesville, Virginia

Tobi Greene, M.D.
General Surgery
Jackson Memorial Hospital
University of Miami
Miami, Florida

Fahim Habib, M.D.
Fellow—Trauma/Surgical Critical
    Care
Ryder Trauma Center
Jackson Memorial Hospital
University of Miami
Miami, Florida

Huntington Hapworth
Medical Student
University of Virginia School of
    Medicine
Charlottesville, Virginia

Teofilo R. Lama, M.D.
Surgery
Jackson Memorial Hospital
Ryder Trauma Center
Miami, Florida

Jana B.A. MacLeod, M.D., MSC
    FRCS (C)
General Surgery
University of Miami
Miami, Florida

Nancy E. Morefield
Medical Student
University of Virginia School of
    Medicine
Charlottesville, Virginia

Mark Mossey
Medical Student
University of Virginia School of
    Medicine
Charlottesville, Virginia

Cherie D. Quesenberry
Medical Student
University of Virginia School of
    Medicine
Charlottesville, Virginia

Moises Salama, M.D.
Resident in General Surgery
University of Miami
Miami, Florida

Carl Schulman, M.D.
Fellow—Trauma/Critical Care
Department of Surgery
University of Miami
Miami, Florida

Akin Tekin, M.D.
Resident in General Surgery
University of Miami
Miami, Florida

Stephanie VanDuzer
Medical Student
University of Virginia School of
    Medicine
Charlottesville, Virginia

Jim Soo Yoo, M.D.
Resident in General Surgery
Duke University Medical Center
Raleigh-Durham, North Carolina

Stephen Yung
Medical Student
University of Virginia
Charlottesville, Virginia

Amer Ziauddin
Medical Student
University of Virginia School of
    Medicine
Charlottesville, Virginia

Contributors to First Edition:

Gina Adrales, M.D.
Stephen Bayne, M.D.
Gauri Bedi, M.D.
Oliver A.R. Binns, M.D.
Lorne H. Blackbourne, M.D.
Carol Bognar
Lee Butterfield, M.D.
Sung W. Choi, M.D.
Jeffery Cope, M.D.
Jennifer Deblasi, B.S.
Matthew Edwards, M.D.
Brian Ferris, M.D.
Anne C. Fischer, M.D.
Kirk J. Fleischer, M.D.
Cynthia Gingalewski, M.D.
Thomas Gleason, M.D.
David D. Graham, M.D.
Sean P. Hedican, M.D.
Stanley "Duke" Herrel, M.D.
Jason Lamb, M.D.
Scott London, M.D.
Tananchai A Lucktong, M.D.
Peter Mattei, M.D.
Addison May, M.D.

Joseph R. McShannic, M.D.
Paul Mosca, M.D.
David Musante, M.D.
Mark J. Pidala, M.D.
John Pilcher, M.D.
Philip Pollice, M.D.
Naveen Reddy, M.D.
Brian Romaneschi, M.D.
Janice Ryu, M.D.
Robert E. Schmieg, Jr., M.D.
Donald B. Schmit, M.D.
Paul Shin, B.A.
Kimberly Sinclair, M.S.
John Sperling, M.D.
Pierre Theodore, M.D.
Steven D. Theis, M.D.
Michael Tjarksen, M.D.
Jeffry Watson, M.D.
Mark Watts, M.D.
Joseph Wells, M.D.
David White, M.D.
Kate Willcutts
Jonathan Winograd, M.D.

Disclaimer

This book is intended to be a study guide for the acquisition of basic surgical facts and should not be used to guide patient care.

Dedication

This book is dedicated to my father, Dr. Brian D. Blackbourne, M.D. and my wife, Patricia Stuart Blackbourne.

Lorne H. Blackbourne, M.D.

Foreword

Advanced Surgical Recall is a study aid for students and residents who have progressed past their introductory experiences in the discipline of surgery. In actuality, this group includes surgical residents, senior medical students, and even junior medical students who have progressed past the usual introductory materials. This book should also serve as a source of questions for teachers of surgery, particularly for the venerable activity of teaching rounds.

The best teachers usually are those individuals who have thought the most about how they themselves learned. The editors of *Advanced Surgical Recall* clearly are teachers who have given an enormous amount of thought to learning and teaching. They have used the principles of the Socratic method and of their own self-education techniques to develop this collection of questions. These editors have a special knack for writing and editing these types of questions and study aids; through their impressive medical and surgical educational trajectories, they have won teaching awards and created a plethora of study aids.

This collection of questions and answers is useful to students of surgery, not only because it will help them learn the answers they need to know, but also because it will help them remember the questions. Knowing the right questions is, in my opinion, more important than knowing the answers, at least in real life. After all, the answers will change over time. The questions are timeless.

Curtis G. Tribble, MD
Professor of Surgery, Vice-Chairman
Division of Cardiothoracic Surgery
University of Virginia
Charlottesville, Virginia

Preface

Advanced Surgical Recall is the perfect tool to help surgical residents and students recall pertinent clinical facts when they most need them—on wards, for the in-service examination, and board exams. As with all titles in the Recall series, the questions are presented in the left column and the answers in the right column. A bookmark is provided to help you cover the answers as you quiz yourself in this rapid-fire format.

The second edition is much more concise and portable than the first edition. The table of contents has been reorganized to make it identical to that of *Surgical Recall*. *Advanced Surgical Recall* in effect is a continuation of *Surgical Recall*, making this the ideal next step for the student who has already begun using and relying upon *Surgical Recall*.

Over 150 new illustrations have been added to help present complicated procedures, concepts, and advanced instruments visually for quick comprehension.

We believe this book will help ensure your success in mastering advanced surgical concepts and we welcome your comments and suggestions to make future editions more concise, complete, and useful at book_comments@lww.com.

In addition to the editors who made the second edition possible, I would also like to thank Kirk Fleischer and his colleagues at Johns Hopkins University for their excellent work on the 1st edition.

Lorne H. Blackbourne, M.D.
University of Miami

Contents

SECTION I. OVERVIEW AND BACKGROUND SURGICAL INFORMATION

SECTION II. GENERAL SURGERY

SECTION III. SUBSPECIALTY SURGERY

Section I

Overview and
Background Surgical
Information

1   Introduction

HOW ADULTS LEARN

Learning is accomplished through **motivation, repetition,** and **association.** Motivation must come from within; most medical students and residents are obviously motivated to learn. Repetition is obtained by reading, rereading, and studying information until it is mastered. Association is obtained by connecting information that has already been mastered to some new knowledge, such as remembering the anatomic order of the trauma neck zones 3,2,1 in conjunction with the Le Fort fractures 3,2,1.

HOW TO STUDY

Always read about your patient's disease while you are taking care of him or her. This habit serves two purposes: you will associate the information to the patient for life, and your increased knowledge will improve that patient's quality of care.

USING THIS BOOK

After completing the surgical basics in *Surgical Recall,* focus your attention on this book. Review the answers on the right until mastered. This book is designed to foster the acquisition of surgical information and will not help you gain experience in test taking; this skill can be learned from other books.

NURSES

Treat nurses with respect and professional courtesy at all times; they often know more than you in any given situation. If your relationship is based on mutual respect, it is also less likely that they will call you at 3 A.M. asking for Tylenol.

SLEEP DEPRIVATION

The best offense to combat sleep deprivation is to be in good physical shape and to be motivated. Staying up for 48 hours is no different than participating in an ultramarathon. Many residents find benefit from caffeine, orange juice, hot showers, brushing their teeth, doing push-ups, running steps, yelling, changing their socks, or listening to loud music. Try not to sit down, because sitting is conducive to falling asleep quickly. Studies have shown that in sleep deprivation physical abilities remain intact until extreme deprivation of sleep occurs. Tell yourself, "I am hardcore and I need no sleep!"

INTERNSHIP

THE PERFECT INTERN

Says only "Yes sir," "No sir," or "My fault, sir" and "Yes ma'am," "No ma'am," or "My fault, ma'am"
Is always honest
Is a team player
Has a "can do" attitude
Always brushes teeth before rounds
Is the first to arrive and the last to leave clinic
Is always clean
Always makes the upper-level residents look good
Teaches the students
Does not scut the students too much
Knows more about the patients than anyone else
Is a physician, and not merely a scribe
Is never late
Never complains
Is never hungry, thirsty, or tired
Is always enthusiastic
Follows the chain of command

Some thoughts for interns to live by:
"They can hurt you but they can't stop the clock." Internship only lasts for 12 months.
"Never trust your brain." Write everything down, do not trust anything to memory, and check off your chores when completed.
"Load the boat." Inform your superiors when a patient is not doing well or if you have any questions. That way, if your patient's condition worsens (the proverbial sinking ship), you have loaded the ship with your superiors and they will go down with you.
"Bad news does not age well." Call right away. (see above)
"Never lie." Honesty is the best policy.

LIVING WITH MISTAKES

You will make mistakes, and many times these mistakes will harm your patients. Mistakes are forgivable if you are **doing your absolute best.** Do not make mistakes that result from laziness.

There is a saying in surgery: "You cannot hurt yourself by getting out of bed." After a mistake is made and you have determined that you were doing your absolute best, you must then **forgive and remember.** That is, forgive yourself for the mistake, but always remember the mistake and try to learn something from it.

RECOVERY ROOM PROTOCOL

Several things need to be done before you can eat some food, so the acronym F.O.O.D.D. is helpful:
Family: Talk to the patient's family.
Operative note: Write in the chart.
Orders: Write postop orders.
Dictate the procedure.
Doctor: Call the primary/referring doctor.

DEALING WITH ACHES AND PAINS IN THE OR

Many residents find that taking NSAIDs before and after long cases helps decrease muscle strains. Others do sit-ups to strengthen abdominal muscles and reduce backache, or use the OSHA back support belts. Support hose can lessen foot edema and the pain associated with venous lower extremity incompetence associated with long periods of standing.

AVOIDING MALPRACTICE

Do the right thing.
Talk to your patients and their families (**never** say "no comment" or "I can't talk about it").
Be nice to your patients and their families.
Honesty is the best policy.
Document everything!
Seek advice from mentor, colleagues, lawyer.

What should you do if you write the wrong word in a chart?

Put a line through the word, but make sure it is still legible, and then initial. Never blot out—it will look as though you are trying to hide something.

HIERARCHY AMONG SURGICAL RESIDENTS

Suggestions and ideas regarding patient care should flow freely among all surgical residents (including interns), but the decisions follow a concrete chain of command.

FOURTH-YEAR MEDICAL STUDENT REQUIRED READING LIST

The fourth year of medical school for future surgery residents allows time for some reading that you will never be able to do again. Read the following books during your fourth year:
Fluids and Electrolytes in the Surgical Patient, by Carlos Pestana
House Officer's Guide to ICU Care, by John Elefteriades, Alexander Geha, and Lawrence Cohen

Cope's Early Diagnosis of the Acute Abdomen, by William Silen
Advanced Trauma Life Support Program for Physicians
Easy ACLS: Advanced Cardiac Life Support Preparatory Manual
Rapid Interpretation of EKGs: An Interactive Course, by Dale Dubin

OBTAINING A RESIDENCY

THE FOURTH YEAR

Research in the Fourth Year

A research elective is highly recommended in the fourth year. It provides a real working relationship with an attending research mentor, builds your curriculum vitae (CV), and gives you some idea of whether you want to pursue research during and after your residency. Research often separates you from the crowd of excellent medical student applicants. Taking your research elective early during your fourth year allows you the time to write one or two papers to add to your CV. It also gives you an opportunity to pursue a clinical study (chart review) while doing subsequent rotations. Also, ask your attending mentor if you can help write a review article or book chapter.

THE INTERVIEW PROCESS

OVERVIEW

Choose an advisor.
Obtain letters of recommendation, dean's letter, and official transcript; prepare CV and personal statement.
Request applications (in writing).
Fill out applications.
Wait for interview requests.
Schedule interviews.
Go to interviews.
Rank list.
Match day.

OFFICIAL TRANSCRIPT

In most cases, the dean submits your official transcript and dean's letter after your application is received. You should send an unofficial photocopy of your grades and board scores with your application. This hastens the arrival of interview acceptance letters, and thus allows you to maximize your scheduling and economize on your trips. Otherwise, your interview invitations may be delayed until the dean's letter arrives with your transcript.

CURRICULUM VITAE

Your CV represents the activities of your life and should include the following data:
Date
Name
Address (school and home)
Social Security number
Phone numbers (school and home)
Facsimile number
Electronic mail
Family information
Education
Military experience
Honors
Positions held
Organizations
Publications
Presentations
Book chapters
Review articles

Sample CV

CURRICULUM VITAE
August 2002

John Cushing
University of Virginia Medical Center
School of Medicine, Box 1145
Charlottesville, Virginia 22909

Home: 2234 Oxford Road
Charlottesville, Va 22909

Phone: Home (804) 983-1111
        School: (804) 924-1212 (and have paged)

Facsimile: (804) 983-1111

Electronic mail: CushingJ@va.edu

SSN: 225-11-1111

Born: October 28, 1974
        Santa Barbara, California

Family: Married Patricia Stuart, July 11, 1999

Education:
    Washington-Lee High School, Lexington, Virginia
    University of Virginia, Charlottesville, Virginia
    Bachelor of Arts, May 1998 (Biology)
    University of Virginia School of Medicine, Charlottesville, Virginia
    Doctor of Medicine, expected May 2002

Military:

   Captain, Medical Corps, United States Army Reserve, 1998-present

Additional Postgraduate Education:

   American Heart Association Advanced Cardiac Life Support, 2001

   Microsurgical Course, Department of Plastic Surgery, University of
      Virginia, 2001

Honors:

   Alpha Omega Alpha

Positions Held:

   Research Assistant, Department of Internal Medicine, University of Virginia,
      1999

   Assistant Instructor, Surgical Techniques Lab, University of Virginia, 2001

Professional Membership:

   American Medical Association

Book Chapters:

   Surgical Nutrition in Blackbourne LH, *Surgical Recall,* 3rd ed, Lippincott,
      Williams & Wilkins, Baltimore, 2002.

Publications:

   Kocher H, Cushing J. A New surgical approach to the posterior pancreas.
      Ann Surg: 116(3):248–254, 2001.

PERSONAL STATEMENT

You should include the following information:

Why you want to go into surgery

Why you are confident you will do a great job in your residency program
   (remember: confident, not arrogant)

Future plans (e.g., research, world missionary work)

   The personal statement is often a focal point in the interview, so be com-
fortable and familiar with the thoughts expressed in your statement. Each person's statement is different, and you need to create yours de novo to assure that
it reflects you and your attributes.

WHAT TO LOOK FOR IN A RESIDENCY PROGRAM

Are the residents happy? (Most important)

Call schedule

Wide exposure to pathology?

Pay/benefits

Parking

Area/crime/housing

Number of fellows to share cases with

Rotations

Moonlighting opportunity

Lab research opportunity

Vacations

What are the graduates doing now? (e.g., fellowships, academics, private practice)

WHERE TO APPLY

Ask your advisor, other attendings, your chairman, and residents at your school. You should apply to a full range of programs (very competitive to less competitive).

INTERVIEWS ON A LOW BUDGET

To minimize costs while on the interview trail:
Drive
Stay with friends, family, medical school alumni (your dean's office should have a list)
Schedule multiple interviews in the same area (i.e., fly in, rent a car)

THE INTERVIEW DAY

Some suggestions:
Wear a traditional dark interview suit (men and women). This is not the time to make a fashion statement. Why stand out? Let your record do that!
Always smile when first introduced to the interviewer. (Actual studies have shown that this is very important!)
Shake hands firmly.
Make eye contact.
Sit up straight.
Be polite to everyone.
Write thank you letters when you get home.

QUESTIONS YOU MIGHT BE ASKED

These are actual questions that students have been asked during interviews:

Personal

Tell me about yourself.
Tell me about your family.
How do you stay in good physical shape?
What do you do in your spare time?
What do you read?
What is the last nonmedical book you read?

Clinical

A 65-year-old man comes into the ER with right upper quadrant pain. How are you going to work him up?
How do you work up a pulmonary embolus?
How many mEq of sodium are in normal saline?

Ethical/Political

Okay, I have a situation for you. You are doing a laparotomy for bowel obstruction and you find a lap pad from a previous lap, but there is no association between the pad and the obstruction. Would you tell the patient? Would you tell the previous surgeon? If you were the previous surgeon who left the lap pad and were informed of your mistake by the subsequent surgeon, would you talk to the patient? What would you say?

Your attending tells you to schedule a patient for procedure A. You have been reading and discover that procedure B is more effective, in addition to having lower morbidity and mortality rates. You inform the attending, but he is adamantly in favor of procedure A. How do you handle the situation?

Academic

Tell me where you went to undergraduate college.

Do you think the college you attended had anything to do with your preclinical grades?

Why did you take Swedish as an undergraduate?

How do you study?

How do you feel about dog labs?

If you could change something about medical school, what would it be?

What is the funniest thing that happened to you during medical school?

Did any patient frustrate you during your surgery clerkship?

During your clinical years, did anything make you uncomfortable?

Tell me about your most interesting patient as a medical student, and tell me what you learned from that case.

Did you do a pediatric surgery rotation? If so, tell me about your most interesting pediatric surgery patient.

To which medical journals do you subscribe? What was the last article you read?

What electives are you taking in the fourth year?

Tell me about your grades in medical school. What were your undergraduate grades like?

Why did you get X (grade) in X (course/clerkship/elective)?

Why didn't you get a PhD?

What were your board scores? What was your overall percentage?

Why did you waive your right to read your letters of recommendation?

Explain this sentence in your personal statement.

Research

Tell me about your research. (Be prepared to answer some fairly in-depth questions regarding your research: basic science questions, clinical applicability, specifics of experiment design, depth of literature review, and occasional pimping. Understand your research thoroughly!)

How did you find the time to do your research?

Do you plan to take time off as a resident to do research?

When do you think it is best to take time off for research?

How do you feel about animal research?

What is it about research that you like and what keeps you motivated?

What percentage of your time as an attending do you plan to spend on research?

What does academic medicine mean to you?

What does it mean to you to be an academic clinician, researcher, or to have your own lab? Why is research important to you?

Residency

Do you have any questions? (Do not ask attendings questions that should be reserved for residents, for example, "What is your call schedule like?")

In our program you have to decide now if you want to do general surgery or cardiac surgery, so what will it be? (It's essential to know about the program beforehand.)

What do you like about our program? Why did you apply here?

What do you like and dislike about our program?

How did you find out about this program?

Why did you choose an academic program over a community program?

Where else have you applied? What programs have you liked?

Are you interested in staying at UVA? What have they told you?

Why didn't you apply to Duke?

Are we your first choice?

What do I have to say to make you come here? (Remember: talk is cheap.)

What would you change about our interview process?

What are you looking for in a general surgery program?

If you could design your ultimate residency program, what would it include?

What would you look for in faculty members?

What if you do not match?

What do you think are the advantages and disadvantages of being on call every third or every fourth night?

What do you think about being on call every other night?

Do you think you will be able to pursue your outside interests as a resident?

What is the worst thing a resident can do?

If you were on my service in June, what clinical weakness of yours would I have to be concerned about?

As an intern, what do you see as your role in teaching medical students?

How do you work with nurses?

How many hours of sleep do you need a night?

How do you know when you're overworked?

Soul-searching

What makes you a better applicant than the other 20 students we are interviewing today?

What makes you different from all those other applicants? Why should I pick you to be one of our residents?

Why should we want you in our program?

What makes you believe that you will be a good doctor?

What skill do you possess that will make you a good doctor?

Do you think that you have leadership potential?

Do you think that surgeons are egotistical or arrogant? Is that a good or bad trait, and why?

If you could describe the ideal attending (or resident) in two adjectives, what would they be?

Why do you like general surgery?

When did you become interested in pediatrics?

So, why do you want to be a surgeon (or neurologist, etc.)?

Are you sure you can give 100% to this residency?

So, why not medicine (or pediatrics, neurology, surgery, etc.)?

Okay, tomorrow you cannot do this residency. What residency would you do then?

What are your weaknesses?

What is your greatest strength/weakness (pick only one for each)? Why is that a strength/weakness?

What do you consider your greatest accomplishment outside of medical school the past 3 years?

What was the most memorable moment of your life outside of your academic career?

What aspect of your life are you most pleased about?

What aspect of your life are you most displeased about?

Who are your role models?

Who has had the greatest impact on you during your lifetime?

What are your two favorite books and why?

Which two books would you bring to a deserted island?

What book would you recommend to a historic figure being brought to the 21st century?

What do you think is the greatest problem in society today?

If you could invite any two famous people (living or dead) to a private dinner party, who would they be? Why?

If you could visit any time and place in history for a day, when and where would it be? Why?

The Crystal Ball

What do you see yourself doing in 10/15/20 years?

How do you think you will be able to balance clinical practice, teaching, research, and family?

What is the greatest challenge to medicine in the next 5 years?

What do you think about the future of general surgery (pediatrics, neurology, etc.), and what do you say to people who feel it's a dying field?

ADVANCED SURGICAL ABBREVIATIONS

ADL   Activities of daily living

AFB   Acid fast bacteria

AIDS	Acquired immunodeficiency syndrome
A.K.A.	Also known as
AKA	Above the knee amputation
ALI	Acute lung injury
AMA	Against medical advice
AMF YOYO	Adios my friend; you're on your own
APS	Acute pain service
ARF	Acute renal failure
ASIS	Anterior superior iliac spine
ATFQ	Answer the first question
AUR	Acute urinary retention
AV	Arteriovenous
AVN	Avascular necrosis
BAL	Bronchoalveolar lavage
BAM	Bilateral augmentation mammoplasty
BCC	Basal cell carcinoma
bid	Twice a day
BMI	Body mass index
BRP	Bathroom privileges
BSO	Bilateral salpingo-oopherectomy
BUN	Blood urea nitrogen
Bx	Biopsy
CAD	Coronary artery disease
CHF	Congestive heart failure

CMV	Cytomegalovirus
CNS	Central nervous system
CRF	Chronic renal failure
CRNA	Certified Registered Nurse Anesthetist
CSF	Cerebral spinal fluid
CT	Computed tomography
DJD	Degenerative joint disease
DOA	Dead on arrival
DOE	Dyspnea on exertion
DVT	Deep venous thrombosis
ECG	Electrocardiogram
ELAP	Exploratory laparotomy
ENT	Ear, nose, and throat
EOMI	Extraocular movement intact
ER	Estrogen receptor
ESRD	End-stage renal disease
ETT	Endotracheal tube (A.K.A. ET)
FDP	Fibrin degradation products
FEV$_1$	Forced expiratory volume in 1 second
FIDO	Forget it; drive on
FOBT	Fecal occult blood test
FOS	Full of stool
FROM	Full range of motion
GB	Gallbladder

G1P1	Gravida (# of pregnancies), Para (# of children)
GI	Gastrointestinal
GIST	Gastrointestinal stromal tumor
GSW	Gunshot wound
hCG	Human chorionic gonadotropin
HIV	Human immunodeficiency virus
HNP	Herniated nucleus pulposus
HOB	Head of bed
ICH	Intracranial hemorrhage
ICU	Intensive care unit
IDDM	Insulin-dependent diabetes mellitus
IHSS	Idiopathic hypertrophic subaortic stenosis
IM	Intramuscular
INR	International normalized ratio
IOC	Intraoperative cholangiogram
IV	Intravenous
IVC	Inferior vena cava
KISS	Keep it simple stupid
KVO	Keep vein open
LAC	Laceration
LMD	Local medical doctor
LOS	Length of stay
LRS	Lactated Ringer's solution
MAP	Mean arterial pressure

MCC	Motorcycle collision/crash
ME	Medical examiner
MI	Myocardial infarction
MODS	Multiple organ dysfunction syndrome
MOF	Multiple organ failure
MRA	Magnetic resonance angiography
MRCP	Magnetic resonance cholangiopancreatography
MRI	Magnetic resonance imaging
MRSA	Methicillin-resistant *Staphylococcus aureus*
MRSE	Methicillin-resistant *Staphylococcus epidermidis*
MVC	Motor vehicle collision/crash
NO	Nitric oxide
OR	Operating room
PCA	Patient-controlled analgesia
PEA	Pulseless electrical activity
PFO	Patent foramen ovale
PFTs	Pulmonary function tests
PO	By mouth (oral)
pRBCs	Packed red blood cells
PSA	Prostate-specific antigen
PSV	Pressure support ventilation
PVR	Pulmonary vascular resistance
QD	Once a day

RBCs	Red blood cells
RHIP	"Rank has its privileges"
RT	Respiratory therapist
RTC	Return to clinic
SDH	Subdural hematoma
SIMV	Synchronized intermittent mandatory ventilation
SIRS	Systemic inflammatory response syndrome
SpO$_2$	Pulse ox O$_2$ saturation
STAT	Immediately
SVC	Superior vena cava
SVR	Systemic vascular resistance
SVT	Supraventricular tachycardia
SW	Stab wound
TAH	Total abdominal hysterectomy
TAPP	Transabdominal preperitoneal (groin hernia repair)
TEPA	Totally extraperitoneal approach (groin hernia repair)
THE	Transhiatal esophagectomy
tid	Three times a day
TLC	Triple lumen catheter
TPN	Total parenteral nutrition
TURB	Transurethral resection of bladder
Ucx	Urine culture

UNOS	United Network for Organ Sharing
VRE	Vancomycin-resistant *Enterococcus*
WBAT	Weight bearing as tolerated
WBCs	White blood cells
WNL	Within normal limits
WWDWWC	"Wound was dry when we closed"
ψ	Psychiatric (Greek letter psi)
μg	Microgram

ADVANCED GLOSSARY

Antecolic	In front of the colon (anterior)
Asplenism	Absence of splenic function
Bezoar	Undigested mass ("hair ball")
Bruit	**Sound** of arterial turbulent flow
Colloid	IV fluid with large molecules (e.g., albumin)
Colonized	Bacteria residing in the anatomic area but not causing infection, inflammation, signs, or symptoms
Demarcation	Line defining borders between two anatomically distinct entities (e.g., between viable and dead tissue)
Epithelialization	Epithelial cells across a wound
Eschar	Thick dead skin seen after 3rd degree burns
Ether screen	Drape between the surgeon and the anesthetist
Granulation	Wound with a surface made of "proud flesh" consisting of collagen/fibroblasts and without an epithelial cover

Montgomery straps	Straps affixed to a patient's abdomen with tape; cloth straps are laced and tied after repeated wound changes, to avoid repeated taping of dressings
Opsonins	Protein particles that bind target cells for phagocytosis
Pulsus paradoxus	Seen with cardiac tamponade; > 10 mm Hg decrease in systolic blood pressure on inspiration
Pyrosis	Heartburn
Retrocolic	Behind the colon (posterior)
Seldinger technique	Placement of a tube over a previously placed wire (e.g., central line placement)
Singultus	Hiccup
Sterile	All microorganisms are killed
Sterile field	The prepped area of the patient, the drapes, and the instrument table: all items touching this area must be sterile
Strike through	Wound drainage penetrating ("striking through") all layers of a wound dressing
Thrill	**Palpable** vibration of arterial turbulent flow

ADVANCED SIGNS

Aaron's sign	Pushing on McBurney's point in patient with acute appendicitis results in **epigastric** pain!
Chandelier's sign	Severe pain upon manual manipulation of the cervix on pelvic exam (patient "jumps for the chandelier")
Claybrook's sign	Pneumoperitoneum (ruptured hollow viscus) results in transmission of breath and heart sounds when abdomen is auscultated.

Danforth's sign	Hemoperitoneum results in shoulder pain on deep inspiration (diaphragm irritation).
Deep sulcus sign	Deep costophrenic angle in supine chest radiograph in patients with a pneumothorax
Dunphy's sign	Abdominal pain with **coughing;** sign of peritonitis
Jiffy Pop sign	Colostomy bag full of air!
Mannkopf's sign	**Increase** in heart rate upon pushing on a point of maximal abdominal tenderness (seen with real pain, not in malingering)
Ransohoff's sign	Yellow umbilicus seen with bile leak (classic in common bile duct injury/rupture)
Ring sign	CSF and blood form rings when dropped on filter paper (or cloth), seen in CSF otorrhea and rhinorrhea.
Soap bubble sign	Retroperitoneal air seen in severe pancreatitis
Ten horns sign	Pronounced tenderness upon manual tension applied to right spermatic cord, seen in acute appendicitis (think **ten horns** will make you go **ten hut**)

MEDICAL STATS YOU NEED TO KNOW

Define the following terms.

Mean	The average value of all data points (e.g., 5, 10, 5, 20; 40/4 = 10 is the mean)
Mode	The most common numeric value of a set (e.g., in the set 2, 3, 4, 4, 4, 5, 6, 7; 4 is the mode)
Median	The middle value within the ordered set (e.g., 4, 4, 5, 6, 6; 5 is the median)
False positive	A data point that is reported as positive but is really negative

False negative

A data point that is reported as negative but is really positive

Distribution

A description of how the data look graphically (i.e., their shape)

Describe some examples of common distributions.

Normal distribution

A bell-shaped curve that is symmetric around the middle.

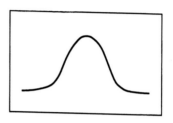

Skewed distribution

Not symmetrical, but slanted to the right or left

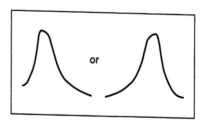

Bimodal distribution

Two graphical peaks of the distribution (i.e., two modes)

Define the following terms.

Sensitivity

$$\frac{\text{True positives}}{\text{True positives + false negatives}}$$

Specificity

$$\frac{\text{True negatives}}{\text{True negatives + false positives}}$$

Blind study

The patient is blind to the clinical intervention

Double-blind study

The patient **and** the care providers are blind to the clinical intervention. (NOT two orthopods trying to read an ECG!)

MEDICAL SPANISH

Translate the following words and phrases:

Hello	Hola (o la)
Good-bye	Adios
Please	Por favor
Sir	Señor
Ma'am	Señora
You	Usted (respectful); Tu (familiar)
Speak	Hablas
English	Ingles
Where	Donde (dohn-day)
Is	Es (esta)
Pain	Dolor (dough-lore)
Worse	Peor
Better	Mejor (mehor)
Nauseated	Mareado or nau`sea
Where is the pain?	Donde esta el dolor?
Is the pain worse?	Es peor el dolor?
Is the pain better?	Es mejor el dolor?
Breathe deeply.	Respiro profundo.
Cough	Tocé (toe say)
Does it hurt to breathe?	Le duele al respiro? (duele = do-el-ay)
Does it hurt if I push here?	Le duele cuando aprieto aqui?

Where does it hurt?	Donde le duele?
Tetanus shot	Inyección de tetano
X-ray	Radiografia
Were you knocked out?	Estuvo inconsciente
Neck	Cuello
Abdomen	Abdomen
Arm	Brazo
Rectum	Rectum
Chest	Pecho
Head	Cabeza
Need an operation	Necesita una operation

2   Surgical Syndromes

Identify the syndromes.

Blue toe syndrome	Painful, **blue** discoloration of the **toes** caused by microcirculatory blockage due to microemboli from aortic plaque
Bouveret's syndrome	**Gallstone** causing obstruction of duodenum
Crouzon's syndrome	Craniofacial dysostosis
DiGeorge's syndrome	Congenital absence of parathyroid glands and thymus
Meigs' syndrome	Pleural effusion, ascites associated with an **ovarian mass**
Morel-Lavallee syndrome	Degloving injury of an extremity after a crush injury (skin and subcutaneous fat are totally separated from muscle)
Münchhausen syndrome	Multiple hospitalizations for acute medical condition although no disease process is found
Nonketotic hyperosmolar syndrome	Severe hyperglycemia **without** ketoacidosis
Plummer-Vinson syndrome	Syndrome of: 1. Esophageal web 2. Iron deficiency anemia 3. Dysphagia 4. Spoon-shaped nails 5. Atrophy of tongue and oral mucosa
Sick euthyroid syndrome	Change in thyroid hormone regulation resulting from severe illness, trauma, or

	stress. Patient has normal thyroid-stimulating hormone (TSH) but has decreased $\downarrow$ T4, $\downarrow$ T3.
Stauffer's syndrome	Hepatic dysfunction in patients with renal cell carcinoma **not** due to metastatic disease that resolves after nephrectomy
Turcot syndrome	Central nervous system (CNS) malignant tumor and colon polyps
Verner-Morrison syndrome	Vipoma
von Hippel-Lindau syndrome	**CAP:** **C**ystic cerebellar hemangioblastoma **A**ngiomatous malformation of the retina **P**heochromocytoma
Waterhouse-Friderichsen syndrome	Adrenal insufficiency caused by bilateral adrenal hemorrhage, classically caused by meningococcal infection
Wernicke-Korsakoff syndrome	Chronic alcohol abuse: Cranial nerve VI palsy (bilateral) Ataxia Delirium Strabismus Nystagmus Diplopia
What is a CN VI palsy?	CN VI = abducens nerve; palsy results in diplopia and inability to look laterally

3

Surgical Most Commons

What is the most common:

Cause of traumatic death in adults?	Brain injury
Tumor causing an adrenal incidentaloma?	Cortical adenoma (nonfunctioning)
Cause of chronic pancreatitis?	Alcohol abuse
Cause of Budd-Chiari syndrome in Western countries?	Prothrombotic state
Benign breast mass in women 18–36 years of age?	Fibroadenoma
Nosocomial infection in surgical patients?	Urinary tract infection (UTI)
Side with a traumatic diaphragmatic rupture?	**Left** (liver protects the right)
Site of GI tract lymphoma?	Stomach
Cause of death in adults < 44 years of age	Trauma
Cause of liver bacterial abscess?	Biliary tract obstruction or disease (used to be appendicitis)
Cause of intraperitoneal fungal infection?	Severe pancreatitis

Small bowel benign tumor?	GIST (gastrointestinal stromal tumors; includes leiomyomas)
Small bowel malignant tumor?	Adenocarcinoma
Site of small bowel adenoma?	Duodenum
Endocrine surgical operation?	Thyroid resection
Cause of spinal cord injury?	MVCs
Cause of a false-positive aortogram for aortic injury in trauma?	Ductus diverticulum
Cause of hypotension?	Hypovolemia
Cranial nerve injured in blunt trauma?	Cranial nerve I (olfactory); easily missed initially!
Benign tumor of the esophagus?	Leiomyoma
Cause of splenic mass?	Pseudocysts (e.g., liquified hematoma)
Cause of a visceral arterial aneurysm?	Splenic aneurysm
Congenital bleeding disorder?	von Willebrand's disease
Cause of postoperative premature labor?	Hypovolemia
Cause of viral transmission with blood transfusions?	Cytomegalovirus
Cause of death of children > 1 year of age?	Trauma
Cause of traumatic death in children?	Brain injury

4   Surgical Percentages

What percentage of spinal cord injuries occur in the cervical spine?

50%

What percentage of clean wounds become infected?

1.5%

What percentage of patients with resolution of mild gallstone pancreatitis will have a common duct stone on intraoperative cholangiogram?

Approximately 5% (i.e., 95% of stones pass)

What percentage of gastrinomas are found in the "gastrinoma triangle"?

80%

What percentage of patients with Crohn's disease will need a laparotomy within 20 years?

75%

What percentage of postop myocardial infarctions are silent (asymptomatic)?

75%

What percentage of patients with antibiotic-associated colitis have pseudomem-branous colitis?

50%

What percentage of patients with pseudomembranous colitis have a positive assay for *Clostridium difficile* toxin?

95%

What percentage of patients with antibiotic-associated colitis without pseudomembranes have a positive assay for *C. difficile* toxin?	Approximately 66%
What percentage of patients who WILL resolve their partial small bowel obstruction (SBO) with conservative treatment do so in 48 hours?	80%
What percentage of patients who have SBO (regardless of treatment) will have a subsequent bout of SBO?	Approximately 33%
In what percentage of cases does a thoracic aortogram to rule out a torn thoracic aorta after blunt trauma yield a positive study?	Approximately 10%
What percentage of patients undergoing laparotomy develop a postoperative SBO at some later time?	Approximately 5%
What percentage of colonic villous adenomas contain cancer?	Approximately 40% (think: **vill**ous = **vill**ain)

5   Surgical History

How are physicians and surgeons in England addressed?

The tradition of addressing physicians as "Doctor" and surgeons as "Mister" persists; it stems from the Medieval era's disdain for surgeons.

Who is widely considered to be the father of experimental surgery?

Hunter (1728–1793), who was born in Scotland

Who was Dominique-Jean-Larrey?

Napoleon's surgeon. He was responsible for the first ambulance and Larrey's point (subxiphoid).

Who was William Beaumont?

A U.S. Army doctor. He studied the gastric physiology of his patient, Alexis St. Martin, who formed a gastrocutaneous fistula from a musket wound in 1822.

Who is responsible for the "germ theory"?

Pasteur (1822–1895)

Who is considered the "father of aseptic surgery"?

Lister (1827–1912)

With what did Lister "disinfect" wounds, hands, and instruments?

Carbolic acid

Who performed the first successful gastrectomy?

Billroth (1829–1894). He also developed the Billroth I and II.

Who performed the first successful end-to-end vascular anastomosis?

Carrel (1873–1944), a Frenchman. His technique made transplantation a technical possibility.

Who is credited with the first cholecystectomy?

Langenbuch, in 1882. The patient endured 5 days of preliminary enemas, but smoked a cigar the day after surgery, got up on the twelfth day, and went home 6 weeks later.

When and at what hospital did McBurney describe the point named after him?

In 1889, at the Roosevelt Hospital in New York City

Who is credited with starting the routine use of sterile surgical gloves during operations?

Halsted, in 1890. His head nurse, Caroline Hampton, complained about dermatitis caused by surgical chemicals. His solution "won her hand," literally!

What role in surgery did Goodyear Rubber Company play?

It manufactured the first thin rubber gloves with gauntlets for Halsted.

On whom did Halsted perform his first gallbladder operation?

His mother, in 1882. He was a pioneer in gallbladder disease research and the first professor of surgery at Johns Hopkins.

What disease did Trousseau, of Trousseau syndrome, die of?

Pancreatic cancer. His syndrome was a deep vein thrombosis (DVT) associated with an abdominal malignancy.

Why was Kocher's (1841–1917) surgical career marked by tragedy as well as triumph?

He perfected the total thyroidectomy by 1898, reducing operative mortality from 13% to 0.5%, but to his horror, produced scores of cretinous and myxedematous patients. He swore thereafter never to remove a complete thyroid again.

Who was Harvey Cushing?

A neurosurgeon who trained at Johns Hopkins. Cushing (1869–1939) was responsible for advances in neurosurgery (Cushing's ulcer), pituitary disease, and intracranial pressure (Cushing's triad).

Why did Cushing insist upon complete silence in the OR?

To minimize droplet infection of wounds. This theory gained increasing acceptance because of the work by Flugge circa 1897, proving that although masks protected the patient against wound infection, they offered little protection if the surgeon was bearded.

Who is considered the "father of the modern residency system" in surgery?	A German named von Langenbeck (1810–1887), who trained Billroth
Who established the first surgical residency program in America?	Halsted, at Johns Hopkins Hospital
With what eponym is Le Fort associated?	The Le Fort fractures were named for him, for experiments he conducted in 1900 in which he dropped cannonballs onto cadaver skulls, resulting in 1 of 3 fracture patterns.
Who set the standard of requiring complete physical examinations of all patients, and started the first of many large clinics staffed with experts from various fields?	The Mayo Brothers. They built their famous clinic in Rochester, Minnesota, in 1910.
Who was Sister Mary Joseph?	The Mayos' nurse. She noticed the paraumbilical adenopathy associated with advanced gastric cancer.
Was Bovie an MD?	No, he was a PhD in physics. He developed the electrocautery in Boston in the 1920s.
Who discovered penicillin?	Fleming, a surgeon, in 1928
Which surgeon performed the first human cardiac catheterization?	Forssmann (1904–1979), in 1929 in Berlin, passed a tube through an arm vein into his **own heart** while watching it on a fluoroscope screen!
Who is credited with developing the heart-lung machine (extracorporeal circulation)?	Gibbon (1903–1973) first used his device in 1953.
Who performed the first heart-lung transplantation?	Reitz, in 1982
Who performed the first successful human pancreas transplantation?	Lillehei and Najarian, in 1966 at the University of Minnesota

Who performed the first human laparoscopic cholecystectomy?

Mouret in Lyon, France, in 1987

Where and when was the first clinical use of general anesthesia?

Massachusetts General Hospital using ether on October 16, 1846 (a dentist, William Morton)

Who performed the first appendectomy?

Claudius Amyand, in 1735

Who designed the ileoanal pull-through?

Sabiston and Ravitch, in 1947

Why was this unusual?

Sabiston is a cardiovascular surgeon.

On whom did Boerhaave first describe the syndrome named after him?

Baron van Wassenaer, admiral of the Dutch fleet

Who was the first to surgically correct Boerhaave's syndrome?

Barrett, of Barrett's esophagus

Which father of American academic surgery used cocaine and opium throughout his career?

Halsted

Which battle was the Battle sign named after?

William Battle (1855–1936) named it. Trick question!

Who developed the first chest tube?

Crosswell Hewett, in 1876

What was the first chest tube?

A rubber catheter

6

Surgical Instruments

Identify the proper technique.

How to cut left to right
with scissors in your right
hand

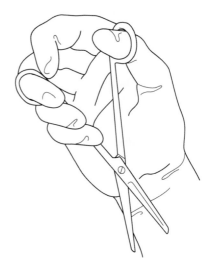

"Palming" an instrument
when you are not using it

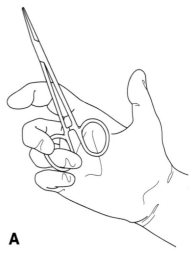

A

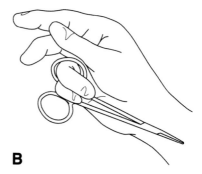

B

**Removing a clamp with
your left hand**

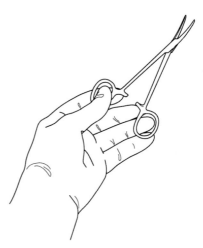

**How do you put a blade
on a scalpel?**

Never with your hands; always use a
clamp

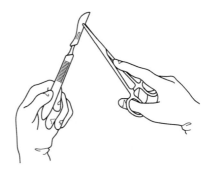

Define the instrument.

**Adson-Brown tissue
forceps**

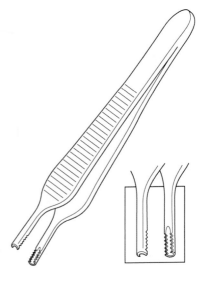

**Angled DeBakey vascular
clamp**

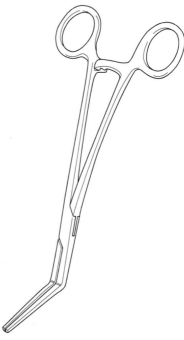

Balfour retractor

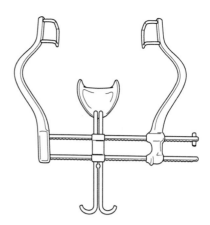

Bandage scissors   Used to cut bandages

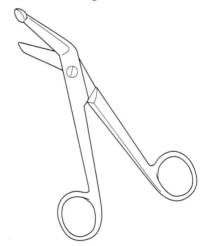

Bayonet forceps

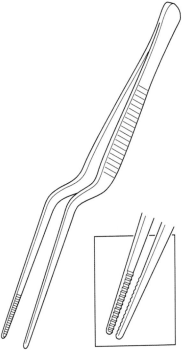

Bone cutting forceps

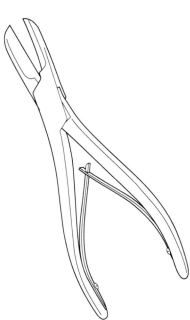

Bookwalter retractor

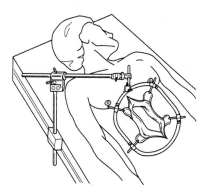

Bulldog clamp

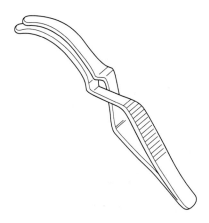

Castroviejo needle holder

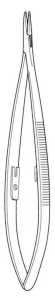

DeBakey aortic clamp

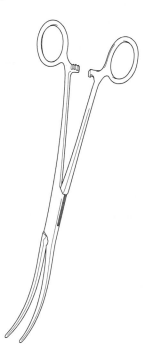

Bowel clamp   Doyen bowel clamp

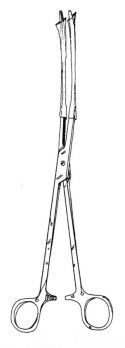

Doyen rib stripper

Periosteal rib elevator

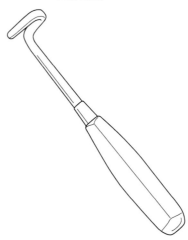

Duvall clamp forceps

Used as a lung clamp (AKA Pennington clamp)

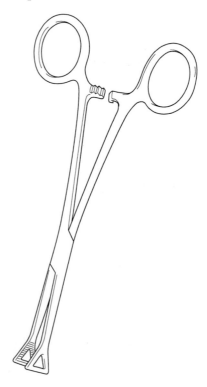

Ferris-Smith tissue forceps

For fascia (often called Ferris Buellers!)

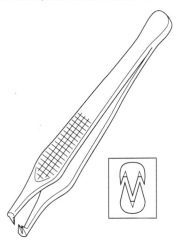

Finochietto rib spreader

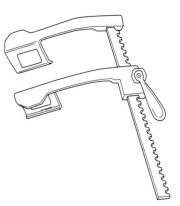

Fish retainer

A sheet of rubber that protects the bowel during laparotomy closure

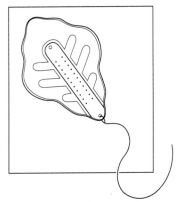

Frazier suction

Designed initially for neurosurgery

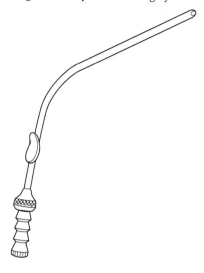

Gelpi retractor

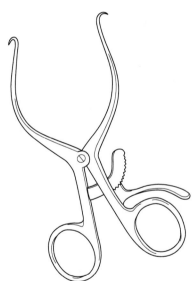

Gigli saw

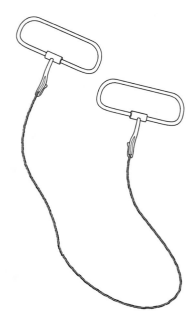

Gomez retractor

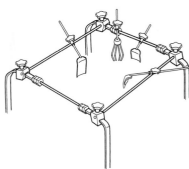

Hegar dilator

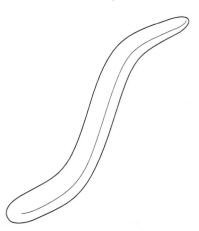

Jamieson scissors

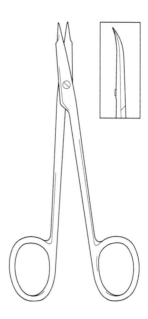

Keuttner   Pronounced "kitner" or "peanut" by most. Basically, a small cloth dressing held by clamp.

Kidney pedicle clamp

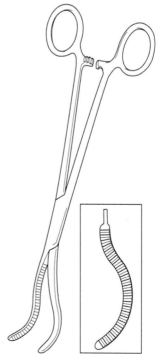

Lahey thyroid clamp

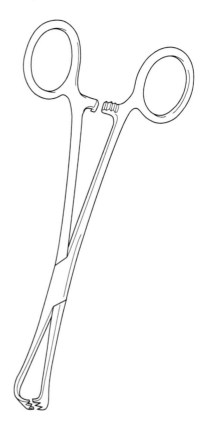

Loupes

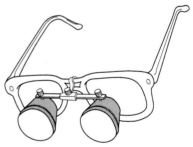

Maryland dissecting forceps

Used for blunt laparoscopic dissection

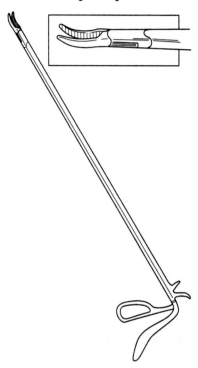

Poole sucker

Used for suctioning fluid (often irrigation) from peritoneal cavity

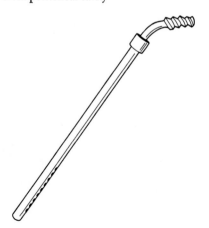

Pratt rectal speculum   Rectal speculum

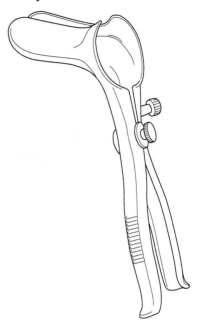

Rat-toothed forceps

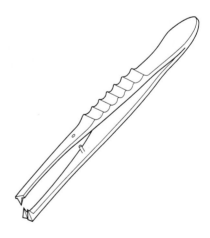

Rongeur

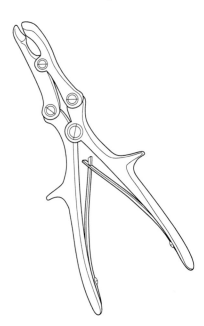

Russian forceps   Used for fascia

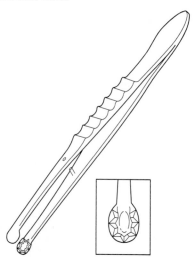

Satinsky

Vascular clamp

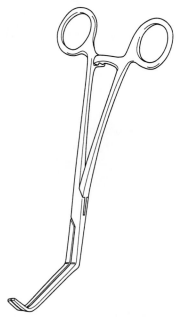

#12 Scalpel blade

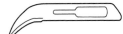

Vein retractor

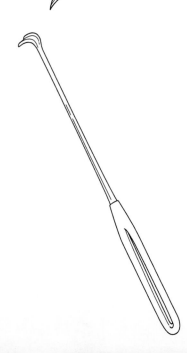

7 Sutures and Stitching

Should the subcutaneous fat be closed with sutures?

No, because fat will not hold sutures, which then become a foreign body, increasing the rate of infection.

SUTURE TECHNIQUES

What is a slip knot?

It slips to tighten but does not hold in place for long.

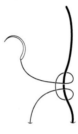

How is a suture removed?

Simply cut one side of the knot and then pull the knot out!

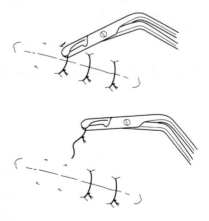

What is a Lembert stitch?   It is a second layer in bowel anastomoses

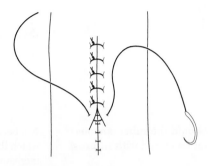

What is a Connell's stitch?   The first mucosa-to-mucosa layer in an anastomoses; basically a running "U" stitch

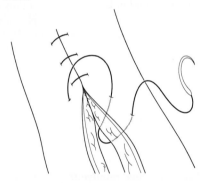

How to remember the order of the Connell's stitch?   "**Into** the bar—have a drink then go **out** of the bar—cross the street and go **into** the bar—have a drink—go **out** of the bar—cross the street. . ."

What is a Gambee stitch?   A one-layer anastomosis

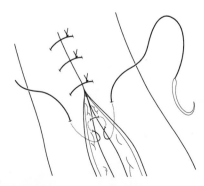

What is a Halsted stitch?

An interrupted horizontal mattress stitch

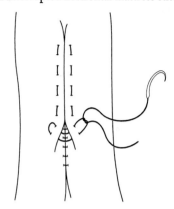

What is the Cushing stitch?

A running horizontal mattress stitch used to approximate 2 adjacent surfaces.

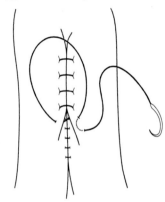

What is a locking stitch?

Used for hemostasis

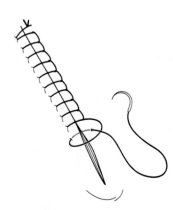

What is a retention suture bridge?

Used to slowly tighten the retention suture as edema resolves

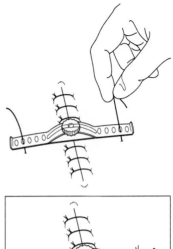

What is a taper needle?

Used in easily penetrated tissues (e.g., bowel)

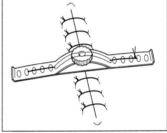

What is a cutting needle?

A needle for getting through tough material (e.g., skin). The edge is on **top** of the needle.

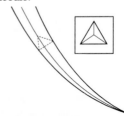

What is a "reverse" cutting needle?	A cutting needle with the edge on the **bottom**

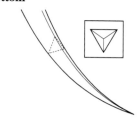

What is a "Keith" needle?	A straight needle

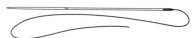

SUTURE MATERIALS

How long do plain and chromic gut sutures retain their tensile strength?	Plain gut: 7–10 days Chromic gut: 10–12 days
How many throws are needed in a Prolene knot?	At least 5 (most use > 6)
What are the following absorbable sutures made of:	
Vicryl?	Polyglactic acid
PDS?	PolyDioxane
Maxon?	Polyglyconate
Dexon?	Polyglycolic acid
Why can PDS or Maxon be used for closing abdominal fascia?	Keeps its strength for > 42 days
Why should silk be avoided in contaminated wounds?	It is nonabsorbable, and its pores can harbor bacteria.
Why do "train tracks" occur with sutures?	Because the suture track epithelializes after 7 days
What type of suture is used to repair the biliary tract or GU system?	**Absorbable** suture; otherwise, the suture material acts as a nidus for stone formation.

8

Surgical Knot Tying

After mastering the instrument knot and two-handed knot tying, now it is time to consider mastering the one-handed knot.

Describe the first throw of the one-hand tie (the "OK" throw).

Grab the suture forming the "OK" sign (A,B). Place the suture between the index finger and the middle finger (C). Use your middle finger to sweep the suture (D,E,F).

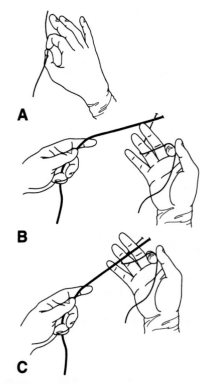

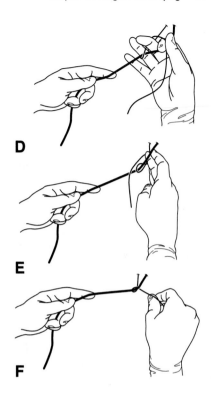

D

E

F

Describe the second half of the one-hand tie (the "snap your finger" throw).

Hold your fingers and the suture like you would snap your fingers (A,B). Put the suture between the index finger and thumb (C). Use the index finger to sweep the suture (D,E,F,G).

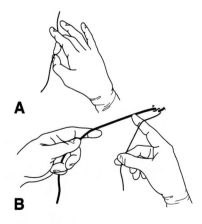

A

B

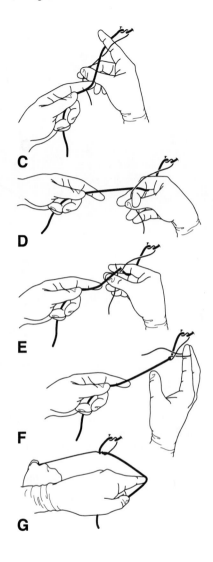

9 _____

Incisions

What is it called if the McBurney or Rocky-Davis incision is extended medially?

Weir extension

What is a Lanz incision?

Right lower quadrant (RLQ) incision following Langer's lines in the RLQ

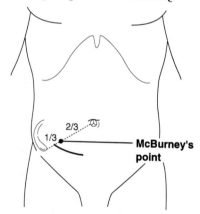

What is a thyroid incision also known as?

The "collar incision"

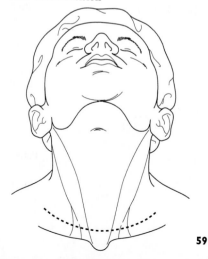

10   Surgical Positions

Describe the following surgical positions.

Sims'

"Semi-prone": patient lies prone with right knee drawn up

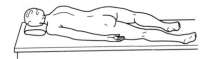

Kidney

Flexed lateral decubitus position; used for nephrectomy and other procedures involving the urinary tract

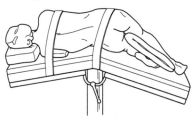

Jack-knife prone

Patient lies prone, with legs lowered and hips raised; used for anorectal procedures

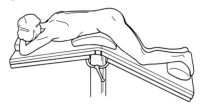

Fowler

Patient lies supine with main body (back) at a 45° incline, with knees flexed and elevated

Durant

Left lateral decubitus with head down; use for patients with air/CO_2 embolus to capture air in the right ventricle/atrium and keep it out of the pulmonary vasculature

11   Surgical Speak

Define the following terms.

Dehiscence	"Splitting open" (e.g., wound dehiscence = skin open, fascial dehiscence = fascia splits open)
Eructation	Belch
Pyrosis	Heartburn

Define the following prefixes.

"Acro-"	Extremity
"Entero-"	Small intestine
"Odyno-"	Painful (e.g., "**odyno**phagia is painful swallowing)

Define the following suffixes.

"-dynia"	Pain
"-itis"	Inflammation (e.g., appendic**itis** is inflammation of the appendix)
"-pexy"	Fixation (e.g., gastro**pexy** is surgical fixation of the stomach to the abdominal wall)

Define these types of surgery.

Enteroenterostomy	Surgical anastomosis between 2 loops of small bowel

Hepaticojejunostomy   Surgical anastomosis of the hepatic duct(s) [but not the common bile duct] to the jejunum

Pancreaticoduodenectomy   Whipple procedure: surgical removal of pancreas (head) and duodenum

Ureteroneocystostomy   Surgical anastomosis between ureter and bladder (at "new" site = neo)

12 _____ Preoperative 201

What should be done before elective surgery for a patient taking a monoamine oxidase inhibitor (MAOI)?	Stop taking the MAOI 2 weeks before the procedure (coordinate with primary care physician).
Why is postoperative MI so feared?	66% mortality!
What is the rate of postoperative MI in the following conditions?	
Previous MI < 3 months	38%
Previous MI > 6 months ago	4%
No previous MI	0.13%
What is the only medication shown to reduce the incidence of postoperative MI?	Beta blocker
What are the 10 Goldman criteria for cardiac risk in patients undergoing noncardiac surgery?	Aortic stenosis, MI within 6 months, jugular venous distention (JVD), S_3 gallop, ectopy, poor medical condition, emergency surgery, thoracic or intraperitoneal procedure, age > 70 years, nonsinus rhythm
Give the points by Goldman criteria for each of the following factors (more points = more risk).	
S_3 gallop or JVD	11

MI within 6 months	10
Ectopy or nonsinus rhythm	7
More than 5 premature ventricular contractions (PVCs)	7
Age > 70 years	5
Emergency surgery	4
Aortic stenosis	3
Intraperitoneal or thoracic surgery	3
Poor medical condition	3

Define *poor medical condition.*	Bedridden, abnormal blood gas ($PO_2 < 60$; $pCO_2 > 50$), abnormal electrolytes ($K^+ < 3.0$; HCO < 20), renal dysfunction (BUN > 50; creatinine > 3.0), chronic liver disease
What is the mortality rate for patients who have less than 5 points according to the Goldman criteria?	0.2%
What is the mortality rate for patients who have more than 26 points according to the Goldman criteria?	50%
What are the 2 major risk factors for perioperative MI?	CHF and recent MI (3 months)
What heart valvular disease is associated with the highest risk for postoperative cardiac complications? Why?	Aortic stenosis, because the heart responds poorly to fluid shifts
What are the signs and symptoms of aortic stenosis?	Systolic ejection murmur, angina, syncope, CHF (think: **a**ortic **s**tenosis **c**omplications = **a**ngina, **s**yncope, **c**ongestive heart failure)

What 2 kinds of noncardiac surgeries are associated with the highest rates of perioperative cardiac complications?

Operations on the aorta, followed by operations on the peripheral vascular system (because of associated CAD)

Is spinal or epidural anesthesia safer than inhalational anesthetics in patients with CAD?

No. Although counterintuitive, the loss of vascular resistance associated with spinal or epidural anesthesia does not result in significantly lower rates of perioperative cardiac events.

Which inhalational anesthetic has the highest degree of cardiac depression?

Halothane

What is the mechanism of cardiac depression with halothane?

It can lead to direct cardiac depression coupled with peripheral vascular dilatation, without the normal compensatory tachycardia.

What are the 2 contraindications for epidural and spinal anesthesia?

1. Hypertrophic obstructive cardiomyopathy
2. Cyanotic congenital heart disease (because of loss of vascular tone and increased venous capacitance)

13

Surgical Operations
You Should Know

BACKGROUND

How should an area be prepped for operation?

Scrub skin with povidone-iodine (Betadine) in an enlarging circular motion from the center to the periphery.

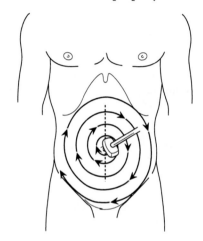

How should you glove yourself?

Never allow the outside of the gloves to touch your skin.
1. Turn gloves upside down on forearm of opposite arm.
2. Grasp back of cuff and turn over other hand.
3. Draw cuff back to wrist.

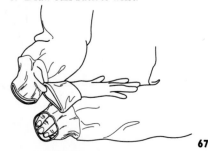

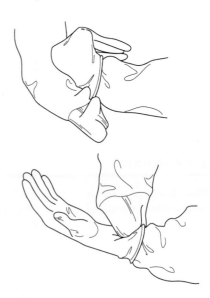

Which drapes do you place first: top and bottom, or sides? Why?

Sides first, because
1. Your gown might touch the sides during placement of towels.
2. If placed last, the side drapes will fall down due to gravity after placement of towel clips (whereas the top and bottom towels will keep the side towels in place).

What is the correct height of the OR table?

Operative field is elbow height.

SURGICAL MANEUVERS

What is the Pringle maneuver?

Occlusion of the porta hepatis; decreases blood flow to the liver to slow bleeding during repair of a traumatic liver injury

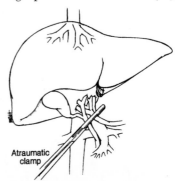

Atraumatic clamp

What is the Kocher maneuver?

Dissection of the lateral peritoneal attachments of the duodenum; allows inspection of the duodenum, pancreas, and other retroperitoneal structures

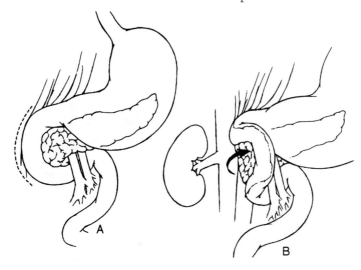

What is the Cattel maneuver?

Mobilization of the ascending colon to the midline. If combined with a Kocher maneuver, exposes the vena cava (think: **C**attel = **K**ocher = right sided).

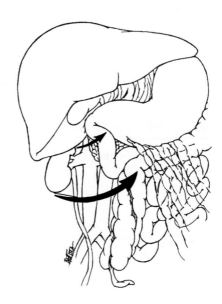

What is the Blaisdell maneuver?

Medial rotation of left sided viscera but leaving left kidney in situ

What is the Mattox maneuver?

Mobilization of the descending colon to the midline; exposes the abdominal aorta

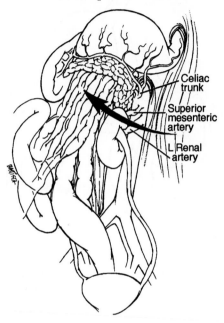

What is the Utley maneuver?

Used in tracheo-innominate fistula hemorrhage; placement of finger into tracheostomy or between innominate and trachea; this provides hemostasis with digital pressure, compressing the innominate artery hole against the sternum

OPERATIVE PROCEDURES

Define or describe the following operative procedures.

Kraske

Transcoccygeal rectal biopsy/resection

Csendes   Gastric resection with long
                                     gastrojejunostomy

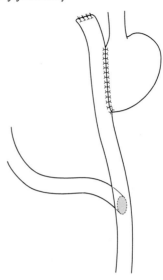

Braun   Enteroenterostomy between the limbs of
                                     a Billroth II

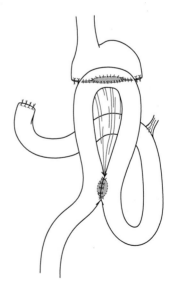

Right hemicolectomy

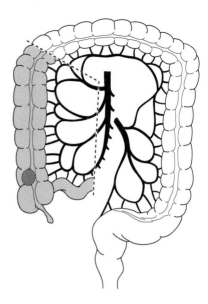

Extended right hemicolectomy

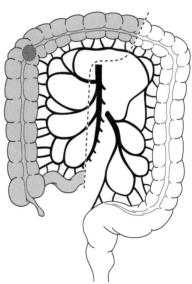

Transverse colectomy

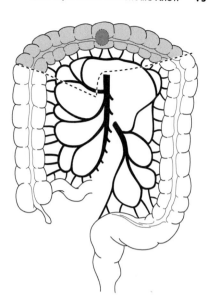

Left hemicolectomy

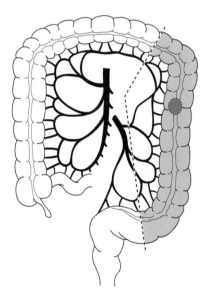

Sigmoid colectomy

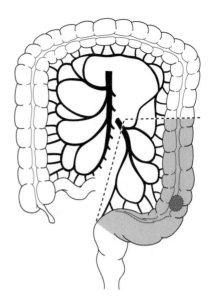

Retrocolic Roux-en-Y   Limb of Roux-en-Y placed behind
                                  transverse colon

Witzel   Wrapping bowel wall around catheter;
                                  used in jejunostomies

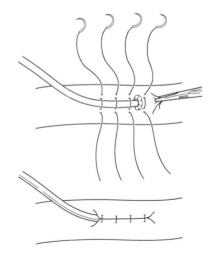

Bogata bag

Abdominal wall closure using plastic
sheet (e.g., urology irrigation bag)

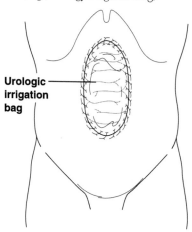

**Urologic
irrigation
bag**

Splenorrhaphy

Surgical repair of the spleen

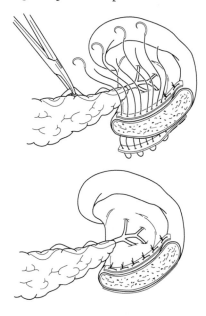

Ripstein

Rectopexy with mesh (think: **Rip**stein = "**rip**" a piece of mesh for repair)

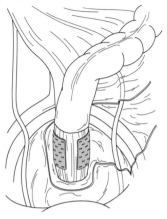

Grillo

Pleural flap for buttressing an esophageal repair

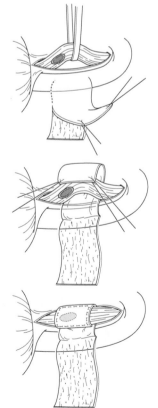

Plug and patch inguinal hernia repair

Plug

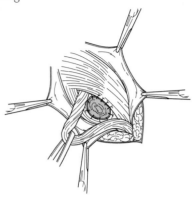

Patch

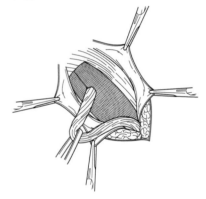

Choledochojejunostomy

Anastomosis of common bile duct to jejunum

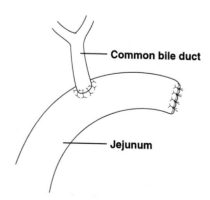

Truncal vagotomy

Transection of vagal nerves (while in the OR, get frozen section to confirm that you actually resected the nerve)

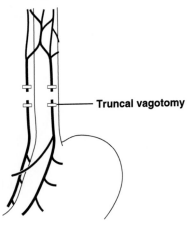

———— **Truncal vagotomy**

Jaboulay pyloroplasty

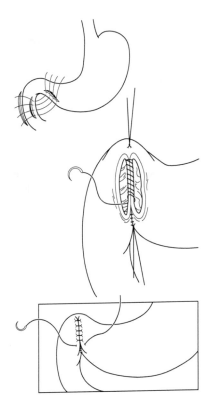

PEG

Percutaneous Endoscopic Gastrostomy

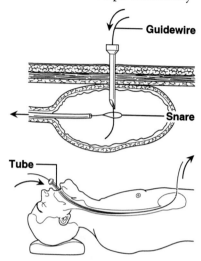

Finney pyloroplasty

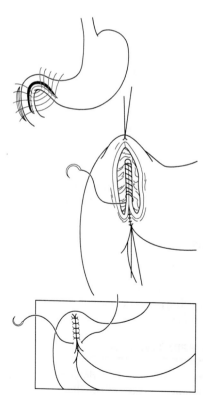

Stamm gastrostomy	Open gastrostomy with purse string suture

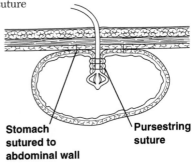

Hasson laparoscopy	Cut down under direct vision and placement of trocar for laparoscopy

FAVORITE TRICK QUESTIONS

What is the most common intraoperative bladder "tumor"?	Foley catheter
How do you describe a wound with pus?	**Purulent,** not **"pus**ie"—if you say it, you **will** be asked to spell it!
How many chest tubes do you put in after a pneumonectomy?	Zero
Describe a stool with melena.	Melenic—not melanotic
When is a rectal exam done after an abdominoperineal resection (APR)?	Never—there is no anus after an APR!
What battle was "Battle sign" named after?	Dr. Battle!
If you have a low BUN, how much BUN is needed to replace it?	None!

OPERATIVE PEARLS

As a last resort, how do you obtain exposure of the iliac vein during trauma surgery?	Transect the iliac artery!

What is the smart operation to perform if you find extensive spread of cholangiocarcinoma at laparotomy?

Cholecystectomy—stents often block the cystic duct, causing cholecystitis!

How do you find the segment III hepatic duct?

Follow the falciform ligament into the umbilical fissure.

How do you advance a dilator when placing a large IV catheter?

Always under fluoroscopic guidance, so the dilator does not have to follow a flimsy guide wire!

What intraperitoneal pressure is needed to release an abdomen to avoid abdominal compartment syndrome?

> 25 mm Hg with compromise. Think: "Release > 25—keeps the patient alive."

Which is closed first: the top or bottom of a laparotomy fascial incision?

Bottom—get the guts in first! (Liver is up top.)

What must be in place before doing a diagnostic peritoneal lavage (DPL) for trauma?

1. Foley catheter
2. Nasogastric tube (NGT) or orogastric tube (OGT)

How do you mark a specimen for orientation?

Short suture = **S**uperior
Long suture = **L**ateral

When should you biopsy an esophageal leiomyoma?

Never

When do you mark varicose veins?

Preoperatively, while the patient is standing. Use nonpermanent ink; otherwise you might tattoo the skin!

Should you ever use a Bovie during a tracheostomy?

Never on the trachea—100% oxygen can result in a **fire**!

When is the best time to cut the peritoneum?

During expiration, because the bowel falls away

Should you close the small bowel longitudinally or transversely?

Transversely—better to shorten than to stricture!

Where must the catheter be placed for a DPL with a pelvic fracture?

Supraumbilical position (pelvic hematoma tracks up the medial umbilical ligaments); even with a supraumbilical approach, there is up to a 20% false-positive rate!

What are the 7 pearls of successfully placing a subclavian central line?

1. Place towels below scapulae transversely or between the scapulae.
2. Place patient in the Trendelenburg position (think: headdownenburg).
3. Keep the needle flat.
4. Go for the left subclavian, if all things are equal.
5. Always have one hand on the wire at all times and never let go.
6. Always go on the side of a chest tube (chest tube treats pneumothorax).
7. Always get a chest x-ray after the procedure, before moving the patient, or **before trying the other side.**

What are the 4 pearls for easy placement of an NGT?

1. Flex the head (chin to chest).
2. Apply mild topical anesthetic (e.g., Cetacaine spray).
3. Apply lubrication.
4. Have the patient drink water.

How many rings on the stapler do you need after a successful end-to-end anastomosis (EEA) with a stapler?

2

What will help open the pylorus and stop the contractions of the stomach/ duodenum during an esophagogastroduodeno-scopy (EGD)?

IV glucagon

What will help retain contrast dye during a biliary cholangiogram?

IV morphine

Can the suprarenal IVC ever be ligated?

No. A mortality rate of approximately 100% is associated with such attempts.

Can the infrarenal IVC be ligated?

Yes, but with a morbidity rate of approximately 50%

How should a through-and-through penetrating injury to the IVC be fixed?

Enlarge the anterior defect, fix the posterior defect, and then close the anterior defect.

Which 3 veins must be ligated during a Warren distal splenorenal shunt for esophageal varices?

1. Coronary vein (left gastric vein)
2. Right epiploic vein
3. Left gonadal vein

If a 12 French Foley catheter cannot be inserted into the bladder, what should be tried next?

1. Larger Foley catheter
2. Lidocaine jelly to anesthetize the urethra
3. Coude catheter

During an inguinal hernia repair, the suture needle goes through the femoral vein or artery. What should be done?

Remove the suture and hold pressure; do not tie the suture down!

How should an anal fistula that goes above the anal sphincters be treated?

Seton suture, which will allow subsequent tightening and scarring down of the sphincter muscles

What test should be performed after a tracheostomy?

Chest x-ray

After the mesoappendix is stapled off during a lap appy, the appendiceal artery continues to pump blood. What should be done?

A metallic clip (as used for lap chole) can be applied or a suture must be placed.

How should the skin be closed after a grossly contaminated abdominal case?

It should be left open, and closed by secondary intention or delayed primary closure.

How should a vas injury be repaired during a procedure to correct an inguinal hernia?

A urologist should be called in to perform an end-to-end repair (unless the patient is elderly).

How should an ilioinguinal nerve transection be repaired during a procedure to correct an inguinal hernia?

A metallic clip should be applied to prevent neuroma formation.

What can help identify the ureters during a difficult pelvic dissection (e.g., postradiation)?

Preoperative ureteral stents placed by a urologist

What can help identify an occult ureteral injury?

IV indigo carmine (collects in urine and most likely will be seen in operative field with ureteral injury)

Why do some surgeons "bowel prep" for gastric cancer surgery?

In case of the unexpected gastrocolonic fistula

Prior to prepping a patient, what mental checklist should be reviewed?

Position? Antibiotics? Clip hair? Sequential decompression device (SCD) boots? NGT? Foley? Special equipment ready and available? Fluoroscopy needed?

What are the 5 intraoperative signs of Crohn's disease?

1. Creeping mesenteric fat
2. Thickened mesentery
3. Thickened bowel wall
4. Serositis
5. Abscesses/fistulae/strictures

Should a frozen section be taken to rule out microscopic disease at the margins before an anastomosis after a small bowel resection for Crohn's disease?

No. Microscopic disease at an anastomosis does not have any effect on the rate of anastomotic healing (1 cm of grossly normal bowel is needed for margins with Crohn's disease).

A stable patient has a chest-penetrating wound in the box formed by the clavicles, nipples, and costal margins. How should this patient be evaluated for cardiac injury?

Subxiphoid pericardial window or echocardiogram if no hemothorax

What is the strongest layer of bowel for an anastomosis?

The submucosa (not the serosa; think **su**bmucosa = **su**perior strength)

What condition contraindicates a hemorrhoidectomy?	Crohn's disease

LAPAROSCOPY PEARLS

What must you do when you use the Argon laser during laparoscopy?	Open a trocar vent; otherwise, intra-abdominal pressure will build up and may result in CO_2 embolus.
What is the appropriate treatment for bladder Veress needle puncture?	Postoperative Foley drainage
What is the appropriate treatment for trocar bladder injury?	Closing by suture and placement of Foley drainage
How can placement of a trocar through an epigastric vessel be avoided?	Transilluminate the abdominal wall and identify the vessels.
Name the options for fixing a bleeding trocar site.	1. Insert a Keith needle into the peritoneal cavity, out the abdomen, under the vessel, and tie over a bolster. 2. Cut down and tie off the vessel. 3. Insert a Foley catheter through the trocar site; pressure should be held with outward traction.

14

Wounds, Drains, and Tubes

How do you get rid of "dog ears" (extra tissue on one side of a wound being closed primarily)?

Pull the extra skin out at the end of the incision and cut it off.

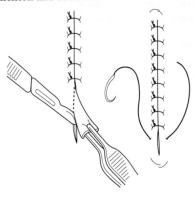

How long before you can débride a brown recluse spider bite?

The area of necrosis may not be demarcated for weeks.

Until the necrotic area is defined, how is a brown recluse spider bite treated?

With dapsone (check for glucose-6-phosphate dehydrogenase [G-6-PD] deficiency)

WOUNDS

DECUBITUS ULCERS

What are decubitus ulcers?

Pressure ulcers due to skin or muscle breakdown and necrosis resulting from prolonged pressure on a bony prominence (e.g., ischial tuberosity, sacrum, occiput)

Describe the stages of decubitus ulcers.

Stage I

Erythema

Stage II	Partial skin thickness loss
Stage III	Full thickness skin loss
Stage IV	Full thickness skin loss and injury to underlying tissues

WOUND CLOSURE AND HEALING

Should you suture the subcutaneous fat closed?	No
How do you treat a large wound with a large subQ space and likely fluid collection?	Insert a drain.
When do you remove drains?	Optimally, when drainage is < 30 mL/day; however, the longer a drain is left in, the higher the infection rate. Remove axillary drains by 2 weeks.
What is a Wound Vac and what is its purpose?	A sponge placed into a wound and covered by an air-tight plastic sheet with suction applied; it is used to help contract and close chronic wounds.
What does a "scab" contain?	Fibrin and blood
Do abrasion wounds heal slower or faster with a scab?	Slower!
Does silver sulfadiazine (Silvadene) slow or speed up abrasion wound healing compared to a dry dressing?	Speeds it up due to moisture and a decreased bacterial wound count
If a skin wound that was sutured closed opens up, when can you reclose it primarily?	If possible to do so in < 8 hours after dehiscence, the wound usually can be reclosed (but, of course, with an increased risk of infection).

WOUND INFECTIONS

What would the Gram stain of a clostridial wound infection show?	Gram-positive **rods**

What does streptococcal or staphylococcal wound infection show on Gram stain?	Gram-positive **cocci**
Name the first and second most common bacterial causes of infection in clean wounds?	1. *Staphylococcus aureus* 2. Streptococcal organisms

When and what antibiotics are used for a clean wound infection?	After opening the wound, if cellulitis or signs of systemic reaction are present, then use anti-staph/anti-strep IV antibiotics:
	    Cefazolin sodium (Ancef)
	    Oxacillin

What is the usual bacterial count necessary for a wound infection?	$> 10^5$
What are the causes of wound infection after perineal or bowel surgery?	Many are mixed infections.
In a nonimmunocompromised patient, when would you treat a wound for a *Candida* infection?	1. Positive culture 2. Antibacterial treatment fails 3. Any coronary artery bypass graft (CABG) patient with a sternal wound infection and culture positive for *Candida*
What is the relationship between risk of wound infection and operation duration?	Infection risk doubles every hour!

DRAINS, CATHETERS, AND TUBES

What is a Cantor tube?	A long intestinal tube with a mercury-filled balloon tip; sometimes used in partial bowel obstruction
How is a Cantor tube removed?	Very slowly—pull out 1 foot every 2 hours
What is a Miller-Abbott tube?	A long intestinal tube

Who invented the Dobbhoff tube?

Not Dr. Dobbhoff. It was actually 2 individuals: **Dobb**ie and **Hoff**meister.

What are some tricks for getting the Dobbhoff tube past the pylorus?

Slack, right lateral decubitus and metoclopramide (Reglan)

What should be given during a T-tube cholangiogram?

IV antibiotics

Is it possible to drain the free peritoneal cavity?

No

Should a drain ever be brought out of the body through a suture line?

No. It should be brought out through a separate incision.

What is the maximum recommended rate of pleural effusion drainage?

Not to exceed 1 L over the first 30 minutes of drainage; a faster rate could result in acute pulmonary edema caused by rapid lung re-expansion (rare).

Have prophylactic oral antibiotics been shown to help prevent drain tract infections after mastectomies?

Yes. Although controversial, antibiotics may help prevent closed-drain tract infections after mastectomy, according to research by Touran and Frost (1990).

What are the 2 indications for intraperitoneal drains?

1. Well-formed abscess cavity
2. To control a fistula

How long after placement are peritoneal drains completely surrounded by omentum?

48 hours

Is a drain needed after a routine appendectomy?

No

Are drains usually needed after a ruptured appendix?

No, unless there is an abscess pocket (**remember:** the free peritoneal cavity cannot be drained).

Should a closed drain be placed after removal of a large sarcoma?

Yes. Always place the drain exit hole close to the incision, for easy postoperative re-excision in case of recurrence.

Is a drain needed after a cholecystectomy?

No

Is a drain needed after an acute rectal perforation?

Yes. Presacral drains (Jackson-Pratt) are necessary, along with a diverting colostomy, if the perforation is intraperitoneal then closure, if easily done.

What is "marsupialization" for a pancreatic abscess?

The practice of packing the wound open with Kerlex or other gauze pads, creating a wound "pouch," following débridement of the pancreas

Are perineal drains indicated after closure of the perineum following an abdominoperineal resection (APR)?

Yes. Closed drainage of the perineum is indicated after primary closure.

Does a drain after splenectomy decrease or increase the intra-abdominal infection rate after a concomitant GI tract injury?

It increases the risk (especially after a colon injury); thus, concomitant GI tract injury is a relative contraindication for postsplenectomy drainage.

For what purpose was the Jackson-Pratt drain initially developed?

For postoperative SDH drainage

What percentage of all pulmonary injuries can be treated definitively with a chest tube?

Approximately 85%

How quickly will a small, stable pneumothorax absorb?

Approximately 1% a day; therefore, 10% by volume will absorb in approximately 10 days.

Does it matter if the chest tube is removed during maximal expiration or inspiration?

No

What treatment is indicated for an extraperitoneal bladder injury?

Drainage of the bladder (with a Foley catheter), in most cases

Currently, which method of draining intraperitoneal abscesses is used most often?

Percutaneous catheter placement, under the guidance of CT or ultrasound

What are 6 relative contraindications for percutaneous drainage of an intraperitoneal abscess?

1. No safe route to the abscess
2. Multiple septations
3. Multiple small abscesses
4. Phlegmon undefined collection
5. Contrast allergy (for CT guidance)
6. Coagulopathy

What is a Hemovac?

A drain with spring suction

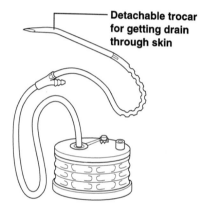

Detachable trocar for getting drain through skin

What is the purpose of a catheter contrast study before removing a percutaneous catheter placed for abscess drainage?

To rule out an enteric abscess cavity fistula to bowel

How often is percutaneous transhepatic cholangiography (PTC) successful:

With dilated biliary ducts?

Approximately 90% successful

With nondilated biliary ducts?

75% successful

What is a Portacath?   A central line with a subQ port for injection over a long period

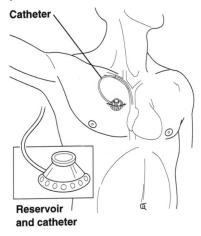

What is a Schrock shunt?   A shunt to bypass the IVC retrohepatic for repair of retrohepatic vena caval injury running from atrium to IVC

What is a Malencott tube?

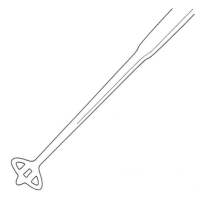

When can a biliary T-tube be removed?   Usually after 3 weeks; if bilirubin level does not increase, no signs or symptoms of cholangitis are seen after clamping, and after obtaining normal T-tube cholangiogram

CATHETERS

What is a pigtail catheter?   A small tube with a curved end (pigtail) placed into pleural cavity to drain fluid by gravity

How long should a peripheral IV be left in place before replacement?	72–96 hours unless obviously infected, at which time they should be removed immediately
How often should IV administration tubing be changed?	Every 96 hours unless TPN-infused, then more frequently
Which IV site has the lowest rate of phlebitis?	The hand
Which site has the highest rate of IV phlebitis?	The lower extremity
Which central line site has the highest infection rate?	The internal jugular (higher than the femoral vein!)
When inserting a central line, does it help to wear a sterile gown and full length sterile drape?	**Yes**—lower central line infection rate if gown, cap, and large sterile drape used
How often should the transparent plastic (polyurethane) central line dressings be changed?	Every 7 days (every 2 days for gauze bandages)
Should you rotate ports of a central line for Hyperal (TPN)?	**No**—use only 1 port exclusively for TPN
Do antiseptic-coated central lines lower the central line infection rate?	**Yes.** Chlorhexidine/silver sulfadiazine-coated catheters lower the infection rate.
What is the most common bacterial cause of central line infection?	Coagulase-negative staphylococci

15

Surgical Anatomy

THYROID

Which nerve travels with the superior thyroid artery approximately 15% of the time?

The superior laryngeal nerve

During a thyroidectomy, should the inferior thyroid artery be transected as close to its origin as possible?

No. The parathyroids receive their blood supply from the inferior thyroid arteries; thus, the inferior thyroid artery should be transected as close to the thyroid as possible.

NECK

Which structure separates the anterior from the posterior neck triangle?

The posterior border of the sternocleidomastoid muscle

Where is Erb's point?

Point in posterior cervical triangle where spinal accessory nerve exits

Which muscle is between the subclavian vein and subclavian artery?

The anterior scalene muscle

Which nerve runs along the anterior border of the anterior scalene muscle?

The phrenic nerve (transection of this nerve paralyzes the diaphragm)

What are the 4 branches of the thyrocervical trunk?

1. Inferior thyroid artery
2. Ascending cervical artery (off the inferior thyroid artery)
3. Transverse cervical artery
4. Suprascapular artery

How can you remember the branches of the thyrocervical trunk?

By the acronym **STAT:**
Suprascapular artery
Transverse cervical artery
Ascending cervical artery
Thyroid artery (inferior)

Which artery does the vertebral artery branch off from?

The subclavian artery, bilaterally

Which artery does the internal mammary artery branch off from?

The subclavian artery, bilaterally

What are the branches of the extracranial internal carotid artery?

None

Where is the thoracic duct located?

It empties into the left subclavian vein.

What is Irish's node?

A node in the left axilla (associated with gastric cancer)

Which muscles lose innervation if the radial nerve is cut at the forearm?

None. Only sensory innervation to the dorsum of the hand is lost.

What is a Langer's arch found in the axilla?

An accessory slip of the latissimus dorsi muscle traversing the axilla; it is a congenital variant.

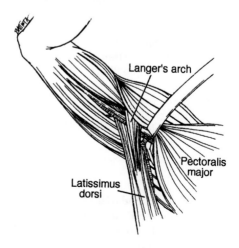

Langer's arch

Pectoralis major

Latissimus dorsi

Where does the subclavian artery turn into the axillary artery?	At the lateral border of the 1st rib
Where does the axillary artery become the brachial artery?	At the inferior border of the teres major muscle
What are the clinical signs of a cut long thoracic nerve during an axillary dissection?	Loss of innervation to the serratus anterior muscle, resulting in a winged scapula
What is the usual distance from the skin at the right internal jugular vein to the pulmonary artery wedge?	50 +/− 5 cm
What is the usual distance from the skin at the right subclavian vein to the pulmonary artery wedge?	45 +/− 5 cm
What is the usual distance from the skin at the left subclavian vein to the pulmonary artery wedge?	55 +/− 5 cm

ABDOMEN

What phrase helps you remember the direction of the external oblique fibers?	"Hands in the pockets"
What phrase helps you remember the direction of the internal oblique fibers?	"Hand over heart"

What are the boundaries of Petit's triangle (inferior lumbar triangle)? (See Chapter 33)	Think: Petit **Lie**
	    Posterior boundary: **L**atissimus dorsi
	    Inferior boundary: **I**liac crest
	    Anterior boundary: **E**xternal oblique
	    (Floor: Internal oblique and transversus abdominis muscle)

What are the boundaries of Grynfeltt-Lesshaft's triangle (superior lumbar triangle)? (See Chapter 33)	Superior: 12th rib Anterior: Internal oblique Floor: Quadratus lumborum

Where is Larrey's point located?

Subxiphoid

What is the criminal nerve of Grassi?

The small posterior branches of the vagus nerve occasionally missed during a truncal vagotomy

What are the veins of Sappey?

The diaphragm veins that drain into the liver

What is Sappey's line?

A line drawn around the abdomen at approximately L2. It is thought that lymph drainage above Sappey's line goes to the axilla and below the line to the groin nodes.

What is the node of Lund?

The cystic node found in the triangle of Calot (also known as Calot's node)

What is the Hartmann's pouch?

The gallbladder infundibulum

What is another name for the supreme artery of Kirk?

The dorsal pancreatic artery

What 3 structures constitute the hepatocystic triangle?

1. Cystic duct/gallbladder
2. Common hepatic duct
3. Lower edge of the liver

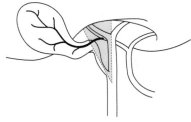

Identify the segments of the liver (French system).

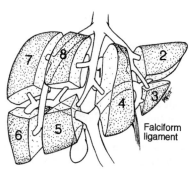

What is the rationale behind the segmental anatomy?

1. Most local and distant metastases to the liver follow the portal venous system.
2. The segmental anatomy is based on the portal and venous systems of the liver.

How many segments are there?

8

What is segment 1?

The caudate lobe (remember, the caudate lobe is caudal to the quadrate lobe)

What is the overall arrangement of the segments in the liver?

Clockwise, starting at segment 1

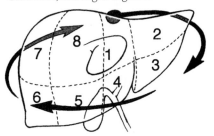

What is segment 4?

Quadrate (named so because it has 4 sides, thus quad = 4)

Which segment is long and often subdivided into parts A and B?

Segment 4

Which segments are divided by the falciform ligament?

It divides segments 2 and 3 from segment 4.

What is Cantlie's line?

An imaginary line drawn from the left of the IVC through the liver, just left of the gallbladder fossa (separates the left and right lobes of the liver)

Which segment is located between Cantlie's line and the falciform ligament?

Segment 4

Which segment is located above the gallbladder?

Segment 5

Which structure lies within Cantlie's line?

The middle hepatic vein

Which segments are separated by Cantlie's line?

Segment 4 is separated from segments 5 and 8

Which segments are resected in the following operative procedures:

Right hepatic lobectomy?

5, 6, 7, 8

Left hepatic lobectomy?

2, 3, 4 (classically, segment 1 is not removed)

Right trisegmentectomy?

1, 4, 5, 6, 7, 8

Left lateral segmentectomy?

2, 3

What is the vein of Mayo?

The vein often seen during a pyloromyotomy for pyloric stenosis over the pylorus

What is the angle of His?

The gastroesophageal angle

What are the boundaries of the gastrinoma triangle?

1. 3rd portion of the duodenum
2. Porta hepatis
3. Neck of pancreas

What is the meandering artery of Gonzalez?

A proximal collateral arterial arcade of the colon that shadows, and is proximal and medial to, the marginal artery

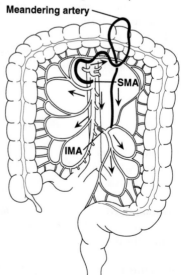

What are 2 advantages of a midline abdominal incision?

1. Wide exposure of peritoneal cavity
2. No major vessel, nerve, or muscle is cut

What is the significance of an arcuate line in the abdominal closure of a midline incision?

Below the arcuate line, all 3 abdominal wall muscle fascias form the **anterior** rectus sheath fascia (i.e., there is no posterior fascia). Above the line, the transversus and half of the internal oblique fascia form a posterior rectus sheath fascia.

Where is the white line of Hilton located?

Between the external and internal anal sphincters

What is the space of Riolan?

The avascular area in the mesentery to the left of the middle colic artery

What are Jackson's veils?

Peritoneal folds across the ascending colon, from the cecum to the right flexure

What are Treves' folds?

Avascular ileocecal peritoneal folds (Treves was also the benefactor of the "Elephant Man")

How long is the average colon?

About 1.5 m

How long is the average length of the adult small bowel?

About 6 m

How long on average is the:

   Anus?

3–3.5 cm

   Rectum?

Approximately 12 cm

Define the amount of peritoneal covering of the rectum by thirds.

   Proximal third

Total peritoneal covering

   Middle third

Anterior surface covered by peritoneum

   Distal third

No peritoneal covering

What is the most common location of an anal fissure? Why?

Posterior due to watershed area of low blood supply

How many anal hemorrhoidal cushions are there?

3—**TROL:**
Two on the **R**ight
One on the **L**eft

What is Griffith's point?

The watershed area between the midgut and the hindgut blood supply to the colon—the area between the proximal two-thirds and the distal third of the transverse colon

What is Sudeck's point?

The watershed between the superior hemorrhoidal artery and the middle hemorrhoidal artery

How do you remember the correct proximal/distal orientation of Sudeck's and Griffith's points?

Just think **G**eneral **S**urgery: **GS** = Griffith's first, Sudeck's second!

What do you call a gallbladder that hangs off the liver and folds in half?

Phrygian cap

Identify the zones of the retroperitoneum.

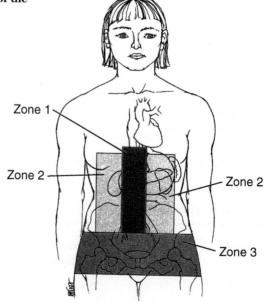

Zone 1

Zone 2

Zone 2

Zone 3

What is the space of Retzius?	The preperitoneal space between the pubis bone and bladder
How much third space fluid would it take to increase the entire peritoneum by 1 mm in thickness?	18 L
What is the node of Rosenmüller?	Node over the greater saphenous vein/femoral vein junction
What is Denonvilliers' fascia?	The fascia between the rectum and the vagina or prostate
What is in Alcock's canal?	1. Internal pudendal artery and vein 2. Pudendal nerve branch (penile or clitoral branch)
Define the boundaries of the femoral triangle.	Acronym **PSA**: 1. **P**oupart's ligament 2. **S**artorius 3. **A**dductor longus
Where does the external iliac artery become the femoral artery?	At the inguinal ligament (Poupart's ligament)
Where does the superficial femoral artery become the popliteal artery?	At the adductor hiatus, where the superior femoral artery leaves the adductor canal and turns into the popliteal fossa
What is another name for the adductor canal?	Hunter's canal
What is the node of Cloquet?	A node in the femoral triangle

LOWER EXTREMITY

Name the 4 compartments of the lower leg.	Anterior, lateral, deep posterior, and superficial posterior

Identify the bones and compartments of the lower leg.

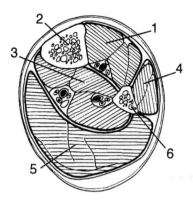

1. Anterior compartment
2. Tibia
3. Deep posterior compartment
4. Lateral compartment
5. Superficial posterior compartment
6. Fibula

What nerve can be injured during lateral lower leg fasciotomy?

The superficial peroneal nerve, which runs in the anterior aspect of the lateral compartment

What does the resulting injury cause?

An inverted foot and loss of sensation of the dorsum of the foot and toes

Why might a patient with CAD go into coronary arrest after clamping the left subclavian?

The patient has an internal mammary artery coronary bypass!

Do only actors have thebesian veins?

No. These are the veins that drain directly into the heart!

Why can one tie off the left renal vein without consequences, but not the right renal vein?

The left renal vein can drain through the left gonadal (testicular/ovarian) vein (the right gonadal vein drains into the IVC).

What is the venous drainage of the adrenal glands?

Usually 1 central vein:
    Right = IVC
    Left = left renal vein
    (+/− accessory vein draining into the inferior phrenic vein)

What is the arterial supply to the adrenal arteries?	3 arteries: 1. **Superior** adrenal artery (branch of the inferior phrenic artery) 2. **Middle** adrenal artery (branch of the aorta) 3. **Inferior** adrenal artery (branch of the renal artery)

GI EMBRYOLOGY

What are the most common sites for heterotopic pancreatic tissue?	The stomach, small intestine, and Meckel's diverticulum
How much does the stomach rotate during development?	90° clockwise; thus, the left vagus is anterior.
How much does the midgut rotate during development?	270° counterclockwise around the superior mesenteric artery, when viewed anteroposteriorly
What is the embryonic origin of a Meckel's diverticulum?	The vitelline duct
To which adult organs does the foregut give rise?	The lungs, esophagus, stomach, and duodenum (up to the ampulla of Vater). The pancreas, liver, bile ducts, and gallbladder are formed from outbuds of the duodenum.
To which adult organs does the midgut give rise?	The duodenum (distal to the ampulla of Vater), small bowel, and large colon (to the distal third of the transverse colon)
To which adult organs does the hindgut give rise?	The distal third of the transverse colon to the anal canal
Which pancreatic bud is connected to the bile duct?	The ventral pancreatic bud
Which pancreatic bud migrates to fuse with another bud?	The ventral bud migrates posteriorly to the left to fuse with the dorsal bud.
What does the ventral pancreatic bud form in the adult pancreas?	The uncinate process and the inferior aspect of the pancreatic head

What does the dorsal pancreatic bud form?

The superior aspect of the pancreatic head, and the body and tail of the pancreas

The small accessory pancreatic duct of Santorini forms from which pancreatic bud?

From the dorsal bud. The main duct of Wirsung forms from the entire ventral pancreatic duct that fuses with the distal pancreatic duct of the dorsal bud.

What abnormality arises if the ventral pancreatic bud migrates posteriorly and anteriorly to fuse with the dorsal pancreatic bud?

Annular pancreas

16

Fluids and Electrolytes

What is the formula for:

Normal total body water?	$0.6 \times$ body wt (kg)
Current body water?	[140/measured sodium (Na^+)] $\times$ body water
Body water deficit?	Normal body water $-$ current body water
Free water deficit with *hypernatremia* (in liters)?	(Patient's Na^+/140) $-$ 1 $\times$ lean body weight $\times$ 0.6 (where 0.6 = total body water)
Na^+ deficit in *hyponatremia*?	$(140 -$ measured $Na^+) \times (0.6 \times$ lean body weight)
Calculated *osmolality*?	$(Na^+ \times 2) +$ (glucose/18) + (BUN/2.8)
Estimating "true" calcium level with low albumin?	For every 1-g deficit of albumin, add 0.8 mg to calcium to correct

Define percentage of total body water in the following.

Men	60%
Women	50%
Older persons	50%
Infants	80%
What 2 electrolyte deficiencies are a sign of a 3rd electrolyte deficiency?	Hypokalemia (refractory to repletion) and hypocalcemia are signs of hypomagnesemia.
What is the primary *intra*cellular cation?	Potassium (K^+), at about 150 mEq (sodium only about 10 mEq!)

106

What is a rough estimate for K+ replacement?

Add 100 mEq = increase in K+ serum level of approximately 0.25!

Name two surgically correctable causes of hypokalemia?

Conn's disease and large colon villous adenomatous polyp secreting mucus high in K+

Why is potassium level important in patients who take *digoxin*?

Potassium and digoxin compete for the same receptors; thus, if K+ is low, the patient is vulnerable to digoxin toxicity.

What electrolyte is decreased in rhabdomyolysis?

Calcium

Should you replace this electrolyte in asymptomatic patients with rhabdomyolysis?

No. Doing so may increase calcium deposition in injured muscles and cause more rhabdomyolysis.

What is the distribution of magnesium?

~50% bone
~50% intracellular
~1% extracellular fluid

What is the primary site of absorbed magnesium loss?

Kidney

Describe the treatment of severe *hyper*magnesemia.

Calcium gluconate IV
Renal dialysis

How much sodium is in 5% albumin?

145 mEq/L

What condition occurs in patients with diabetes insipidus?

Hypernatremia

Define diabetes.

Basically, polyuria

Define insipidus.

Insipid means "tasteless," in contrast with the "sweet" urine of diabetes mellitus!

Which common medication causes nephrogenic diabetes insipidus in the ICU?

Amphotericin B

What condition occurs with the syndrome of inappropriate secretion of antidiuretic hormone (SIADH)?

Hyponatremia

What is the pH of the following:

Lactated Ringer's solution (LRS)?

6.5

Normal saline?

4.5

What is A-line "cycling"?

In intubated patients with **hypovolemia,** the A-line (arterial line) tracing baseline has a wave form (up, then down).

17

Blood and Blood Products

Which blood component is the most common source of bacterial infection in a transfusion?

Platelets, because they are stored at room temperature and staphylococci or streptococci from the donor's skin may be incubated

What percentage of a unit of packed RBCs can be hemolyzed in the first 24 hours after transfusion?

Up to 25%!

How much will the platelet count increase with 1 unit of platelets?

Approximately 5000

How many units of platelets are usually transfused?

6 or 10 (6 or 10 "pack")

What is the risk of receiving a unit of blood infected with hepatitis C?

Approximately 1 in 100,000

Briefly describe hemostasis in a cut vessel.

First, vasoconstriction occurs. Platelets adhere and form a "white thrombus," and then 1 of the coagulation pathways adds fibrin.

Describe the extrinsic coagulation pathway.

$7 \rightarrow 10 \rightarrow$ thrombin (from prothrombin) to fibrin (from fibrinogen)—think 7, 10, T, F (test the extrinsic pathway with prothrombin time [PT])

Describe the intrinsic coagulation pathway.

12 → 11 → 9 → 8 → 10 → thrombin (from prothrombin) to fibrin (from fibrinogen)—think 8–12, T, F (test the intrinsic pathway with partial thromboplastin time [PTT])

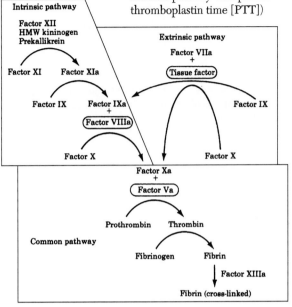

From Ewald GS, McKenzie CR, eds. *Manual of Medical Therapeutics,* 28th ed. Boston: Little, Brown, 1995, with permission.

Which molecules are responsible for platelet aggregation?

Adenosine diphosphate (ADP), thromboxane, and serotonin

Which enzyme is responsible for thromboxane formation?

Cyclooxygenase

What are the 2 main products of arachidonic acid?

1. Thromboxane
2. Prostacyclin (PGI_2)

Which enzymes are responsible for:

Thromboxane?

1. Cyclooxygenase
2. Thromboxane synthetase

Prostacyclin?

1. Cyclooxygenase
2. Prostacyclin synthetase

What is the major source of thromboxane?

Platelets

What is the major source of prostacyclin?

Endothelial cells

Is thromboxane a vasodilator or vasoconstrictor?

A vasoconstrictor

Is prostacyclin a vasodilator or vasoconstrictor?

A vasodilator

What is the effect of prostacyclin on platelet function?

Inhibits platelet aggregation

How can you remember the function of thromboxane compared with that of prostacyclin?

Thromboxane = **thrombo**sis, thus causes vasoconstriction and platelet aggregation

Prosta**cyclin** = **cycling** of platelets, thus causes platelet cycling by inhibiting thrombosis through vasodilation and inhibition of platelet aggregation

What is the function of platelet-derived growth factor?

It is released from platelets and causes growth and migration of fibroblasts and smooth muscle cells.

What effect does nitric oxide have on platelets?

Inhibits platelet aggregation

What do fibroblasts make?

Collagen

How does von Willebrand factor (vWF) work?

It binds the platelet to subendothelial collagen.

What is the role of DDAVP on coagulation?

It causes release of vWF and procoagulant factor VII:C from tissue stores.

When should IV calcium be administered following a massive blood transfusion?

Most experts believe that calcium should be infused after 10 units of packed RBCs because of the citrate (a calcium binder).

Do packed RBCs have any clotting factors?

No

What percentage of patients receiving IV heparin develop antiplatelet antibodies?	Up to 10%!
What does the abbreviation "HIT" stand for?	Heparin-induced thrombocytopenia
How should HIT be treated?	By stopping the administration of heparin (always monitor platelet counts in patients receiving heparin)
Can heparin prolong prothrombin time (PT), as well as partial thromboplastin time (PTT)?	At very high doses, PT can also be prolonged with heparin.
How does heparin work?	It activates antithrombin III.
What side effect is associated with prolonged (> 2 months) heparin infusion?	Osteoporosis
What disorder may inhibit heparin anticoagulation?	Antithrombin III deficiency
What factors can cause the oxyhemoglobin dissociation curve to shift to the right?	Acidosis, elevated 2,3-diphosphoglycerate (2,3-DPG), fever, elevated pCO_2
Give the normal life span for polymorphonuclear neutrophil (PMN) leukocytes.	1 day
Which test—PT or PTT—measures the extrinsic clotting system?	PT (think: pet = extrinsic)
Which test—PT or PTT—measures the effect of heparin on the clotting system?	PTT (often reported by the lab as "heparin PTT")
What substance binds platelets to each other?	Fibrinogen

What binds platelets to collagen?	vWF
What substance binds platelets to vWF?	Platelet glycoprotein Ib (GpIb) [think: **Gp**Ib = **G**rab **p**latelet]
What is Bernard-Soulier syndrome?	A bleeding disorder caused by decreased levels of GpIb, factor V, and factor IX
What is Glanzmann thromboasthenia?	A defect in platelet aggregation caused by the absence of GpIIb and GpIIIa, which bind platelets to fibrinogen and thus to each other
What lab findings are associated with hemolysis?	Increased indirect bilirubin, normal direct bilirubin, decreased hematocrit, decreased haptoglobin
What disorder (other than hemolysis) can cause decreased haptoglobin levels?	Liver disease. Haptoglobin, which is synthesized by the liver, is increased in inflammatory reactions (i.e., acute phase reactant).
What is the function of haptoglobin?	It binds hemoglobin and then is cleared by macrophages.
Which enzyme causes fibrinolysis?	Plasmin
What substance activates plasmin?	Tissue plasminogen activator (tPA) activates plasmin from plasminogen.
How does ε-aminocaproic acid (εACA) work?	εACA is an antifibrinolytic that inhibits plasminogen-to-plasmin conversion, thereby inhibiting fibrinolysis by plasmin.
How does aprotinin work?	1. Inhibits fibrinolysis by inhibiting plasmin and kallikrein 2. Promotes platelet adhesion receptors
What does the abbreviation ACT stand for?	Activated Clotting Time
What is ACT?	A widely used measure to assess heparin anticoagulation in the OR
What is an abnormal ACT?	> 120 seconds

What type of medications increase the breakdown of warfarin?	Medications that increase cytochrome P-450 liver microsomal enzyme metabolism (e.g., barbiturates, carbamazepine)
What is Christmas disease?	Hemophilia B
What is hemophilia C?	A deficiency of factor XI
Which type of hemophilia is more common in the United States?	Hemophilia A is 4 times more common than other types.
Which blood product, cryoprecipitate or fresh frozen plasma (FFP), has the highest concentration of vWF?	Cryoprecipitate
What is lupus anticoagulant?	An antibody associated with systemic lupus erythematosus (SLE), procainamide, phenothiazine, hydralazine, quinidine, and HIV infection. It can prolong PTT in vitro, but does not inhibit hemostasis in vivo, and can actually cause thrombotic problems.
What effect does uremia have on platelets?	Inhibits platelet function
How should uremic platelet dysfunction be treated?	With dialysis or DDAVP, or both
What can cause a coagulopathy in brain-injured patients?	Brain thromboplastin
What are the 3 main inhibitors in coagulation regulation?	Antithrombin, protein C, and protein S
What does antithrombin do?	Binds factors (heparin accelerates this process)
What does protein C do?	1. Inhibits factors V and VIII 2. Possibly releases tPA

What does protein S do?

Stimulates and enhances the effects of protein C (think protein **S** = **s**timulates protein C)

How should protein C deficiency be treated in the acute thrombotic setting?

Although counterintuitive, fresh frozen plasma (FFP) is the best source of protein C and heparin, and should be supplemented with antithrombin III, as needed. (Consult a hematologist.)

If a patient has a deficiency in protein C, S, or antithrombin III, what is the effect on the coagulation system?

A hypercoagulable state

Which renal disease is associated with a hypercoagulable state?

Nephrotic syndrome with the wasting of proteins, including proteins C and S

What is the effect of hypothermia on clotting?

It inhibits clotting factors and platelet function.

Does double gloving lower the incidence of finger blood soilage in the OR?

Yes (so do it!)

On average, how many HIV particles are transmitted on a solid bloody needle:

    Through 1 glove?

10 HIV particles per puncture

    Through 2 gloves?

1 HIV particle per puncture!

Which antibiotic can have the side effect of anticoagulation?

Cefotetan

How does ticlopidine work?

Inhibits platelet aggregation by disrupting adenosine diphosphate (ADP)-induced fibrinogen binding to platelet membrane. Ticlopidine is an aspirin substitute, but it has side effects: neutropenia and agranulocytosis.

What is post-transfusion purpura?	Thrombocytopenia and purpura due to antiplatelet antibodies after a platelet transfusion (patient has had a previous transfusion)
Who can get O$^+$ blood as a universal donor?	Males
What is the risk of death from a blood transfusion?	1 in approximately 650,000
What is the risk of HIV from a blood transfusion?	1 in 500,000
What is the risk of nonfatal hemolytic transfusion reaction?	1 in 6000

18   Surgical Hemostasis

What is the motto of surgical hemostasis?

"Charcoal doesn't bleed."

What is bipolar electrocautery?

Coagulation between 2 electrocautery electrodes

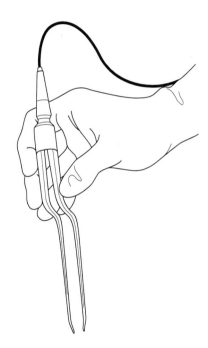

What 2 factors need to be in place before bipolar coagulation will work?

1. Gap between the metallic electrodes
2. Electrolyte-containing fluid between electrodes

Does bipolar coagulation require a grounding pad?

No

What antibiotic is associated with causing a coagulopathy?

Cefotetan. A side chain (methylthiotetrazole, if you must know) increases partial thromboplastin time (PTT).

What IV colloid fluid is associated with a coagulopathy?

Hespan (if > 1500 mL infused)

Define the following.

Avitene

Collagen powder or sheets; act as a matrix for clotting factors/platelets

Argon beam coagulator

Argon gas coagulator for topical hemostasis by heat; excellent for liver oozing

CUSA

Cavitron **U**ltrasonic **S**urgical **A**spirator. Acoustic vibrator breaks up tissue and then aspirates the debris; it is used to dissect liver parenchyma while sparing vessels that are then coagulated.

19

Surgical Medications

**Define the mechanism of
action for each of the
following medications.**

Quinolones	Inhibit DNA gyrase
Promethazine	Antinausea agent; affects medullary chemoreceptor trigger zone
Haloperidol	Competitive blocker of postsynaptic dopamine receptors in the brain (contraindicated in patients with Parkinson's disease)
Misoprostol	Prostaglandin analog for gastric cytoprotection
Cyclosporine	Inhibits interleukin (IL)-2
FK-506	Inhibits secretion of IL-2 and blocks IL-2 receptors
Bacitracin	Inhibits bacterial cell walls, mostly gram-positive coverage; used for peritoneal irrigation and topically only because it causes severe nephrotoxicity if given systemically
Digoxin	Inhibits the Na^+-K^+-ATPase, which leads to an increase in intracellular Ca^+ (positive inotrope and negative chromotrope)
Streptozocin	Selective uptake and death of pancreatic β-cells

| Sulfasalazine | Cleaved into 2 compounds: 5-aminosalicylate (5-ASA) and sulfapyridine (which is absorbed). The 5-ASA stays in the gut and most likely wreaks havoc with the arachidonic pathways. |

ENDOCRINE MEDICATIONS

What is the most common cause of adrenal insufficiency in surgical patients?	Suppression of the hypothalamic-pituitary-adrenal axis by therapeutic steroid administration
How long after the discontinuation of chronic steroid use is a patient at risk for adrenal insufficiency?	Up to 1 year
What is the treatment of choice for acute adrenal insufficiency?	100 mg of hydrocortisone, every 8 hours
What are the medical options in the treatment of diabetes insipidus?	Free access to water DDAVP (10 to 40 μg via nasal spray, qd) Pitressin (IM administration of 5 to 10 U every 24 to 48 hours)
What is the major difference between DDAVP and pitressin?	DDVAP has **no** vasoconstriction effect! (Pitressin does.)

MISCELLANEOUS AGENTS

How long would it take to replenish depleted stores of iron with typical Fe therapy (200–400 mg/day of elemental Fe)?	3 to 6 months
Which nebulized medication is contraindicated in patients allergic to sulfa?	Acetylcysteine, which contains sulfa
Who should not receive cephalosporins?	Patients with a history of anaphylaxis, swelling/edema, or hives after receiving penicillin, because cross reactivity occurs in approximately 8% of cases

Give the relative anti-inflammatory potency of the following substances, with cortisol as 1.0.

Hydrocortisone	1.0
Prednisone	4.0
Prednisolone	4.0
Methylprednisolone	5.0
Dexamethasone	30.0 (Think: Dex = 10 = > 10 × potency)

Which drug is used to treat refractory hiccups?

Thorazine

Does acetaminophen affect platelet function?

No

Which medications increase the metabolism of warfarin?

Any drugs that increase the cytochrome P-450 microsomal enzyme system in the liver (e.g., barbiturates)

Classically, what 2 types of patients should avoid β-blockers?

Patients with asthma or reactive airway disease, because β-blockers can cause bronchospasm (albuterol is a β-agonist)
Patients taking a calcium channel blocker I.V.

What is the major side effect of imipenem?

Seizures

Which electrolyte will cause muscle/skin necrosis if infused subcutaneously (i.e., IV infiltration)?

Calcium

When a patient does not respond to a dose of furosemide, should the dose be repeated? Increased? Decreased?

Double the dose if the patient does not respond to the initial dose.

Why can shortness of breath be alleviated more quickly than diuresis in patients with CHF who are being treated with furosemide?

Because furosemide is a venodilator and thus increases the venous capacitance faster than the diuresis

Which medication is used to treat promethazine-induced dystonia?	IV administration of diphenhydramine hydrochloride
How is theophylline administered intravenously?	It is not; there is no IV form of theophylline. Give IV aminophylline, instead.
What is the antidote for acetaminophen overdose?	Acetylcysteine
What drug is used to treat malignant hyperthermia?	Dantrolene
What drug is used to treat a brown recluse spider bite?	Dapsone
What must be ruled out before starting dapsone?	Glucose-6-phosphate dehydrogenase (G-6-PD) deficiency
What antibiotic can be an anticoagulant?	Cefotetan
What is the treatment for β-blocker overdose?	Glucagon (Yes, glucagon!)
Which vitamin deficiency is often seen with long-term antibiotic use?	Vitamin K
What is the dose of epinephrine 1:1000?	1 g in 1 L, or 1 mg/mL
What is the dose of epinephrine 1:10,000?	1 g in 10 L, or 100 µg/mL (1 mg per 10 mL)
How should most patients (not older persons) be dosed for gentamicin these days?	Once daily
Why the change in gentamicin dosing?	Same efficacy, but less nephrotoxicity in younger persons
What is the usual dose for once daily or "extended interval dosing" for gentamicin?	5–7 mg/kg; then check blood levels and adjust by nomogram.

20 Complications

ATELECTASIS

Why would high levels of inspired oxygen cause atelectasis?	High levels of oxygen eliminate the nitrogen in the normal alveoli that help keep them open.

PULMONARY EDEMA

What are the symptoms of pulmonary edema?	Dyspnea, cough productive of frothy sputum, tachypnea, rales, and cyanosis
What are Kerley B lines?	On chest radiograph, **straight lines** (not curly!) from fluid thickening of the lung interstitium (B lines horizontal)
What is cephalization on a chest radiograph?	Increased pulmonary vascular markings superiorly (toward the head) resulting from increased pulmonary venous pressure
What is the appropriate treatment?	1. Oxygen 2. Furosemide (diuresis) 3. If ventilated, continuous positive airway pressure/positive end-expiratory pressure (CPAP/PEEP) 4. Vasodilators and dobutamine as needed (prn) 5. Treatment of the underlying cause
In chronic heart failure, why does furosemide begin to work before the resulting diuresis?	It also causes systemic venous dilation and a subsequent decrease in preload.

THYROID STORM

What is thyroid storm?	Severe hyperthyroidism
What is the risk factor?	Hyperthyroidism
What events trigger this condition?	Infection, acute abdomen, surgery, trauma, any severe stressor in an already thyrotoxic patient
What are the signs and symptoms?	Fever, tachycardia, psychosis, delirium/confusion, abdominal pain, nausea/vomiting, diaphoresis, CHF, pulmonary edema, tremors, hypertension, fever
What is the appropriate treatment?	1. Supportive therapy (oxygen, fluids, fever reduction) 2. Propranolol 3. Propylthiouracil, iodide 4. Hydrocortisone
What is the mortality rate?	10 to 20%

FAT EMBOLI SYNDROME

What is fat emboli syndrome?	Embolization of fat particles
What are the risk factors?	Fractures of the long bones, trauma
What are the signs?	**Bergman's triad** (mental status changes, petechiae, and dyspnea); chest radiograph picture similar to acute respiratory distress syndrome (ARDS) because fat particles cause pneumonitis
What are the complications?	Respiratory failure, disseminated intravascular coagulation (DIC)
What is the treatment?	Ventilatory support with PEEP as necessary, ± steroids, and treatment of DIC (if it develops)

GASTROINTESTINAL COMPLICATIONS

BLIND LOOP SYNDROME

What are the differential diagnoses of blind loop syndrome?	Stricture of the intestine, Crohn's disease, postvagotomy syndromes, scleroderma, small bowel diverticula, decreased gastric acid secretion, incompetent ileocecal valve
What are the signs/ symptoms?	Diarrhea, steatorrhea, malnutrition, abdominal pain, hypocalcemia, megaloblastic anemia, vitamin B_{12} deficiency, iron deficiency
What is the treatment?	Surgical correction of the underlying disorder causing the stasis, if feasible; otherwise, antibiotics to inhibit bacterial overgrowth

POUCHITIS

What is pouchitis?	Inflammation of the pouch of an ileoanal pull-through anastomosis (usually after a colectomy for ulcerative colitis)
What are the signs/ symptoms?	Fever, abdominal cramping, increased frequency of liquid stools
What is the treatment?	Metronidazole PO

POSTGASTRECTOMY COMPLICATIONS

What is a postgastrectomy syndrome?	A syndrome of complications following gastrectomies
Name the 8 types of postgastrectomy syndromes.	1. Afferent loop syndrome 2. Efferent loop syndrome 3. Postvagotomy diarrhea 4. Dumping syndrome 5. Roux stasis syndrome 6. Alkaline (bile) reflux gastritis 7. Chronic gastric atony 8. Small gastric remnant syndrome

AFFERENT LOOP SYNDROME

What is afferent loop syndrome?

Obstruction of the afferent loop of a Billroth II (afferent loop is the proximal duodenum/jejunum loop draining bile toward the gastrojejunostomy)

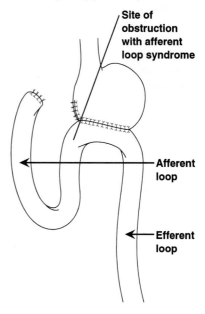

Site of obstruction with afferent loop syndrome

Afferent loop

Efferent loop

What is the efferent loop?

The distal loop draining away from the stomach (think: **e**fferent = **e**gress)

What is the incidence?

Less than 1%

What are the causes?

Kinking, intussusception, adhesions, volvulus, hernias of the afferent loop

What are the associated risks?

Long afferent loop
Antecolic anastomosis
Anastomosis to a lesser curvature of the stomach

What are the signs/ symptoms of acute onset?

Abdominal pain, epigastric mass, nonbilious (usually in 1st week), vomiting, nausea, fever

What are the signs/ symptoms of chronic disease?

Abdominal pain relieved by pure bile emesis (from decompression of the obstructed afferent loop)

What is the dreaded complication?	Duodenal stump blowout
What mortality rate is associated with acute onset?	Approximately a third! (surgical emergency)
How is the diagnosis of acute disease confirmed?	Fluid-filled epigastric mass on ultrasound or CT
How is the diagnosis of chronic disease confirmed?	Esophagogastroduodenoscopy (EGD; to rule out alkaline reflux gastritis)
What is the appropriate treatment?	Convert Billroth II to a Roux-en-Y of the afferent loop 40 to 50 cm from the gastrojejunostomy on the efferent limb

EFFERENT LOOP SYNDROME

What is efferent loop syndrome?	Obstruction of the efferent loop, or at the anastomosis of the gastric remnant to the efferent loop
What causes it?	Adhesions, volvulus, hernia, omental wrap with fibrosis of the omentum, tight mesocolon tunnel, anastomotic stricture
How is the diagnosis confirmed?	Upper GI barium series, esophagogastroduodenoscopy (EGD)
What is the appropriate treatment?	Surgical correction of the obstruction or balloon dilatation of stricture

POSTVAGOTOMY DIARRHEA

What is postvagotomy diarrhea?	Diarrhea after a truncal vagotomy
What causes it?	It is thought that after truncal vagotomy, rapid transport of unconjugated bile salts to the colon causes osmotic inhibition of water absorption in the colon, resulting in diarrhea.
What is the incidence?	Approximately one-third of patients will have diarrhea after a truncal vagotomy, but only about 1% will have severe diarrhea.

What are the associated signs/symptoms?   Diarrhea

What is the appropriate medical treatment?   Cholestyramine (binds bile salts), Lomotil (after ruling out *Clostridium difficile*)

What is the appropriate surgical treatment?   Reversed interposition jejunal segment or Roux-en-Y for refractory cases

What is a reversed interposition jejunal loop?

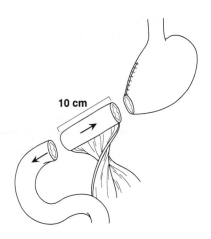

10 cm

DUMPING SYNDROME

What is dumping syndrome?   Delivery of hyperosmotic chyme to the small intestine (normally the stomach will decrease the osmolality of the chyme prior to its emptying). Late dumping is thought to be caused by hypoglycemia.

With what conditions is it associated?   Any procedure that bypasses the pylorus or compromises its function (i.e., gastroenterostomies or pyloroplasty), thus "dumping" of chyme into the small intestine

What are the associated signs/symptoms?   Postprandial diaphoresis, tachycardia, abdominal pain/distention, emesis, increased flatus, dizziness, weakness, weight loss, mental status changes

What is the appropriate medical treatment?   Small, multiple, low-fat, low-carbohydrate, high-protein meals
Avoidance of liquids with meals to slow gastric emptying

Lying down after eating
Octreotide
Ingestion of carbohydrates to raise blood
    glucose (for late dumping syndrome)

What percentage of patients with dumping syndrome resolve with medical treatment?

Approximately 75% in < 1 year

If medical therapy fails, what is the appropriate surgical treatment?

1. Roux-en-Y
2. Henley jejunal interposition
3. Billroth II converted to a Billroth I

ROUX STASIS SYNDROME

What is Roux stasis syndrome?

Stasis of chyme in the gastric remnant

What causes it?

Loss of normal gastric motility (loss of migration of the normal pacemaker motor waves)

What are the associated signs/symptoms?

Abdominal pain, nonbilious vomiting, nausea postprandially

How is the diagnosis confirmed?

Endoscopy (rule out outlet obstruction/ ulcer)
Emptying study

What is the appropriate medical treatment?

Metoclopramide (Reglan), erythromycin

What is the appropriate surgical treatment?

Subtotal gastrectomy with > 75% stomach removed

ALKALINE (BILE) REFLUX GASTRITIS

What is alkaline reflux gastritis?

Reflux of bile into the stomach after a Billroth I, Billroth II, or pyloroplasty

What are the associated signs/symptoms?

Epigastric burning, abdominal pain, nausea, weight loss, anemia, bilious vomiting

How do the symptoms compare with those of afferent loop syndrome?

With reflux gastritis, the bilious vomiting does not relieve the symptoms as it does in chronic afferent loop syndrome.

What is the major risk factor for alkaline reflux gastritis?	Billroth II
How is the diagnosis confirmed?	EGD reveals gastritis/bile Biliary scan (pooling in stomach remnant)
What is the appropriate medical treatment?	H_2 blockers, cholestyramine, metoclopramide, sucralfate
What is the appropriate surgical treatment?	1. Conversion to Roux-en-Y 2. Braun enteroenterostomy 3. Henley jejunal interposition

CHRONIC GASTRIC ATONY

What is chronic gastric atony?	Delayed gastric remnant emptying following vagotomy
What are the associated risk factors?	Diabetes, smoking, alcohol, Roux-en-Y
What are the associated signs/symptoms?	Epigastric pain, nausea, early satiety, weight loss, anemia, postprandial exacerbation
How is the diagnosis confirmed?	EGD (to rule out ulcer/obstruction) Gastric emptying study
What is the appropriate medical treatment?	Small meals, cessation of smoking and/or alcohol, metoclopramide/cisapride
What is the appropriate surgical treatment?	Near total gastrectomy with Roux-en-Y (Roux-en-Y without gastric resection is disastrous)

SMALL GASTRIC REMNANT SYNDROME

What is small gastric remnant syndrome?	Loss of gastric reservoir and vagal-mediated receptive gastric relaxation in patients with > 80% gastric resection and vagotomy
What are the associated signs/symptoms?	Early satiety, epigastric pain, weight loss, anemia, malnutrition
How is the diagnosis confirmed?	EGD (to rule out obstruction, ulcer, bezoar, cancer)

What is the appropriate medical treatment?	Small meals, liquid supplements
What is the appropriate surgical treatment?	Jejunal pouch reconstruction

MISCELLANEOUS

What nutritional problems can follow gastrectomy?	Deficiencies of vitamin B_{12} (by loss of intrinsic factor), folate, iron, and calcium; weight loss caused by poor food intake; bacterial overgrowth; steatorrhea because of loss of pancreatic enzymes (loss of vagal stimulation)
What is the incidence of gastric cancer following a partial gastrectomy?	Probably slightly increased, usually after 20 years
What is the incidence of cholelithiasis after truncal vagotomy?	Increased, most likely because of decreased emptying of the gallbladder and decreased opening of the sphincter of Oddi; higher incidence after truncal vagotomy with total gastrectomy

21

Common Causes of Ward Emergencies

CARDIAC EMERGENCIES

How can you remember the advanced cardiac life support (ACLS) protocols?

Carry a copy of ACLS protocols with you at all times!

What is the treatment for asystole?

Think asystol"**TEA**":
Transcutaneous pacing
Epinephrine
Atropine

What is PEA?

Pulseless **E**lectrical **A**ctivity (i.e., no pulse, but ECG tracing)

What are the common ACLS manual causes of PEA?

"5 HT"
5 H: **H**ypoxia, **H**ypovolemia, **H**yperkalemia (or Hypokalemia), **H**ypothermia, **H**ydrogen ion (acidosis)
5 T: **T**ension pneumothorax, **T**amponade, **T**hrombosis (CAD), **T**hrombosis (pulmonary embolism), **T**ablet (i.e., medications)

What is the treatment of PEA?

Think **PEA**:
Primary and secondary surveys: fix mechanical problem
Epinephrine
Atropine

What is the mnemonic for pulseless ventricular tachycardia/ventricular fibrillation (VT/VF)?

Think **DIVA**:
Defibrillate
Intubate
Vasopressin
Amiodarone

What is the treatment of pulseless VT/VF?

Simplified: Defibrillate, maintain airway, then give vasopressin or epinephrine, then amiodarone or lidocaine

TRACHEOSTOMY COMPLICATIONS

Describe the mechanism of tracheoesophageal fistula formation.	Pressure necrosis by tracheostomy tube in apposition to nasogastric tube (NGT)
What are the symptoms?	1. Marked increase in tracheal secretions 2. Gastric distention 3. Hypoxia
What diagnostic test is indicated?	Bronchoscopy
What is the appropriate treatment?	Surgical repair
Describe the mechanism of tracheoinnominate artery fistula formation?	Pressure necrosis by tracheostomy tube against the innominate artery
What symptom is associated with the disorder?	Tracheal bleeding—ranging from minor to exsanguinating (known as a "herald" bleed)
What diagnostic test is indicated with minor bleeding?	Bronchoscopy
What is the Utley maneuver?	Direct digital innominate artery pressure through the tracheostomy stoma (with finger in or anterior to trachea), to control massive tracheostomy bleeding
What else can be tried to control bleeding?	Hyperinflation of the tracheal cuff
What is the appropriate treatment?	Surgical repair

ENDOCRINE EMERGENCIES

DIABETIC KETOACIDOSIS

Who is at risk for diabetic ketoacidosis (DKA)?	Patients with type I diabetes mellitus, following cessation of insulin therapy or stress that renders an insulin dose inadequate

What are the possible precipitants?

Infection, traumatic injury, MI, surgery

What is the pathogenesis?

The ratios of glucagon, growth hormone, catecholamines, and cortisol to insulin increase, causing unrestrained glycogenolysis, gluconeogenesis, and ketogenesis.

What are the symptoms?

Vomiting, polyuria, thirst, weakness, altered mental status, abdominal pain, orthostasis, and hyperventilation

What diagnostic laboratory results are typical?

1. Hyperglycemia
2. Ketoacidosis
3. Pseudohyponatremia
4. Elevated serum potassium
5. Urine ketones

What is the appropriate treatment?

1. Administer insulin and glucose to maintain serum glucose levels between 200 and 300 mg/dL.
2. Administer isotonic saline until hypovolemia is corrected, then one-half normal saline.
3. Administer potassium when levels are < 4.5 mEq/L.
4. Administer phosphorus, as needed.
5. Administer bicarbonate when DKA is accompanied by shock, when pH is < 7.1, or with severe hyperkalemia.

What are the possible complications?

1. Shock caused by hypovolemia or acidosis
2. Vascular thrombosis
3. Cerebral edema
4. Hypokalemia
5. Hypophosphatemia

NEUROLOGIC COMPLICATIONS

SEIZURES

Define status epilepticus.

Continuous seizure activity beyond 5 minutes, or at least 2 sequential seizures without full recovery of consciousness

What initial actions should be taken when a patient experiences a seizure?	Use the ABCs of life support: 1. Administer oxygen by nasal cannula or mask. 2. Position head for optimal airway patency; intubate if necessary. 3. Monitor ECG. 4. Establish IV access and order appropriate laboratory tests. 5. NGT to decompress the stomach and decrease the chance of massive aspiration.
What laboratory tests should be ordered immediately?	Electrolytes, antiepileptic drug levels (if applicable), arterial blood gases, hemogram, urinalysis, bicarbonate (low levels associated with seizures secondary to local areas of anaerobic metabolism)
What is the initial treatment?	Benzodiazepines and phenytoin (Dilantin) [in different IVs]
What is secondary treatment if refractory?	1. Propofol 2. Phenobarbital
Name the 5 most common precipitants of status epilepticus in adults.	1. Cerebrovascular phenomena (cerebrovascular accident, tumor, subarachnoid hemorrhage, etc.) 2. Medications (e.g., imipenem) 3. Anoxia 4. Alcohol or drug withdrawal 5. Metabolic/electrolyte imbalances

DIGOXIN TOXICITY

What are the symptoms?	1. Fatigue, visual disturbances, anorexia 2. Bradyarrhythmias (2nd- or 3rd-degree atrioventricular block) 3. Tachyarrhythmias (VT or VF) 4. Hypokalemia
What is the frequency?	2% to 5% of hospitalized patients on digoxin
What is the emergent treatment for life-threatening toxicity?	Digoxin-specific antibody fragments

ALCOHOL WITHDRAWAL

What are the symptoms of alcohol withdrawal at the following intervals:

After 6 to 8 hours?   Tremulousness and irritability

At 8 to 12 hours?   Hallucinosis (usually auditory)

At 12 to 24 hours?   Generalized withdrawal seizures

At 3 to 4 days?   Delirium tremens: confusion, delusions, hallucinations, tremor, agitation, autonomic overactivity (dilated pupils, fever, tachycardia, diaphoresis)

How is it treated?
1. Supportive therapy: fluids, thiamine, and folate
2. Benzodiazepines (e.g., chlordiazepoxide, lorazepam [Ativan])
3. +/− Clonidine

DELIRIUM

Describe delirium.   A patient is disoriented to person, place, or time with fluctuating levels of consciousness. Hallucinations, usually visual, may also occur.

What is the usual perioperative timing of onset?   Onset occurs at approximately the 3rd postoperative day, although it can obviously occur at any time, depending on the patient and the circumstances.

What is the treatment approach?
1. Check electrolytes, obtain complete blood cell count (CBC), urinalysis, and oxygen saturation to assure that mental status changes do not have a simple organic cause.
2. If the patient is not frankly psychotic or agitated, reassurance may be all that is needed.
3. If restlessness continues, sedate the patient with haloperidol (Haldol).

With what ECG finding is haloperidol contraindicated?   Prolonged QT interval

When is a CT scan indicated?	If the condition persists with no identifiable systemic cause, or with focal findings of any type

ANAPHYLAXIS

What is anaphylaxis?	An acute allergic response mediated by immunoglobulin (Ig)E-stimulating release of histamine, leukotrienes, kinins, and prostaglandins from mast cells and basophils
What are the precipitants?	1. Drugs 2. Transfusions 3. Contrast agents 4. Insect stings 5. Foods 6. Latex
What are the symptoms?	Pruritus, urticaria, angioedema, laryngeal edema, laryngeal spasm, **bronchospasm,** and vascular collapse
What is the appropriate treatment?	1. Airway control 2. Epinephrine 0.5 mg (5 mL of 1:10,000 solution) IV, repeat as needed 3. Oxygen 4. Fluids to maintain blood pressure 5. Diphenhydramine 6. Steroids

How much epinephrine is in 1 mL of:

Epi 1:10,000?	100 µg (1 g/10 L = 100 mg/1 L)
Epi 1:1000?	1 mg (1 g/1 L = 1 mg/1 mL)

EPISTAXIS

What is the most common site of epistaxis?	In the inferior portion of the nasal septum, in Kiesselbach triangle (90% of bleeds occur here)
Define the Kiesselbach triangle.	A plexus of vessels in the anteroinferior part of the septum

What is the appropriate treatment of bleeds at this site?

Simple pressure and a topical vasoconstrictor

What is the appropriate treatment for a patient bleeding from the posterior nasal cavity?

1. Patients can swallow a great deal of blood while bleeding from this site; first assess their overall volume status to assure that they are not in shock.
2. Obstruct the bleed with an inflated Foley balloon, or with a nasal pack of gauze and 2–0 silk. Give prophylactic antibiotics to prevent sinusitis and otitis media. Obtain ENT consult.

What is the usual relationship between hypertension and epistaxis?

When they occur together, hypertension is often the result of patient anxiety. Rarely is it the cause of the bleed, but an ongoing bleed may persist until pressure is lowered.

STEVENS-JOHNSON SYNDROME

What are the signs and symptoms?

Blistering skin rash on mucous membranes and extensor surfaces, fever

What are the major causes?

Medications

What is the urgent treatment?

Stop medications; give steroids

22

Surgical Nutrition

ASSESSMENT

What is the Harris-Benedict equation?	An equation for calculating basal energy expenditure (BEE) in kcal/day
What is the Harris-Benedict equation for men?	$66 + (13.7 \times \text{wt/kg}) + (5 \times \text{ht/cm}) - (6.8 \times \text{age})$
What is the Harris-Benedict equation for women?	$65 + (9.6 \times \text{wt/kg}) + (1.7 \times \text{ht/cm}) - (4.7 \times \text{age})$
What is the formula for respiratory quotient (RQ)?	$RQ = \dot{V}CO_2/\dot{V}O_2$
What does an RQ < 0.7 indicate?	Starvation or underfeeding (ketosis)
What does an RQ of 0.7 indicate?	The majority of substrate oxidized is fat.
What does an RQ of 0.8 to 0.85 indicate?	A balanced mixture of substrates are oxidized.
What does an RQ of 1.0 indicate?	The majority of substrate oxidized is carbohydrate.
What does an RQ > 1.0 indicate?	Lipogenesis or overfeeding
What is nitrogen balance?	The difference between the amount of nitrogen ingested and the amount excreted
What is the formula for nitrogen balance?	**Nitrogen in** (dietary protein divided by 6.25) − **Nitrogen out** (urinary nitrogen + GI nitrogen loss + skin nitrogen loss)

What is average daily GI nitrogen loss?	2 to 4 g
What is the average daily skin nitrogen loss?	1 to 4 g
What does a positive nitrogen balance indicate?	More protein ingested than excreted, indicating net anabolism
What does a negative nitrogen balance indicate?	More protein excreted than ingested, indicating net catabolism
What is the nitrogen balance goal?	In critical illness, equilibrium is the goal. Positive nitrogen balance is more likely during recovery.

MISCELLANEOUS

When does refeeding syndrome manifest?	Within 2 days after starting parenteral nutrition, and about 5 to 7 days after starting enteral nutrition
What conditions or (non-nutritional)treatments can increase serum prealbumin?	Renal failure; corticosteroid use
What is "immunonutrition"?	Nutrition fortified with nucleotides, arginine, omega-3 fatty acids, and glutamine to augment immune function (efficacy under study)
Define Kwashiorkor syndrome.	**Protein** deficiency
What is marasmus?	Semistarvation (calories and protein deficiency)
With a normal gut mucosa, is there any advantage to using elemental tube feeding?	No, except elemental tube feeding has a lower incidence of tube clogging!
What feeding route has been shown to hasten the closure of a enterocutaneous fistula?	TPN

What are the best amino acids for patients with liver failure?

Controversial: Branched-chain amino acids (aromatic amino acids are thought to convert to false neurotransmitters)

What is the formula for estimating daily caloric need?

Oxygen consumption (VO2) $\times$ 7

23

Shock

What is the classic Dr. Gross quote on shock?	Shock is the "rude unhinging of the machinery of life." (Samuel Gross, 1872)
Define the following.	
Gastric tonometry	Evaluation of shock by monitoring gastric intramucosal pH via a modified nasogastric tube
Inflammatory shock	Shock caused by release of inflammatory factors (e.g., septic shock, reperfusion injury, trauma)
Tissue oximetry	Measures tissue oxygen levels **directly** from peripheral tissue bed (e.g., muscle) by percutaneously placed probe
Washout phenomenon	Increased lactic acid levels with improved perfusion due to "washout" of lactic acid from previously underperfused tissue beds (conflicting laboratory vs clinical pictures)
SIRS	**S**ystemic **I**nflammatory **R**esponse **S**yndrome; manifested by fever, leukocytosis, increased heart rate, increased respiratory rate
Sepsis	SIRS plus documented infection
Septic shock	Sepsis with hypotension refractory to fluid resuscitation
Can a patient be *hyper*tensive and *hypo*volemic?	Yes; with increased vascular tone from increased sympathetic release

Can a patient have normal blood pressure and be in shock?	Yes, especially if the patient is normally hypertensive
What is the most common cause of hypotension in patients with closed head injury?	Hypovolemic shock; **NEVER** assume that hypotension is due to head injury
At what pH would most give bicarbonate IV for acidosis?	7.2 (especially when CO_2 pulmonary elimination is not impaired)
What is the lethal triad in shock?	ACH: **A**cidosis, **C**oagulopathy, **H**ypothermia
Describe the basic moves to rewarm a patient.	Warmed IV fluids/blood, warm room (hot lights, thermostat), warmed gases in ventilator, Baer hugger
What is a Baer hugger?	A plastic blanket with hot air circulating inside
What is the mortality of septic shock?	50%
What is the cause of gram-negative septic shock?	Endotoxin = lipopolysaccharide (LPS), which then causes release of inflammatory factors and subsequent decrease in vascular tone
In septic shock, what is the classic cardiac output?	**Elevated** due to increased heart rate, but with **decreased** contractility
What pressors are used for septic shock?	Norepinephrine, dopamine
Is a lower body temperature (< 35.5°C) a good sign in septic shock?	**No.** It is associated with higher mortality rate.
What pressors are used in refractory neurogenic shock?	Phenylephrine, norepinephrine (always only after fluid administration)

LACTIC ACID

What are the laboratory "end points" of resuscitation?	Lactic acid and base deficit are most commonly used.
What base deficit is associated with a 25% mortality in trauma patients?	-12 mmol/L
What base deficit is associated with a 50% mortality in trauma patients?	-15 mmol/L
In trauma patients, what is the associated mortality until normalization of lactic acid for the following times postinjury?	
< 24 hours	Approximately 0% mortality
24–48 hours	22% mortality
> 48 hours	86% mortality
In *anaerobic* metabolism (glycolysis) how many adenosine triphosphates (ATPs)are produced?	2 ATPs
In *aerobic* metabolism (glycolysis) how many ATPs are produced?	36 ATPs
What is lactate produced from?	Glycolysis of **glucose** during anaerobic glycolysis (glucose $\rightarrow$ 1 lactate + 2 ATP + H_2O)
In what organs are lactate and lactic acid metabolized?	Mostly the liver and kidney, but all cells can metabolize lactic acid except RBCs
How is lactic acid metabolized?	Back to glucose or CO_2 + and H_2O (lactate $\rightarrow$ pyruvate $\rightarrow$ glucose)

24

Surgical Infection

BACKGROUND AND GENERAL INFORMATION

What is the most common:

Nosocomial infection?

Urinary tract infection (UTI)

Cause of death from a nosocomial infection?

Pneumonia

Bacteria causing upper respiratory tract infection (URTI)/pneumonia < 5 days in the intensive care unit (ICU)?

Gram-positive

Bacteria causing pneumonia in the ICU > 5 days?

Gram-negative

Cause of UTI in surgical patients?

Escherichia coli (second: *Pseudomonas*)

Cause of pneumonia in surgical patients?

Pseudomonas aeruginosa (second: *Staphylococcus aureus*)

Cause of wound infections?

S. aureus (second most common: tie between *E. coli* and *Enterococcus*)

Cause of bacteremia in surgical patients?

Coagulase-negative *Staphylococcus* (second: *S. aureus*)

Cause of intra-abdominal *Candida* infections?

Severe pancreatitis

Device associated with nosocomial bacteremia?

Intravascular catheters in > 75% of cases!

| When should you systemically treat a fungal wound infection? | 1. Positive *Candida* blood culture
2. Failure of antibacterial agents to clear the wound of infection
3. All sternal wound infections with positive *Candida* cultures |

ANTIBIOTICS

What are the indications for antibiotics with wound infections?	First, always open the incision. Antibiotics are indicated if cellulitis/induration are present around the open wound.
What antibiotic is commonly used for wound infection after clean operation?	Cefazolin (Ancef)
What is the common IV antibiotic for wound infections after bowel surgery?	Cefoxitin or cefotetan
What new antibiotic is used for vancomycin-resistant enterococcal (VRE) infection?	Linezolid (Zyvox)
Generally, how long should antibiotics be administered for surgical infections?	General principle: Until the patient demonstrates obvious clinical improvement with a normal temperature for at least 48 hours
How do β-lactam antibiotics work?	They bind to one of several penicillin-binding proteins (PBP) and inhibit bacterial cell-wall synthesis.
What are 2 potentially serious side effects of carbenicillin and ticarcillin?	1. High sodium load 2. Inhibition of platelet aggregation
What is the only β-lactam antibiotic that does not crossreact in patients who are allergic to penicillins or cephalosporins?	Aztreonam
What class of antibiotics is aztreonam in?	It is a monobactam.

What type of bacteria is aztreonam effective against?

Gram-negative

What is the representative drug of the carbapenem class of β-lactams?

Imipenem

With what other drug is imipenem always combined? Why?

Cilastatin (enzyme inhibitor), because it prevents hydrolysis of the active form of the drug in the kidneys

What side effect of imipenem is important to remember?

It is associated with a significantly higher incidence of **seizures.**

Compared with first-generation cephalosporins, what type of spectrum do second-generation cephalosporins have?

Expanded gram-negative activity

Can second-generation cephalosporins be used for empiric treatment of hospital-acquired gram-negative rod infection?

No. They are generally effective against community-acquired gram-negative rod infections with known susceptibility patterns.

Which cephalosporins have good anaerobic activity?

Second-generation cephalosporins: cefoxitin and cefotetan

Which has a longer half-life, cefoxitin or cefotetan?

Cefotetan

What is the potentially serious side effect unique to cefotetan?

Prolonged clotting time

What antibiotic is associated with gallbladder sludge and cholestatic jaundice?

Ceftriaxone

Which bacteria do third-generation cephalosporins have increased activity against?

Gram-negative rods

Which third-generation cephalosporins have increased activity against *Pseudomonas*, *Acinetobacter*, and *Serratia*?	Cefoperazone and ceftazidime
What is the mechanism of action of trimethoprim-sulfamethoxazole?	Trimethoprim is a structural analog of folic acid and competes with dihydrofolic acid for the binding site of dihydrofolate reductase. Sulfamethoxazole is an analog of para-aminobenzoic acid (PABA), which is required for the synthesis of folic acid.
What is the mechanism of action of quinolones?	They inhibit DNA gyrase, thus inhibiting DNA replication.
What type of antibiotic is vancomycin?	A glycopeptide
What is the mechanism of action of vancomycin?	Cell-wall inhibitor; inhibits the transfer of subunits to peptidoglycan by binding to D-alanine residues of penta-peptide moiety
What is the mechanism of action of amphotericin B?	Complexes with fungal sterols (predominantly ergosterol) in plasma membrane, alters membrane permeability
What are the adverse effects of amphotericin B?	**Nephrogenic diabetes insipidus** Dose-dependent **nephrotoxicity** (in up to 80% of patients) Fever, hypotension, chills Anemia Hypokalemia
What is the dosage range and dosing interval of amphotericin B?	IV administration of 0.25 to 1 mg/kg daily, depending on the type of infection and renal function
What electrolyte problem is associated with amphotericin administration?	Hypokalemia

SPECIFIC MICROORGANISMS

What are common bacterial causes of infection after a clean operation?	*S. aureus* Streptococcal species Or both staph and strep

What are the common bacterial causes of superficial wound infections after bowel surgery/groin surgery?

Mixed: aerobic and anaerobic

In most cases, how long is it before responsible bacteria and their sensitivities are known?

Bacteria: at least 24 hours
Sensitivities: 48 to 72 hours

How are enterococcal infections usually treated?

Although no single antibiotic reliably eradicates enterococcal infections or bacteremia, the most effective antibiotic combination is gentamicin **combined** with either a penicillin or with vancomycin.

What antibiotic combination is used to kill *Enterococcus*?

1. Penicillin or vancomycin **and**
2. An aminoglycoside

What broad class of bacteria are the most numerous inhabitants of the GI tract, including the mouth?

Anaerobes

What is the most common anaerobic isolate from surgical infections?

Bacteroides fragilis

What would a Gram stain of clostridia recovered from a soft-tissue infection look like?

Gram-positive rods

True or false: *Candida* organisms recovered from open wounds usually represent true invasion and infection?

False; usually only contamination (but treat all sternal wounds positive for fungus)

Which types of *Candida* are not treated by fluconazole?

C. glabrata and *C. kruzeii* (think "**G**lad to **C**ruise" = **g**lab **k**ruz)

What is the most common cause of breast abscess?

S. aureus; often in nursing mothers

What is lymphangitis and how does it present?

Inflammation of lymphatic channels in subcutaneous tissues

Visible red streaks; may lead to lymphadenitis (inflammation of lymph nodes)

What bacteria can cause splenic abscess in patients with sickle cell anemia?

Salmonella

Infection with which microorganism commonly mimics acute appendicitis?

Yersinia enterocolitica

What are the 3 most common pathogens in suppurative thyroiditis?

S. aureus, Streptococcus pyogenes, Streptococcus pneumoniae

What is the treatment for pelvic inflammatory disease (PID)?

Ceftriaxone 250 mg IM (antigonococcal) and doxycycline 100 mg po bid for 7 days (antichlamydial); treat both

What is a common cause of upper GI bleeding in HIV-infected individuals?

Kaposi sarcoma lesions

What is the most common cause of stomach/duodenal perforation in patients with HIV?

Local CMV infection

What is the most common infectious agent causing colon lesions in patients with HIV?

CMV

How is CMV small bowel perforation treated in patients with HIV?

1. Resect area of perforation
2. Small bowel stomas—no anastomosis!

Do asymptomatic HIV-infected patients undergoing elective surgical procedures exhibit significantly more problems with wound healing and infection than their uninfected counterparts?

No

TOXIC SHOCK SYNDROME

What is toxic shock syndrome?	A syndrome of fever, hypotension, skin rash, and multiple organ failure (MOF). Other symptoms include diarrhea and headache.
What causes it?	Exotoxin from *S. aureus*
What are the associated risk factors?	Tampons, pelvic infection, and sinusitis (nasal packing)

MISCELLANEOUS

What is the most common organism causing osteomyelitis of the foot after a nail puncture through a shoe?	*Pseudomonas*
Which bacteria are associated with infections after dog or cat bites?	*Pasteurella multocida*
Which bacteria are associated with infections after a human bite?	*Eikenella*
How often are central lines changed in burn patients?	Every 3 days
What is generally accepted as the number of contaminating bacteria that must be present to establish a clinical infection in a nonimmunocompromised host?	10^5
How do fluid collections and edema increase the likelihood of infection?	They act as culture media and inhibit phagocytosis and white blood cell (WBC) migration ("WBC can't swim").
By what percentage does hair removal by shaving increase the infection rate when compared with removal by clippers or no removal at all?	100%

What is the classic history of an epidural abscess?	Status postoperative, epidural/spinal anesthetic with **fever** and **back pain**
What is BAL?	**B**roncho**a**lveolar **l**avage (irrigate and aspirate the alveolus by a bronchoscope or sterile tubing through the ETT)
What colony-forming unit (CFU) number do you need for a positive BAL?	> 10,000 CFUs
Why treat *Pseudomonas* infections with 2 antibiotics?	It is thought that 1 antibiotic will rapidly result in antibiotic resistance.
What is the best diagnostic test for sinusitis?	Sinus CT scan
What serologic marker is positive after successful immunization against hepatitis B?	Anti-hepatitis B surface antigen (HBsAg)
Is hand washing able to stop the spread of *Clostridium difficile*?	No. Hibiclens and gloves are needed.

25

Fever

What regulates body temperature?	Anterior hypothalamus
Do all patients with postoperative infections develop fever?	**No.** Only about 50% develop a significant fever.
After GI surgery, what can cause tachycardia and fever specific to the type of surgery?	Anastomotic leak
What acid-base abnormalities are associated with malignant hyperthermia (MH)?	Acidosis
What electrolyte abnormality is associated with MH?	Hyperkalemia
What medications are used to treat MH?	**Dantrolene,** sodium bicarbonate
What should you do if in the middle of a procedure a patient develops MH?	Halt until hyperthermia is corrected, change to different anesthetic, and then when stable and afebrile, continue with procedure.
What are 2 common endocrine causes of fever?	Pheochromocytoma, thyroid storm
What is the risk of surface cooling in a patient with fever?	May cause vasoconstriction and shivering (which will make more heat)

What is the cause of postoperative fever within 48 hours due to *Staphylococcus aureus*?

Toxic shock syndrome

26

Surgical Prophylaxis

What medication lowers the mortality (for up to 2 years postop) for patients with CAD?

β-blockers (e.g., atenolol) before and after operation

What measures may help patients with asthma and chronic obstructive pulmonary disease (COPD)?

1. Stop smoking 4 weeks before operation
2. Administer bronchodilator (e.g., albuterol) preoperatively

What treatment lowers renal failure before, during, and after IV radiocontrast dye?

1. IV fluid alone (dopamine, diuretics are no help)
2. Acetylcysteine (Mucomyst) PO

What medication provides protection against seizures in patients with brain injury?

Phenytoin (Dilantin) × 1 week

What antibiotic provides protection against pancreatic abscess in cases of pancreatic necrosis?

Imipenem IV

What IV antibiotic provides protection from endocarditis in patients with vascular graft and heart valves?

Cephazolin (Ancef)

What IV antibiotic should be used if patients are allergic to penicillin?

Vancomycin

What antibiotic provides protection from infection:

> **During colon surgery?**

Cefoxitin

> **In patients with abdominal trauma?**

Cefoxitin; cefotetan; ampicillin and sulbactam (Unasyn); (or clindamycin/gentamicin if patient is allergic to penicillin)

> **In patients with acute appendicitis?**

Cefoxitin or cefotetan

What antibiotic provides protection from endocarditis in endoscopy, incision and drainage, or bronchoscopy (rigid) in patients at risk for endocarditis?

Amoxicillin 2 g PO, or ampicillin IV

What hand scrub is the best?

Chlorhexidine (povidone-iodine hand scrub results in systemic absorption of iodine!)

What risk is associated with overly hard scrubbing?

Dermatitis, which harbors bacteria!

How may an upper extremity (arm) sequential compression device (SCD) provide some prophylaxis against lower extremity DVT?

SCD activates tissue plasminogen activator (tPA)—but this is an urban legend and there is no adequate data to support it.

What measures provide protection against urinary tract infection (UTI)?

Remove catheters ASAP
Never open catheter drainage system
(i.e., never disconnect tubing system, because doing so doubles the UTI rate)
Take all urine samples with a needle

27 Surgical Radiology

GENERAL

What is the risk of IV contrast?

Contrast-induced nephrotoxicity (3–7% risk)

Anaphylaxis: Urticaria, hypotension, facial or laryngeal edema, bronchospasm

How do you figure out the orientation of the arteries below the knee on an angiogram?

LAMP:
  Lateral = **A**nterior tibial
  Medial = **P**osterior tibial

ABDOMEN

What is the "parrot's beak" or "bird's beak" sign?

Evidence of sigmoid volvulus on barium enema

Evidence of achalasia on barium swallow

What are the differential diagnoses of retroperitoneal calcification?

Pancreatitis, abdominal aortic aneurysm, generalized aortic calcification, kidney stone, renal-cell carcinoma, renal artery aneurysm (phleboliths, if seen in the pelvis)

What is meant by a "cut-off sign"?

Seen in obstruction, bowel distention and air-fluid level are "cut off" from the normal bowel.

What are sentinel loops?

Distention and/or air-fluid levels near a site of abdominal inflammation (e.g., in the right lower quadrant with appendicitis)

What is pneumatosis intestinalis?

Air in the bowel wall

What signs of small bowel obstruction are visible on abdominal x-ray (AXR)?	1. Distended loops of the bowel 2. Air-fluid levels 3. String of beads 4. Step-ladder appearance of distended small bowel 5. Paucity of gas in the colon
What is the "step-ladder" appearance on AXR associated with small bowel obstruction?	Dilated small bowel loops lining up on top of each other from the right lower to the left upper quadrant
What is the "string of beads" on AXR?	Seen with small bowel obstruction; small air bubbles (beads) trapped and separated by the plicae circulares, giving the appearance of a string of beads
What are the best studies to further evaluate small bowel obstruction after AXR?	Abdominal CT scan, contrast studies (small bowel follow through—SBFT)
What AXR finding is associated with a diffuse ileus?	Distended loops throughout, with gas in the small bowel and colon
What is a "string" sign?	Contrast GI study that reveals a stricture; contrast appears as a "string" outlining the narrowing
What is the most common cause of calcifications above the kidney?	Adrenal calcifications (make sure they are not pancreatic calcifications)
What is the best x-ray for diagnosing an abdominal aortic aneurysm (AAA)?	Cross-table lateral; reveals AAA in more than two-thirds of cases by eggshell calcifications
Can there be free air after a successful percutaneous endoscopic gastrostomy (PEG) procedure?	Yes
What is a "lead pipe" on barium enema (BE)?	Seen with chronic ulcerative colitis owing to haustral obliteration and smooth narrowing of the colon. The contrast looks like a smooth lead pipe.

What are "collar button" ulcers on BE?	Asymptomatic deep ulcers associated with Crohn's disease
What is an "apple core" lesion on air contrast BE?	A circumferential lesion of the colon (the vast majority owing to colon cancer)
What do aphthous ulcers look like on BE?	Punctate ulcers with a "lucent halo" of surrounding edema
What is the "double bubble" sign?	Seen on AXR with duodenal obstruction, a duodenal bubble in addition to the gastric bubble
What is a "Meckel's scan"?	A nuclear medicine scan for ectopic Meckel's gastric mucosa
What is the falciform ligament sign?	Free air outlines the falciform ligament
On ultrasound of the liver, what is the "double barrel shotgun" sign?	Dilated intrahepatic duct with the paired portal vein branch; looks like a double barrel shotgun (due to distal biliary duct obstruction)
What is the double duct sign?	Dilated pancreatic and biliary ducts caused by obstruction of the distal common bile duct/ampulla
What test is used for localizing a pheochromocytoma?	A metaiodobenzylguanidine (MIBG) scan (a norepinephrine analog)
What diagnostic study is used to evaluate rectal cancer invasion preoperatively?	Transrectal ultrasound (US)
What diagnostic studies are used to localize the parathyroid glands with hyperparathyroidism?	1. US 2. MRI 3. Sestamibi scintigraphy (CT and thallium-technetium scans are losing favor)

What radiologic studies should be considered for a patient in the ICU with a fever of unknown origin?

1. Chest x-ray (CXR; to rule out pneumonia)
2. Sinus films/CT (to rule out sinusitis)
3. Lower extremity US, Doppler, venogram (to rule out DVT)
4. Abdominal CT (to rule out abscess)
5. Gallbladder US (to check for acalculous cholecystitis)

Where does peritoneal fluid accumulate in the upright position?

The pouch of Douglas, the space anterior to the rectum and posterior to the uterus (women) or bladder (men)

What is the Mickey Mouse sign?

Orientation of common bile duct (right ear), portal vein (head), and hepatic artery (left ear) looks like a Mickey Mouse head and ears

TRAUMA RADIOLOGY

What can be missed on an anteroposterior CXR in trauma?

Anterior pneumothorax

What is a FAST exam?

Focused Assessment Sonogram for Trauma

What 4 areas are examined?

Pericardial sac, bladder, Morison's pouch, and spleen

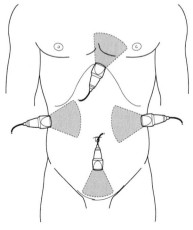

In a trauma patient, what is the significance of fracture of the 3 lower ribs?

Increased risk of liver or splenic injury

How long should it take for a 10% pneumothorax to reabsorb without a chest tube?

A pneumothorax reabsorbs approximately 1% of its measured percentage volume per day; therefore, a 10% pneumothorax should reabsorb in 10 days.

How long after a laparotomy can free air be seen on AXR?

Approximately 1 week

What is the study of choice to evaluate for head trauma?

Unenhanced head CT (blood "lights up")

Give 4 CT scan signs of increased intracranial pressure.

1. Effacement of the ventricles
2. Flattening of the brain sulci
3. Loss of the gray-white matter interface
4. Loss of cisterns

What is DAI?

Diffuse **a**xonal **i**njury, or brain shear injury

What is the best test for DAI?

MRI

What is the falx sign?

Seen with subarachnoid hemorrhage as blood tracts along the falx, it results in a "thickened" falx on unenhanced head CT.

CERVICAL SPINE

What 3 x-ray views must be taken to evaluate the bony cervical spine (c-spine) in trauma?

1. Anteroposterior
2. Lateral
3. Odontoid

What should you look at when evaluating a c-spine film?

1. Adequacy of film
2. The 4 parallel lines
3. Soft tissue thickness
4. Atlantodental interval
5. Disc spaces
6. Bones

What does an adequate c-spine film include?

All of C1–C7 and at least top of T1

What are the 4 parallel lines to check?

SPAT:
1. **S**pinolaminar line
2. **P**osterior vertebral line
3. **A**nterior vertebral line
4. **T**ips of spinous processes

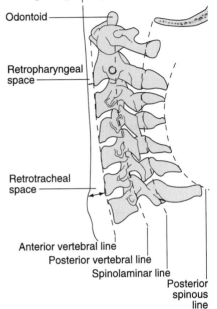

Odontoid

Retropharyngeal space

Retrotracheal space

Anterior vertebral line
Posterior vertebral line
Spinolaminar line
Posterior spinous line

From Gay SB, Woodcook Jr. RJ: Radiology Recall. Philadelphia: Lippincott, Williams & Wilkins, 2000, p. 301.

What are the typical prevertebral soft tissue measurements for normal c-spines?

< 5 mm from C1–C3 and < 20 mm at C4–C7 (easy way to remember basic measurements: < 6 mm at C2 and < 22 mm at C6, or "6 at 2 and 22 at 6")

What is the atlantodental interval?

The distance between the arch of C1 and the odontoid process of C2 (normal adult: < 3 mm)

What injury may cause an increased atlantodental interval?

Transverse ligament tear

What x-rays are used to evaluate for ligamentous c-spine injuries in awake patients?

Lateral flexion and extension c-spine films

CHEST

What is the "deep sulcus" sign?	Deep costophrenic angle sulcus on anterior CXR due to hidden pneumothorax
What is the "fuzzy border" sign?	On CXR, a bullet in the heart has a fuzzy border because the heart is always in motion.
What can cause a cold leg after a thoracic GSW?	Bullet embolus from the heart to the femoral artery!
How many lung lobes are on the right?	3
How many lung lobes are on the left?	2
The lingula is part of which lobe?	The left upper lobe
What is the normal heart size?	The transverse heart diameter is normally less than half of the transverse diameter of the chest.
What are the signs of fluid overload on CXR?	1. Large heart 2. Cephalization (distended large vessels in upper lung fields) 3. Pulmonary edema 4. Kerley B lines 5. Pleural effusion
What are Kerley B lines?	Horizontal lines < 2 cm long that are found at the lung bases, usually signifying pulmonary edema (**B** lines = **B**ases)
What is an air bronchogram?	The outline of an airway made visible by fluid or inflammatory exudates filling the surrounding alveoli
How do you recognize a tension pneumothorax?	**Clinically,** but on CXR: pneumothorax with mediastinal shift away from the affected side and a small heart

What x-ray indicates whether a pleural effusion is free or loculated?

An ipsilateral lateral decubitus CXR; free fluid will "layer out"

If an ETT is placed down too far, which bronchus will it most likely be in?

The right mainstem bronchus

What is the ideal position for a:

Swan-Ganz catheter?

Tip in the right or left pulmonary artery, usually no more than 1 cm lateral to the mediastinal margin

Central venous catheter?

Tip in the SVC, below the brachiocephalic veins and above the right atrium

ETT?

Tip at or below the clavicles and at least 2 cm above the carina

What x-ray must be taken after a tracheostomy is performed?

CXR (to rule out pneumothorax)

What x-ray should be obtained after a central line placement?

CXR to confirm placement and rule out pneumothorax

What x-ray must be taken after a bronchoscopy?

CXR (to rule out pneumothorax, collapsed lobe)

28   Anesthesia

What is the American Society of Anesthesiologists (ASA) Physical Status Classification? What is its purpose?

It is a status rating (I-VI) assigned to each patient prior to receiving anesthesia. It allows for assessment of anesthetic outcome, but is not meant to predict anesthetic risk and is independent of the surgery planned.

Describe the following ASA Physical Status categories.

ASA I

Healthy patient

ASA II

Patient with mild to moderate systemic disease without significant impairment of activity

ASA III

Patient with moderate to severe systemic disease that limits activity

ASA IV

Patient with severe, life-threatening illness

ASA V

Patient who is critically ill and is not expected to live more than 24 hours

ASA VI

A transplant donor

What does the suffix "E" denote in ASA Physical Status rating?

Patients undergoing emergency surgery, regardless of the type of operation or their ASA classification (e.g., emergency appendectomy on an otherwise healthy, young patient: ASA IE)

What is the classification for tongue to mouth size used to assess "airway adequacy"?

Mallampati classification

According to the Mallampati classification, what is:

Class I?

Can see soft palate, anterior and posterior tonsillar pillars, and uvula

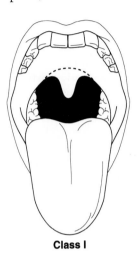

Class I

Class II?

Cannot see tonsillar pillars

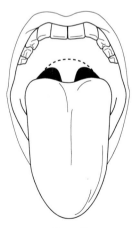

Class II

Class III?   Only uvula base can be seen

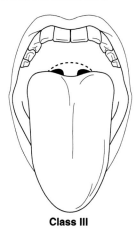

Class III

Class IV?   Cannot see uvula at all

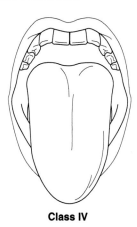

Class IV

What is a Miller blade?   Straight laryngoscope used for intubation
                                  (Think: Miller = 2 letter l's that are
                                  straight)

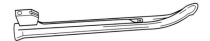

What is a Macintosh blade? Curved laryngoscope blade used for intubation (Think: curved, like the "**c**" in Macintosh)

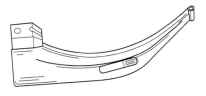

How do you intubate with a Miller blade? Blade is used to hold up the epiglottis (posterior to the epiglottis)

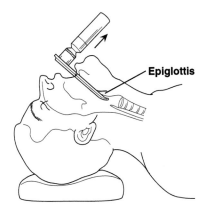

How do you intubate with a Macintosh blade? Blade is used anterior to the epiglottis

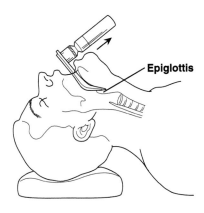

MUSCLE RELAXANTS

What are the sedative or analgesic properties of neuromuscular blockers (NMBs)?	None; patients are unable to move, but they can be fully aware of their surroundings!
What are the 2 classes of NMBs?	1. Depolarizing 2. Nondepolarizing (A.K.A. competitive)
What is the class, onset, and duration of succinylcholine (Sch)?	Depolarizing, onset < 1 minute, duration 5–10 minutes
What is the primary indication for Sch?	Rapid muscle relaxation for endotracheal intubation or treatment of laryngospasm
What are the potential side effects of Sch?	1. Hypertension 2. Cardiac arrhythmias 3. Tachycardia 4. Bradycardia 5. Increased intracranial pressure 6. Hyperkalemia (usually a 0.5–1 mEq/L increase) 7. Prolonged paralysis (in patients with atypical plasma cholinesterase) 8. Malignant hyperthermia 9. Increased intraocular pressure
Which patients are at greatest risk for Sch-induced hyperkalemia (and for whom is the use of Sch contraindicated)?	Patients with: 1. Burns 2. Massive soft-tissue trauma 3. Spinal cord injury 4. Neurologic/neuromuscular disorders 5. Intraperitoneal sepsis 6. Renal failure (relative contraindication)
Is there a safe period for the use of Sch in patients with acute spinal cord injury?	Yes, in the first 24 hours
What is the primary drug for treating malignant hyperthermia (MH)?	Dantrolene

Name 2 long-acting nondepolarizing muscle relaxants (NDMRs).	1. Pancuronium 2. Metocurine
Name 3 intermediate-acting NDMRs.	1. Atracurium 2. Vecuronium 3. Rocuronium
Name 1 (relatively) short-acting NDMR.	Mivacurium
Which NDMRs cause histamine release?	1. Curare 2. Metocurine 3. Atracurium
What is the principal hemodynamic effect of histamine release?	Decreased blood pressure (and reflex tachycardia)
Which NDMR causes sympathetic nervous system stimulation?	Pancuronium
How is it manifested?	A 10–15% increase in heart rate and blood pressure
What is the advantage of rocuronium?	Rapid onset gives adequate muscle relaxation for rapid sequence intubation in patients with a contraindication to Sch.
What drugs are used to reverse NDMR?	Anticholinesterase drugs (neostigmine or edrophonium), which inhibit the breakdown of acetylcholine
What drugs must be combined with these reversal agents (and why)?	Anticholinergic drugs (glycopyrrolate or atropine) are used to counteract systemic cholinergic effects of the anticholinesterases.
What are the systemic cholinergic effects of anticholinesterases?	Vagotonic effects can cause severe bradycardia, as well as crampy abdominal pain and vomiting.

INTRAVENOUS ANESTHETICS

Which 3 agents are most commonly used for induction? Which 3 agents are less commonly used?	Most common: Thiopental (Pentothal), propofol (Diprivan), and etomidate Less common: Methohexital, ketamine, and midazolam

What are some advantages and disadvantages of thiopental?

It is inexpensive and predictable. It causes dose-dependent blood pressure decreases that can be especially dangerous in hypovolemic patients and in the elderly.

What is the advantage attributed to etomidate?

It produces little hemodynamic change and may be well suited for hemodynamically unstable patients (trauma, hypovolemic, frail, elderly patients; patients with CAD).

What are the advantages of propofol (Diprivan) compared with benzodiazepines or barbiturates when used for sedation?

High lipid solubility allows for:
1. Rapid changes in the level of sedation (when administered by continuous infusion) by simply changing infusion rate
2. Rapid recovery (usually within 10–15 minutes) after a bolus dose or after infusion is stopped
3. Physical dependence does not seem to occur
4. Antiemetic properties (suggested by some studies)
5. Bronchodilation

What is the nutritional value of Diprivan?

It is suspended in a carrier of 10% intralipid, providing 1.1 kcal per mL (as fat).

What are the CNS effects of ketamine?

It produces a state of "dissociative anesthesia," which is accompanied by amnesia and analgesia. Patients who receive large doses of ketamine can have hallucinations and unpleasant dreams.

What are the respiratory effects of ketamine?

Respiratory drive is largely preserved and laryngeal protective reflexes remain intact.

INHALATION ANESTHETICS

What does "minimum alveolar concentration" (MAC) mean?

It is the concentration of an inhalation agent (at 1 atm) at which 50% of patients do not move in response to surgical stimulation (similar to the ED_{50}).

What are the 5 most widely used inhalation anesthetics?	1. Nitrous oxide (gas) 2. Halothane 3. Sevoflurane 4. Isoflurane 5. Desflurane
What is the principal intraoperative risk of nitrous oxide?	Diffusion of nitrous oxide into closed gas spaces can cause complications related to the anatomic area involved. The doubling time of the volume of gas in closed or obstructed loops of bowel is about 3–4 hours, whereas the doubling time for gas volume in a pneumothorax can be as little as 10 minutes.
What does "diffusion hypoxia" mean?	At the cessation of nitrous oxide therapy, the nitrous oxide diffuses rapidly from blood into the alveolar space and can dilute the concentration of inspired oxygen, particularly if the patient is placed on room air. Placing the patient on 100% oxygen for 3–5 minutes can prevent this hypoxia.
Which of the volatile inhalation agents is commonly used for mask (or inhalation) induction? Why?	Halothane, because it has the least pungent odor of the volatile agents and tends to be the least irritating to the respiratory tree
Which of the volatile inhalation agents is most commonly associated with cardiac dysrhythmias? Why?	Halothane, because it sensitizes the myocardium to endogenous (and exogenous) catecholamines

REGIONAL ANESTHESIA

What are the 4 types of regional anesthesia?	Local (infiltration) or topical Peripheral nerve blocks (including ganglionic and plexus blocks) Epidural Spinal
What are the 2 most commonly used regional anesthetic agents?	Lidocaine and bupivacaine; other less commonly used agents include tetracaine, mepivacaine, procaine, 2-chloroprocaine, prilocaine, etidocaine, and ropivacaine

What are the signs of systemic toxicity from the injection of local anesthetics (in ascending order of toxicity)?

1. Lingual numbness (tongue numbness), metallic taste
2. Visual and hearing disturbances
3. Sedation
4. Unconsciousness
5. Seizures
6. Respiratory depression
7. Cardiac arrhythmias
8. Cardiovascular collapse

What is the most common cause of toxic plasma levels of local anesthetics?

Inadvertent intravascular injection

Which local anesthetic is the most cardiotoxic?

Bupivacaine is approximately 16 times more cardiotoxic than lidocaine.

How does the addition of epinephrine alter the peak plasma levels of absorbed local anesthetics?

It decreases the peak level, presumably by causing local vasoconstriction and thus slowing absorption.

How does the addition of epinephrine affect the duration of local anesthetics?

It increases the duration, also presumably by local vasoconstriction and decreasing the blood to washout the anesthetic.

In what cases is the addition of epinephrine to local anesthetics discouraged?

1. Uncontrolled hypertension
2. Cardiac arrhythmias
3. Unstable angina
4. Uteroplacental insufficiency
5. Local infiltration into tissues with poor or absent collateral blood flow (digits, ears, tip of nose, penis)
6. Regional IV anesthesia

What is a Bier block?

Regional anesthesia of an extremity by placing a tourniquet and then infusing local anesthetic into a **vein.**

Why are infected tissues difficult to anesthetize with the infiltration of local anesthetics?

Local tissue acidosis present in infected tissues tends to ionize the local anesthetics, preventing their spread and penetration into nerve sheaths.

SPINAL AND EPIDURAL ANESTHESIA

What dermatomes innervate the peritoneal?

T6–T12

What is a "high spinal"?	An excessively high level of spinal anesthesia resulting in respiratory depression. Symptoms range from difficulty breathing to apnea.
What are the risk factors for spinal headache/ postdural puncture headache (PDPH)?	1. Younger patients (< 50 years) 2. Gender (women > men, especially parturients) 3. Use of larger needles (22 ga vs. 25 ga)
What are the characteristics of a PDPH?	Severe frontal or occipital headache that worsens with sitting up. With increasing severity, the headache becomes circumferential and can result in visual, auditory, or vestibular disturbances.
What are the differential diagnoses of severe headache after epidural or spinal anesthesia?	1. PDPH 2. Caffeine withdrawal 3. Migraine headache 4. Meningitis 5. Cortical vein thrombosis 6. Intracranial hematoma
What is the appropriate treatment of PDPH?	1. Bed rest 2. Adequate hydration 3. Caffeine (IV) 4. Analgesics 5. Epidural blood patch (usually for headaches lasting longer than 24 hours)
What is an epidural blood patch?	Blood is injected into the epidural space to form a "patch" over the dural puncture.
What is a "saddle block"?	A low spinal anesthetic affecting primarily the perineum (i.e., the parts that would touch a saddle); performed using hyperbaric (heavier than CSF) anesthetic solutions with the patient sitting up to facilitate caudal spread of the anesthetic
What is a caudal block?	An epidural block obtained by accessing the epidural space via the sacral hiatus. The epidural space can be cannulated, or a single dose of anesthetic can be delivered through the needle.

What are the advantages of propofol?

Bronchodilator, low nausea, quick "on and off"

Why not use pancuronium in trauma patients?

May cause **tachycardia,** confusing the hemodynamic status of the patient

Name a common error when providing conscious sedation.

Not waiting at least 2 minutes between sedative doses (can lead to oversedation = unconscious sedation!)

What is EMLA cream?

A topical cream of lidocaine and prilocaine that causes skin anesthesia, but may take 2 hours to work

What is the Sellick's maneuver?

The use of **cricoid** pressure during rapid sequence intubation

29

Surgical Ulcers

What is a "crack ulcer"?

Small punctate gastric ulcer seen in crack cocaine users

Define the different types of gastric ulcers.

Type I

An ulcer in the body of the stomach proximal to the incisura and not near the gastroesophageal junction; most are on a lesser curvature.

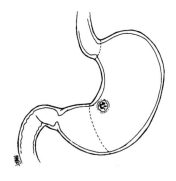

Type II

A type I ulcer and a duodenal ulcer in the body of the stomach (think: type II = 2 ulcers)

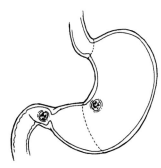

Type III   An ulcer in the pyloric or prepyloric area
                                (think: type III = prepyloric, or 3 = pre)

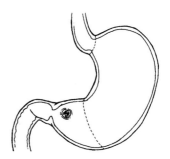

Type IV   An ulcer near the gastroesophageal
                                junction (think: 4 near the "door" to the
                                stomach)

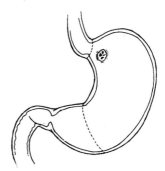

30 Surgical Oncology

Define the following terms.

IORT	**I**ntra**O**perative **R**adiation **T**herapy
Aneuploidy	Abnormal amount of DNA/chromosomes
Malignant potential	The ability of a tumor to invade and metastasize
Hyperplasia	Increased number of cells
Atypical hyperplasia	Increased number of abnormal cells
Metaplasia	Change in cell type from one type to another
On average, how many cell doublings must take place for a cell to become a tumor of 1 cm³ in volume?	Approximately 30
What is flow cytometry?	Stained DNA passed through a laser beam to identify abnormal DNA of tumor cells
What is the duration of the cell cycle of tumors?	2 to 5 days

Name the tumors associated with the following oncogenes.

C-myc	Breast and lung cancer
N-myc	Neuroblastoma (think: **N**-myc = **N**euroblastoma)

L-myc	Lung cancer (think: **L**-myc = **L**ung)
Erb B-2	Breast and ovarian cancer
K-ras	Pancreatic and colon cancer
How does radiation therapy work?	1. Causes breaks in DNA 2. Forms free radicals that damage DNA and intracellular components

TUMOR MARKERS

Name the tumors often associated with the following tumor markers:

Carcinoembryonic antigen (CEA)	Colon cancer
Alpha-fetoprotein (AFP)	Hepatoma
CA 19–9	Pancreatic cancer
CA 125	Ovarian cancer
Human chorionic gonadotropin (β-HCG)	Testicular cancer
PSA	Prostate cancer
CA 50	Pancreatic cancer
Neuron-specific enolase	Small-cell lung cancer
CA 15–3	Breast cancer
Ferritin	Hepatoma

MISCELLANEOUS TUMOR FACTS

Has the monitoring of postoperative CEA levels proved to prolong survival in colon cancer patients after resection?	No

What is the most common primary site with metastatic axillary lymph nodes in women?	Breast cancer
What is the most common malignant cause of axillary adenopathy?	Lymphoma
What is the most common site of sarcoma metastasis?	Lungs (via blood)
What is the most important factor in the prognosis of sarcomas?	Tumor grade
What are the Lynch tumors?	Familial colon cancer syndromes not associated with polyposis
How many types of Lynch syndrome have been identified?	2
What is Lynch syndrome I?	Autosomal-dominant inheritance Early onset of colon cancer Location of tumor in proximal colon (think: Lynch 1 = 1 cancer)
What is Lynch syndrome II?	Colon cancer and Stomach cancer and/or Ovarian cancer and/or Endometrial cancer
Lynch syndrome colon cancers account for what percentage of all colon cancer?	Approximately 7%
In addition to prostate cancer, what other type of cancer must be ruled out in men with elevated PSA levels?	Breast cancer
Which bacteremia is associated with colon cancer?	*Clostridium septicum*

Which tumors are associated with left supraclavicular adenopathy?	GI tumors (the thoracic duct is right there!)
Why is meperidine contraindicated for long-term pain control in cancer patients?	Because of the buildup of normeperidine, a toxic metabolite that causes seizures and myoclonic movements
What infamous toxicity is associated with bleomycin?	Pulmonary fibrosis (dose related; 1% of patients treated with bleomycin will die from this complication)

CHEMOTHERAPY

METHOTREXATE

Describe its mechanism of action.	A folic acid analog that inhibits dihydrofolate reductase (DHFR), an enzyme that reduces dihydrofolate (FH_2) to tetrahydrofolate (FH_4). FH_4 is necessary for the 1-carbon transfers that occur in the synthesis of purines, glycine, methionine, and thymidylate. Without it, DNA, RNA, and protein synthesis is impaired. The most important and lethal effect is the inhibition of thymidylate synthesis.
What is leucovorin "rescue"?	Leucovorin is folinic acid. It bypasses the need for FH4, thus alleviating the lethal inhibitory effects of MTX. Normal cells with intact transport systems take up the leucovorin and are rescued. Resistant tumor cells with decreased active transport do not take up leucovorin, and die. (Kills bad cells, saves good cells!)

MERCAPTOPURINE (6-MP) AND THIOGUANINE (6-TG)

Describe their mechanism of action.	Purine analogs that are converted to nucleotides. They inhibit both de novo purine synthesis and interconversion of precursor molecules into dATP and dGTP, thus decreasing synthesis of DNA, RNA, and proteins.

FLUOROURACIL (5-FU)

Describe its mechanism of action.	A fluorinated analog of the pyrimidine precursor uracil. Its active form, F-dUMP, forms a covalent complex with FH4 and thymidylate synthetase (TS), inhibiting TS and decreasing DNA synthesis.
What type of cancer is interleukin-2 (IL-2) approved to treat?	Renal cell cancer metastases
Identify the unique toxicities.	
Bleomycin	Pulmonary fibrosis
6-MP	Cholestasis
MTX	GI bleeding and GI perforation
Cisplatin	Hearing loss
Cyclophosphamide	Cystitis

Section II

General Surgery

31   GI Hormones and Physiology

GLUCAGON

What is its general role?	Energy utilization
What is its source?	**α-islet cells of the pancreas**—pancreatic glucagon **Stomach**—gastric glucagon **Intestines**—enteroglucagon
What stimulates its release?	Hypoglycemia Elevated serum amino acids (alanine, arginine) Cholinergic (neural stimulation; β-adrenergic; stimulate weakly) Gastric-inhibiting peptide (GIP; only in vitro, not in vivo) Gastrin-releasing peptide (GRP)
What inhibits its release?	Hyperglycemia Insulin Somatostatin α-adrenergic (neural stimulation) Glucagon-like peptide 1 (GLP-1; feedback control)
What does it target?	Liver adipose tissue
How does it act?	Increases hepatic glycogenolysis and gluconeogenesis (i.e., mobilizes glucose into the bloodstream) Increases lipolysis and ketogenesis
What other actions is it associated with?	Inhibits gastric acid secretion Causes relaxation and dilatation of stomach and duodenum Increases intestinal motility and transit time Inhibits pancreatic secretion of water and bicarbonate

What are its clinical uses?	Decreases motility of stomach and duodenum for endoscopy and radiography

GASTRIC INHIBITORY PEPTIDE (GIP)

What is its source?	K Cells of the duodenal glands, jejunum, terminal ileum
What stimulates its release?	Duodenal amino acids Glucose Long-chain fatty acids Hyperglycemia
What does it target?	Pancreas islet cells Stomach
How does it act?	Enhances insulin release Inhibits gastric acid secretion

VASOACTIVE INTESTINAL POLYPEPTIDE

What is its source?	Diffuse pattern of cells throughout the gut and pancreas Peripheral nerve fibers
What stimulates its release?	Intragastric fat Vagal input
What are its effects?	Vasodilation Smooth-muscle cell relaxation General increase of water and electrolyte secretion by gut mucosal cells Inhibits gastric acid secretion Inhibits gallbladder contraction

PANCREATIC POLYPEPTIDE

What is its source?	Islet cells of the pancreas and of other tissues of the pancreas
What stimulates its release?	Food, vagal input, hypoglycemia, and other GI hormones (e.g., cholecystokinin)
How does it act?	Inhibits pancreatic water and bicarbonate secretion in postprandial state Inhibits gallbladder contraction May help regulate intestinal motility Causes a change from fasting to digestive patterns

What is its clinical significance?	Tumor marker for pancreatic apudoma tumors

PEPTIDE YY

What is its source?	Cells in the distal ileum, colon, and rectum
What stimulates its release?	Intraluminal fat in the intestine
What does it target?	Stomach
How does it act?	Inhibits gastric emptying Inhibits gastrin-stimulated acid secretion Inhibits pancreatic exocrine secretion stimulated by cholecystokinin May mediate the "ileal brake"

NEUROTENSIN

What is its source?	N cells in distal small intestine (ileal mucosa)
What stimulates its release?	Intraluminal fat
How does it act?	Inhibits gastric acid secretion Inhibits intestinal motility Stimulates pancreatic secretion of water and bicarbonate Triggers mesenteric vasodilation Has trophic effects for small- or large-bowel mucosa

MOTILIN

What is its source?	Cells throughout the gut (highest concentration is in the duodenum and jejunum)
What stimulates its release?	Duodenal acid and food Vagal tone Gastrin-releasing peptide
What inhibits its release?	Somatostatin Secretin Pancreatic polypeptide Duodenal fat or mixed meal

How does it act?	Increases interdigestive gut motility (think: **M**otilin = **M**otility = MMC) Initiates MMCs
What is an MMC?	**M**igrating **M**yoelectrical **C**omplex
What is its clinical significance?	Erythromycin and other macrolides may stimulate gastric motility as motilin receptor agonists.

GASTROINTESTINAL PHYSIOLOGY

What are the histologic layers of the gastrointestinal tract?	Mucosa (epithelium, lamina propria, muscularis mucosae) Submucosa Muscularis externa (inner circular, outer longitudinal) Serosa
What is the strongest structural layer?	Submucosa (**S**trongest = **S**ubmucosa)
Where are the intramural neural plexi located?	**Meissner's**—submucosal **Auerbach's**—myenteric (between the circular and longitudinal layers)
Which neurotransmitters are associated with external innervation to the gut?	Acetylcholine (parasympathetic) Norepinephrine (sympathetic)
What structures are associated with sympathetic innervation of the gut?	Cell bodies of postganglionic adrenergic neurons located in the prevertebral and paravertebral plexi (celiac, superior mesenteric, inferior mesenteric, hypogastric plexi)
What is the effect of sympathetic stimulation of the gut?	Inhibits motility Causes vasoconstriction Stimulates contraction of sphincters
What is the effect of parasympathetic stimulation of the gut?	Stimulates motility, secretion, and digestion
What are the major dietary sources of carbohydrates?	Starches from plants (e.g., amylose and amylopectin) Lactose from milk Fructose from fruits

What are the steps in carbohydrate digestion?

Mouth—salivary amylase
Stomach—amylase inactivated by acid
Intestines—pancreatic amylase
Intestinal brush border—
  oligosaccharidases (e.g., sucrase,
  lactase, maltase)

What are the products of starch digestion by amylase?

Amylase hydrolyzes the α-1,4-glycosidic
linkages, and basically results in maltose
(gluc-gluc)and maltotriose (gluc-
gluc-gluc).

DIGESTION

What are the essential fatty acids?

Linoleic (18-carbon)
Linolenic (20-carbon)
(**Lif**e = **Li**noleic and **Li**nolenic)

What is the first enzyme to hydrolyze fat?

Lingual lipase is the first enzyme that
hydrolyzes dietary triglycerides and is
stable at pH 2.2–6.0.

Describe the digestion of lipids.

Start as fat droplets
Emulsification by bile salts and
  phosphatidylcholine to form micelles
  occurs in the duodenum.
Lipids in micelles are hydrolyzed by
  pancreatic lipase, cholesterol esterase,
  and phospholipase A2.
Lipids in micelles diffuse across the
  luminal membrane of enterocytes.

What are the types of lipoproteins and what function is each responsible for?

VLDL (very low density lipoprotein)—
  transport of triglycerides from liver
IDL (intermediate density lipoprotein)—
  formed in plasma by degradation of
  VLDL
LDL (low density lipoprotein)—formed
  in plasma from IDL; transports
  cholesterol esters to body tissues
HDL (high density lipoprotein)—
  transports cholesterol to liver

Where are most lipids absorbed?

In the proximal 2/3 of the jejunum

What are the essential amino acids?

Histidine
Isoleucine
Leucine
Lysine
Methionine
Phenylalanine
Threonine
Tryptophan
Valine
(Think: **HIS ISO**lated **L**over **L**ied; **M**ike **P**ushed **TH**en **TR**ipped **VAL**erie)

Describe the digestion of proteins.

Stomach—denatured by acid; hydrolyzed by pepsin
Pancreas—secretes multiple endopeptidases and carboxypeptidases into the intestine; trypsin, chymotrypsin, and carboxypeptidase hydrolyze protein to small peptides and amino acids
Approximately half of protein digestion and absorption is completed in the duodenal intestinal brush border.
Dipeptides, tripeptides, and free amino acids are formed by the action of aminopeptidases and dipeptidases.

Describe the absorption of protein digestion products.

Enterocytes absorb dipeptides, tripeptides, and free amino acids. Dipeptidases and tripeptides are digested to free amino acids by cytosolic enzymes. Protein digestion and absorption are completed by the mid-jejunum.

What are the characteristics of pepsin?

Stored as inactive proenzyme (pepsinogen) in chief cells as zymogen granules
Secreted from chief cells by exocytosis at apical surface
Secretion stimulated by gastric acid and by stimulators of gastric acid secretion
Acts upon approximately 20% of intragastric proteins
Requires acidic environment for enzymatic action
Permanently inactivated in neutral duodenal environment

What are the characteristics of enterokinase?	Secreted by duodenal mucosa Activates trypsinogen, chymotrypsinogen, and procarboxypeptidase
What are the characteristics of trypsin?	Secreted by pancreatic acinar cells Activates proenzyme trypsinogen In turn activates chymotrypsin, elastase, and carboxypeptidases
What are the characteristics of chymotrypsin?	Secreted by pancreatic acinar cells Inactivates proenzyme chymotrypsinogen Activated by trypsin Hydrolyzes proteins to free amino acids
What are the characteristics of carboxypeptidase?	Secreted by pancreatic acinar cells Inactivates proenzyme procarboxypeptidase Activated by trypsin Hydrolyzes proteins to free amino acids

GASTRIC ACID SECRETION

What 3 main agonists act on parietal cells to secrete acid?	Acetylcholine at muscarinic cholinergic receptors Histamine at H_2 receptors Gastrin at gastrin receptors
What are the phases of gastric acid secretion?	Cephalic Gastric Intestinal
What stimulates the cephalic phase?	Thought, smell, taste, or presence of food in the mouth (classic Pavlov experiments)
What are the pathways of the cephalic phase of acid secretion?	1. Telencephalon nucleus tractus solitarius → dorsal motor nucleus → vagal muscarinic cholinergic efferent fibers → parietal cell (cholinergic receptors) → secrete acid 2. Vagus nerve to G cells → secrete gastrin → to parietal cells (gastrin receptors) → secrete acid (chief cells also increase secretion of pepsinogen in cephalic phase)
What stimulates the gastric phase?	Gastric distention

What are the pathways of the gastric phase of acid secretion?	Local and vagovagal reflexes → G cells → gastrin → parietal cells (gastrin receptors) → secrete acid Local and vagovagal reflexes → parietal cells (cholinergic receptors) → secrete acid Gastric mast cells → histamine → parietal cells (histamine-2 receptors) → secrete acid
What inhibits the gastric phase?	Antral acidification
How is gastric secretion measured?	Basal acid output (BAO)—4 to 6 mEq/h Maximal acid output (MAO)—30 to 40 mEq/h

COLON

Through what networks is the colon innervated?	Two intramural plexi: 1. Submucosal (Meissner's) plexus; innermost between the muscularis mucosa and the circular muscularis propria 2. Myenteric (Auerbach's) plexus; outermost between the circular and the outer longitudinal muscle layers

What are the major types of colon motility and how do they function?	Ring contractions:
	  Mix contents
	  Move contents (either antegrade or retrograde)
	  Enhance surface contact with contents
	  Left colon—sustained giant migrating contractions:
	  Propel stool toward rectum
	  Empty colon of luminal contents

What stimulates colonic motility?	Fatty acids, bile acids, undigested food particles, luminal distention, cholinergic stimulation
What is the function of the bacterial load of the colon?	Breakdown of carbohydrates to short-chain fatty acids, which can then be absorbed

32

Acute Abdomen and Referred Pain

"The general rule can be laid down that the majority of severe abdominal pains which ensue in patients who have been previously fairly well, and which last as long as 6 hours, are caused by conditions of surgical import."

Sir Zachary Cope
(1881–1974)

What are the possible causes of diffuse abdominal pain?

Uremia, porphyria, diffuse peritonitis, gastroenteritis, inflammatory bowel disease (IBD), diabetic ketoacidosis (DKA), early appendicitis, small bowel obstruction (SBO), sickle cell crisis, ischemic mesenteric disease, aortic aneurysm, lead poisoning, black widow spider bite, pancreatitis, perforated viscus

Of patients < 50 years of age, what are the 3 most common causes of surgical abdominal pain?

1. Acute appendicitis
2. Cholecystitis
3. SBO

Of patients > 50 years of age, what are the 3 most common causes of surgical abdominal pain?

1. Cholecystitis
2. Acute appendicitis
3. SBO

What percentage of patients presenting to a physician with abdominal pain need surgery?

Approximately 33%!

What are the classic sites of anterior referred abdominal pain?

A: Esophagus
B: Stomach
C: Gallbladder
D: Duodenum/Pylorus
E: Early appendicitis
F: Colon
G: Kidneys
H: Ureter

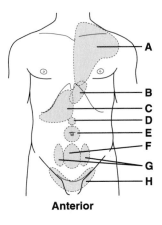

Anterior

What are the classic sites of posterior referred abdominal pain?

A: Diaphragm
B: Biliary colic
C: Renal colic/Pancreatitis
D: Uterus/Rectum

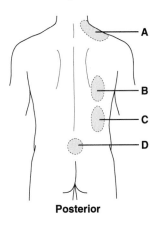

Posterior

SIGNS OF ACUTE ABDOMEN

What is Markle's sign?

"**Jar**" abdominal tenderness, elicited by shaking the bed, foot, or pelvis; sign of peritoneal inflammation

What is Blumberg's sign?

Rebound tenderness

What intra-abdominal conditions can result in death within minutes?

All involve massive bleeding: ectopic pregnancy with rupture, ruptured abdominal aortic aneurysm, aortic-enteric fistula, ruptured splenic aneurysm, splenic rupture (usually after mononucleosis, malaria, trauma, etc.), ruptured dissecting aorta into the abdomen (very rare), ruptured uterus (during pregnancy), ruptured liver hemangioma (most common benign tumor of the liver), ruptured subcapsular liver hematoma, abdominal trauma

What signs/symptoms are associated with gastroenteritis?

Vomiting, followed by abdominal pain, with or without diarrhea. Symptoms usually resolve in < 12 hours.

What is the classic position to decrease abdominal pain in patients with pancreatitis?

Pain is often relieved by sitting up.

What is the classic sequence of vomiting and abdominal pain in acute appendicitis or other surgical abdominal conditions?

Pain followed by vomiting, in most cases. The pain activates vomiting via the medulla.

What is the most common type of MI associated with abdominal pain, nausea, and vomiting?

Inferior MI

Name the possible unique cause of nonsurgical abdominal pain in the following scenarios:

African-American with a history of joint pain

Sickle cell crisis

Child who eats paint, and has a history of recurrent right lower quadrant pain with no evidence of true right lower quadrant tenderness or peritoneal signs

Lead poisoning

Patient with abdominal pain and high porphobilinogen in the urine	Acute porphyria, usually in women 30–40 years old with a history of recurrent abdominal pain radiating to the back out of proportion to abdominal exam findings; fever; elevated WBC count (often)
Patient on preoperative steroids	Addisonian crisis (acute adrenal insufficiency)
Abdominal wall pain in a patient on warfarin	Rectus sheath hematoma
Patient with a DVT	Pulmonary embolus
Patient with skin hyperesthesia in a dermatomal distribution	Herpes
Individual of Jewish or Armenian background with a history of recurrent epigastric abdominal pain; status post 2 negative exploratory laparotomies; fever to 39°C	Familial Mediterranean fever (autosomal recessive inheritance)
What are the differential diagnoses of gynecologic causes of lower quadrant pain?	Mittelschmerz, ovarian cyst, endometriosis, fibroids (with or without necrosis; found in approximately 20% of women < 40 years old), ovarian torsion, pelvic inflammatory disease (PID), ovarian tumor (e.g., Krukenberg tumor/teratoma), ectopic pregnancy, adhesions in the pelvis, pregnancy, infection of uterus following gynecologic procedures, threatened abortion, round ligament pain secondary to pregnancy
What is round ligament pain?	Lower quadrant pain secondary to stretching of the round ligament attached to the uterus (remember, the round ligament, instead of the spermatic cord, travels through the inguinal canal in women); may be confused with appendicitis in pregnancy

What are the symptoms of endometriosis?	Classic triad of 3 **D**s: 1. Dyschezia (painful defecation) 2. Dyspareunia (painful sexual intercourse) 3. Dysmenorrhea (painful menstruation); also, spotting, pain, and infertility

PELVIC INFLAMMATORY DISEASE (PID)

What are the associated signs/symptoms of PID?	Bilateral lower quadrant abdominal pain, vaginal discharge, cervical motion tenderness, fever
When during the menstrual cycle does PID most commonly occur?	Usually the first half
What organisms are most commonly responsible for PID?	1. *Neisseria gonorrhea* 2. *Chlamydia*
What long-term complications are associated with PID?	1. Pelvic pain 2. Ectopic pregnancy 3. Infertility

33   Hernias

**Define the following types
of hernias:**

Petit's	Hernia through Petit's triangle (rare)
Grynfeltt's	Hernia through Grynfeltt's triangle
Properitoneal	Intraparietal hernia between the peritoneum and the transversalis fascia
Cooper's	Hernia involving the femoral canal and tracts into the scrotum or labia majus
Velpeau's	Hernia through the Gimbernat's ligament (also known as Laugier's or lacunar ligament hernia)
Hesselbach's	Femoral hernia that passes laterally to the femoral vessels
Sciatic	Hernia through the sacrosciatic foramen in the pelvis
Cloquet's	Femoral hernia that penetrates the pectineus muscle fascia (thigh muscle lateral to the adductor longus muscle)
Parastomal	Hernia through the same fascial opening created for a colostomy or ileostomy
Serafini's	Femoral hernia that travels underneath the femoral vessels
"Herald"	A hernia that "warns" of a more serious medical condition such as colon cancer, prostate cancer, benign prostatic hyperplasia, or lung cancer; due to increase in intra-abdominal pressure (e.g., straining at stool, cough)

What are the boundaries of Petit's triangle?

Think: "petite **LIE**" (just a "little lie"):
  Latissimus dorsi
  Iliac crest
  External oblique

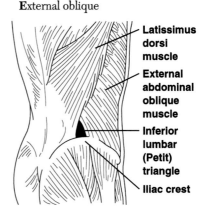

What are the boundaries of the Grynfeltt's triangle?

Think: Petit's lie and Grynfeltts "**SIT**":
  Sacrospinal muscle
  Internal oblique muscle
  Twelfth rib

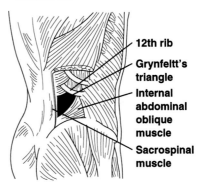

What is the most common complication that arises after inguinal hernia repair?

Urinary retention

What is the plug and patch inguinal hernia repair?

1. **Plug** (See Chapter 13)
2. **Patch**

Which inguinal hernia repair involves merely a tightening up of the internal inguinal ring?

Marcy treatment

Who first described "pants over vest" repair for umbilical hernias?

Mayo (most surgeons now repair the "umbo hold the mayo")

In what type of patient are infantile umbilical hernias most common?

African American infants

Why can a reduced incarcerated abdominal wall hernia still progress to strangulation?

The hernia is out of the fascia defect but still in the hernia sac! (aka reducing **en masse**)

Why ligate transected nerves?

If a neuroma develops, it will develop in the nerve sheath and thus be less symptomatic.

What is the most common causative factor for an incisional hernia?

Wound infection

34

Laparoscopy

When should a trocar site be sutured?	Suturing of sites > 0.7 cm is recommended.
What is the appropriate treatment of CO_2 embolism?	Stop CO_2 insufflation, release the pneumoperitoneum, and use Trendelenburg and left lateral decubitus positions (Durant's position). Also, hyperventilation should be followed by central venous access to extract the CO_2.
How can CO_2 embolus be prevented when using the laparoscopic argon laser coagulator?	With an open port, so that the intraperitoneal pressure does not build up
Define the measures that will help prevent common bile duct injuries during a laparoscopic cholecystectomy.	
Type of scope	30° (especially in obese patients)
Fundus retraction	Firm cephalad
Infundibulum retraction	Lateral retraction
Gallbladder neck dissection	Complete identification and mobilization of the neck
Junction of the gallbladder and cystic duct	Complete identification of the gallbladder and cystic duct junction with 360° view
Porta hepatis bleeding	No blind clips or electrocautery
Unclear anatomy	Open incision

Why is electrocautery contraindicated for transection of tissue between clips?	Because of the potential for thermal injury to surrounding tissue and arcing of the current
What is the most common cause of common bile duct injury?	Mistaking the common bile duct for the cystic duct
Is there any evidence that routine intraoperative cholangiography decreases the risk of common bile duct injury?	No
Which laparoscopic instrument is responsible for the most visceral injuries?	The Veress needle
What action should be taken if a major vascular structure is injured by a cannula trocar?	Opening of the abdomen through a midline incision
How should a bleeding trocar site be repaired?	1. Insert a Keith needle into the peritoneal cavity and out the abdomen under the vessel and tie over a bolster. 2. Insert a Foley catheter through the trocar site and hold pressure with outward traction. 3. Cut down and tie off the vessel. 4. Coagulate under direct laparoscopic vision.
How should a Veress needle bladder puncture be treated?	Postoperative Foley drainage
How should a trocar bladder injury be treated?	Suturing and Foley drainage
What is the most common cause of a postoperative periumbilical trocar site urine leak?	Transection of a patent urachal sinus

How can placement of a trocar through an epigastric vessel be avoided?

Transilluminate the abdominal wall and identify the vessels before placing the trocar

What cardiac problem is associated with pneumoperitoneum and distention of the peritoneum?

Vagal stimulation and bradycardia

What complication is associated with a "mill wheel" murmur?

CO_2 embolus

Can the camera endoscope light cause small bowel injury?

Yes. The xenon light source can become quite hot and burn a hole in the bowel wall.

What is the advantage of lasers over electrocautery?

None. Lasers actually have an increased expense, longer operating time, and less efficient hemostasis; in addition, they may be associated with more injuries to surrounding tissues.

What is the "trapezoid of doom" associated with inguinal hernia laparoscopic repair?

The trapezoid lateral to the femoral vessels and below the iliopubic tract in which several nerves run; if a staple is placed in this region, a painful neuralgia may occur postoperatively.

What nerves are located in the "trapezoid of doom"?

Femoral branch of the genitofemoral nerve
Lateral cutaneous nerve of the thigh
Femoral nerve

What complication is more common with the Hasson technique?

Wound infection is more common due to more dissection and more manipulation

What complication is more common with the Veress needle trocar placement than with Hasson trocar placement?

Major vascular injury (due to relatively blind placement)

35

Trauma

HISTORY

What is the blunt trauma history acronym?

Rat's Lamps:
    Restraint?
    Airbag?
    Tetanus status?
    Seat in car? (e.g., driver vs back seat passenger)

    Loss of consciousness?
    Allergies?
    Meds?
    Past medical history (PMH)
    Speed of collision?

PEDIATRIC TRAUMA BASICS

What is the age limit for intraosseus (IO) IV access?

6 years or younger only

What is the ratio of needle cricothyroidotomy ventilation?

1 on, 4 off

Give a rough estimate of ET size in children.

Approximately the size of child's pinky

Define the "20, 20, 10" rule of pediatric fluid resuscitation.

20 mL LR /kg, then 20 mL LR /kg; if still unstable, then 10 mL pRBCs/kg

What is the primary physiologic clinical response to hypovolemic shock in children?

Tachycardia

Describe the Glasgow Coma Scale (GCS) verbal scoring for young children.

5	Words, social smile, fixes and follows
4	Consolable cry
3	Irritable (persistently)
2	Restless, agitated
1	No response

| **What is the formula for normal systolic blood pressure (SBP) in pediatric patients?** | 80 plus twice the patient's age (e.g., in a 5-year-old, normal SBP should be around $90 = 80 + [5 \times 2]$) |

CIRCULATION

| **How should the results of a fluid challenge be monitored clinically?** | Urine output, mental status, capillary refill, heart rate, SBP, respiratory rate |
| **What are the laboratory "end points" of resuscitation to follow?** | Lactate, base deficit |

GUNSHOT WOUNDS (GSWS)

What is a hollow-point bullet?	A bullet with a hollow end that "mushrooms" out upon impact with a solid object (e.g., a human)
What is larger: a 22-caliber bullet or a 44-caliber bullet?	A 44-caliber bullet; caliber is a rough estimate of bullet size in inches (i.e., a 44-caliber bullet is about 0.44 inch in diameter)
What is a shotgun?	A large-bore long firearm that shoots multiple pellets per shot (up to 50)
What is larger: a 28-gauge shotgun or a 12-gauge shotgun?	A 12-gauge shotgun barrel is larger. (Gauge is determined by the number of lead balls the same diameter as the barrel that it takes to equal 1 pound; for a 12-gauge, 12 lead balls equal 1 pound, and for a 28-gauge, 28 lead balls.)

Which pellets are larger: number 8 shot or number 2 shot?	Number 2 shot (the larger number is smaller)
What is bullet yaw?	Deviation of the bullet from its longitudinal projection
What is bullet tumble?	Head-over-heel somersaults
What material must be sought in all shotgun wounds?	The plastic or cardboard wadding: a small "cup" that holds the pellets
Can the entrance and exit wounds be reliably determined?	Exit wounds are generally larger than entrance wounds. The entrance wound can be reliably determined only by evidence of gunpowder tattoos.
What is cavitation?	When a high-powered bullet enters the body, it transfers its kinetic energy to the surrounding tissues, which are then violently thrown out from the bullet's path in a radial direction, forming a "cavity" and thus injuring tissues not in the bullet's actual path.

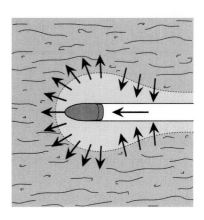

EMERGENCY DEPARTMENT (ED) THORACOTOMY

Why perform an ED thoracotomy?	As a last-ditch effort to save a patient in severe extremis

What are the indications for an ED thoracotomy?

No vital signs (no pulse, no blood pressure) or severe hypotension (SBP < 60) and in extremis:
1. Penetrating injury with signs of life in ED or in the field
2. Blunt trauma with signs of life in ED (most surgeons also require witnessed loss of vital signs in the ED)

Define signs of life.

PERM:
    Pupillary reaction
    ECG electrical activity
    Respirations
    Movement

What is the mortality for ED thoracotomy??

Over 95%

What incision is used?

Left anterolateral thoracotomy (5th intercostal space)

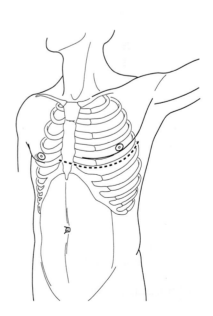

What is done after entering the chest?

Clamp aorta.
Open pericardium.
Ligate internal mammary artery!

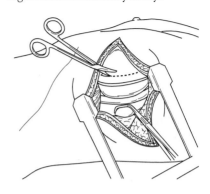

Where do you open the pericardium?

Anterior to the phrenic nerve (think: **AP** = **A**nterior-**P**osterior = **A**nterior to **Ph**renic)

What if you need to get to the right chest?

Perform a clam shell incision.

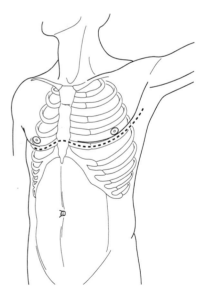

Describe the outcomes after ED thoracotomy for:

Blunt trauma, no vital signs.

< 1% survive (0.03%)

Penetrating stab wound, no vital signs.	7% (5% for GSWs)

TRAUMA MANAGEMENT

Why should the leg of a trauma patient be prepped in the field?	For access to a saphenous vein for vascular procedure
What percentage of patients with penetrating trauma to the pancreas will have an elevated serum amylase?	Only approximately 15%
What is the appropriate treatment of each of the following wounds?	
Pancreatic contusion from a GSW cavitation injury	Hemostasis and wide external closed drainage
Distal pancreatic duct transection from a GSW	Distal pancreatectomy (almost always with splenectomy)
Proximal pancreatic duct injury	1. Distal pancreatectomy, or 2. Roux-en-Y pancreaticojejunostomy (especially if distal resection would leave < 15% pancreatic remnant)
Small laceration to the small bowel from a GSW	Close in 2 layers in a transverse fashion (better short than narrow).
What is the appropriate treatment of 2 small-bowel perforations that are side by side?	Make into one perforation, and close transversely.
Which types of retroperitoneal hematoma from a GSW should not be explored?	Stable retrohepatic hematoma Stable renal hematoma with preoperative imaging that reveals adequate function
What is the appropriate treatment of pelvic hematoma from penetrating trauma?	Open it up after proximal (aorta/vena cava) and distal (iliac vessels) control, in contrast to blunt trauma.

Can the portal vein be ligated?	Repair if at all possible; otherwise, it can be ligated if the injury is isolated, but with a mortality of at least 50%.
What major operative and postoperative complications can follow ligation of the portal vein?	1. Massive fluid sequestration in the splanchnic vascular bed; massive amount of crystalloid resuscitation 2. Bowel necrosis
Can the common or proper hepatic artery be ligated?	Yes, especially proximal to the gastroduodenal branch, because this artery then provides collateral flow from the superior mesenteric artery via the pancreaticoduodenal arcades
Can the right or left hepatic artery be ligated?	Yes, especially if the portal vein is intact, because the portal vein delivers approximately 50% of the liver O_2
Can a lobar bile duct be ligated?	Yes, and without jaundice in most patients
How do you close a stomach laceration?	2 layers: 1. Absorbable running 2. Silk Lembert outer layer

What is the appropriate treatment of the following wounds?

Popliteal vein-penetrating injury	Repair; do not ligate
Suprarenal vena caval injury	Repair; do not ligate
Infrarenal vena caval injury	Repair if at all possible; otherwise, ligate
Internal jugular vein injury	Lateral venography, if possible; otherwise, ligate
Bilateral internal jugular vein injury	Must repair at least one internal jugular vein

Transection of the femoral vein	Repair if possible; otherwise, ligate
Transection of a single artery of the lower leg	Ligate
How many trifurcation arteries need to be patent to the foot for a viable foot?	1
What procedure must be performed with a common or proper hepatic artery ligation for trauma?	Cholecystectomy
In the patient with penetrating wounds to both the stomach and the diaphragm, what should be done besides closing the holes?	Irrigate pleural cavity via the diaphragm hole or via a chest tube, because empyema is often a problem after this combination of injuries
In penetrating trauma, should a perirenal hematoma be opened?	Yes, unless a preoperative CT/intravenous pyelogram (IVP) reveals an intact kidney
Define lower chest wound.	Below the nipple and above the costal margin
What is a safe treatment of a lower chest GSW?	Abdominal exploration, because of frequent diaphragm injury
What percentage of penetrating solitary lung parenchymal injuries are treated solely by a chest tube?	> 85%
What are the options for treatment of severe retrohepatic venous hemorrhage?	1. Vascular isolation with direct suture repair 2. Atriocaval shunt 3. Retrograde balloon catheter vena caval occlusion

What is the atriocaval shunt?

Usually, a modified chest tube that is placed into the right atrium and descends in the IVC past a retrohepatic vena caval injury; allows treatment of retrohepatic venous injury, control of blood loss, and venous return to the heart (associated with significant mortality)

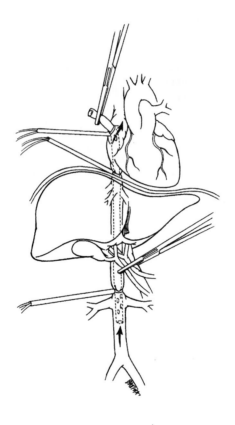

Define the signs and symptoms of the following injuries with penetrating neck trauma.

Esophageal neck injury

Odynophagia
Dysphagia
Subcutaneous crepitus
Hematemesis

Vascular neck injury	Expanding/stable hematoma
	Bleeding
	Shock
	Loss of pulse
	Focal neurologic deficit
Laryngeal/tracheal injury	Subcutaneous air/crepitus
	Change in voice
	Hemoptysis
	Dyspnea
What determines peritoneal penetration from an abdominal stab wound more accurately: probing or local exploration?	Local exploration
After penetrating trauma to the abdomen, is there any benefit to administering perioperative antibiotics for > 24 hours?	No. As long as the antibiotics have anaerobic and aerobic coverage, 24 hours is satisfactory.
How long do you give IV antibiotics after a penetrating colon injury (regardless of soilage)?	Only 24 hours!
Are sternal fractures in patients who were wearing shoulder seat belts associated with aortic injury?	No
What is the difference between exposure for left vs right "proximal control" in proximal subclavian injuries?	Right = median sternotomy
	Left = 2nd intercostal thoracotomy

TRAUMA INJURY SCALES

Which trauma scales do you most need to know?	**Liver**
	Spleen

Which 2 types of injuries define most of the liver and spleen grades?

1. Hematoma
2. Laceration

LIVER INJURY SCALE

Define the following.

Grade 1 liver injury

Hematoma—subcapsular blood < 10% of surface area of the liver (nonexpanding)
Laceration < 1 cm deep, capsular tear (nonbleeding)
(Think: Grade **1** = **1** cm deep and **10**% surface area)

Grade 2 liver injury

Hematoma—subcapsular, < 50% of surface area; intraparenchymal, < 10 cm in diameter (both nonexpanding)
Laceration 1–3 cm deep and < 10 cm long

Grade 3 liver injury

Subcapsular hematoma, > 50% of surface area (nonexpanding); or expanding; or ruptured with active bleeding
Intraparenchymal hematoma, > 10 cm in diameter, or expanding
Laceration > 3 cm deep (think: **3** = **3**)

Grade 4 liver injury

Laceration—massive parenchymal destruction: 25–75% of hepatic lobe or 1–3 Couinaud segments (Couinaud segments are segments in the French system; See Chapter 15)

Grade 5 liver injury

Laceration—massive parenchymal destruction > 75% of hepatic lobe, or > 3 Couinaud segments
Vascular injury—retrohepatic venous injury (i.e., IVC, major hepatic vein injury)

Grade 6 liver injury

Vascular injury—total hepatic avulsion

What is the "finger fracture" technique for liver hemostasis?

"Fracture" away liver parenchyma with fingers to expose bleeding liver vessels, which are then ligated

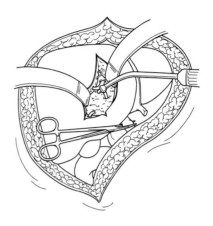

SPLEEN INJURY SEVERITY SCALE

Define the following.

Grade 1 spleen injury

Subcapsular hematoma, < 10% surface area, nonexpanding (just like liver Grade 1)

Laceration < 1 cm deep with capsular tear, but nonbleeding (just like liver Grade 1)

Grade 2 spleen injury

10–50% surface area subcapsular hematoma; < 5 cm intraparenchymal hematoma

Laceration—capsular tear 1–3 cm deep, but must not involve a trabecular vessel

Grade 3 spleen injury

> 50% subcapsular hematoma or expanding subcapsular hematoma; ruptured subcapsular or parenchymal hematoma; contained hematoma > 5 cm; or contained expanding subcapsular hematoma > 3 cm deep parenchymal laceration, or involving trabecular vessels

Grade 4 spleen injury

Ruptured intraparenchymal hematoma with active bleed. Laceration involving segmental or hilar vessels with major devascularization (> 25% of spleen)

Grade 5 spleen injury

Laceration—shattered spleen (massive) Vascular injury—hilar injury that completely devascularizes the spleen

What ligaments need to be transected prior to spleen mobilization?

1. Splenorenal (sharply)
2. Phrenosplenic (sharply)
3. Splenocolic: ligated due to large vessels, then brought into midline by **non**dominant hand

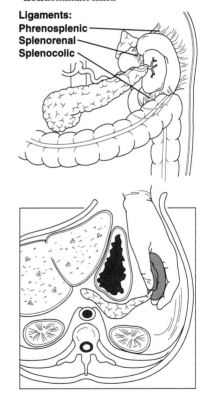

Ligaments:
Phrenosplenic
Splenorenal
Splenocolic

RETROPERITONEAL TRAUMA

Define the retroperitoneal trauma zones.

Zone 1

Central and medial aspects of the retroperitoneum

| **Zone 2** | Flanks |
| **Zone 3** | Pelvis |

Should a pelvic hematoma be opened:

| **In blunt trauma?** | No |
| **In penetrating trauma?** | Yes |

URETHRAL TRAUMA

| **What percentage of patients with urethral injuries have pelvic fractures?** | 95% (usually involve rami or symphysis) |

DUODENAL INJURIES

| **What is the appropriate treatment of an intramural duodenal hematoma?** | May be treated conservatively if perforation is excluded (i.e., nasogastric tube decompression, IV fluids, and TPN) |
| **What is pyloric exclusion?** | 1. Close pylorus (stapled or sutured)
2. Gastrojejunostomy |

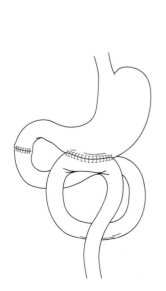
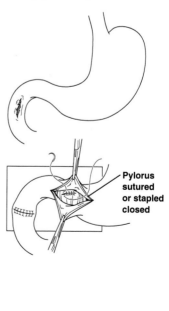

Pylorus
sutured
or stapled
closed

What is duodenal diverticulization?

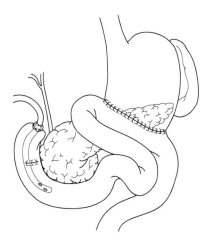

What is the best surgical treatment for severe duodenal injury with significant tissue loss?

Duodenal augmentation: Roux-en-Y side to side anastomosis to injury.

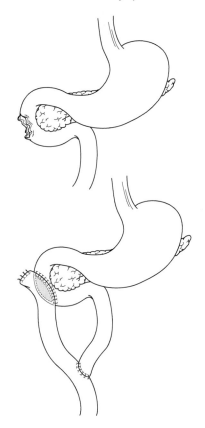

MISCELLANEOUS TRAUMA FACTS

Are prophylactic antibiotics helpful for chest tubes placed for chest trauma?	EAST (Eastern Association for the Surgery of Trauma) guidelines: 24 hours of first-generation cephalosporin (e.g., cefazolin [Ancef])
What is the RICE treatment for extremity injuries?	**R**est **I**ce **C**ompression (e.g., Ace bandage) **E**levation
Name a memory aid for remembering the arm position of decorticate vs decerebrate?	Decorticate: the arms and hands form an "**o**" as in dec"**o**"rticate (or hands towards the "core")
What is the "tertiary" exam?	Physical exam looking for missed injuries after the trauma work up. Studies have found up to 40% of patients have missed injuries (usually extremity).
What are the "deadly dozen" thoracic injuries?	**Lethal 6:** obstructed airway, tension pneumothorax, cardiac tamponade, massive hemothorax, flail chest, open pneumothorax **Hidden 6:** severe cardiac contusion, pulmonary contusion, esophageal rupture, thoracic aortic injury, tracheobronchial injury, diaphragmatic rupture
Which timing has a higher rate of pneumothorax after chest tube pull: end expiration or end inspiration?	**No** difference!
What is a sciwora?	**S**pinal **c**ord **i**njury **w**ith**o**ut **r**adiographic **a**bnormality
When does a chest wound become a "sucking" chest wound?	When the area of the chest wall injury becomes larger than the cross-sectional area of the trachea!

What is the major risk factor for infection after colon injury?

Blood transfusions!

Define pulsus paradoxus.

> 10 mm Hg drop in systolic blood pressure with inspiration (seen with pericardial tamponade)

Define a "Marcus Gunn" pupil.

Clinically, placing light intermittently into both eyes ("swing light test") results in **dilation** of pupil with severe retinal or optic nerve injury.

What is the McKenney score on a FAST exam?

The anteroposterior depth of the largest abdominal fluid collection plus the number of all other areas positive for fluid (score > 3 equals 85% chance of therapeutic laparotomy)

What is Waddle's triad?

Pedestrian hit by car (PHBC) triad of injuries:
1. Tibia-fibula fracture
2. Truncal injury
3. Head injury

What are the signs of infection with postoperative leukocytosis from trauma splenectomy?

1. WBC > 15
2. Platelet to WBC ratio < 20

What is the "box"?

Clavicles, nipples to line across costal margin (aka "Box of Death")

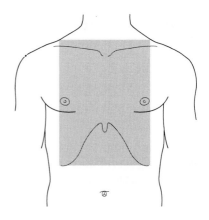

What if a patient has a penetrating injury to the Box and is *unstable*?

Pericardial window or FAST (if positive medial sternotomy)

What if a patient has a penetrating injury to the Box and is *stable*?

FAST evaluation of pericardium

Should you probe a thoracic penetrating injury?

Never—may cause a pneumothorax!

36

Burns

After a major burn, what burn-specific labs need to be ordered?

How do you treat cyanide toxicity?

Where do you make classic escharotomy incisions?

Cyanide, carbon monoxide

1. Sodium nitrite
2. Sodium thiosulfate

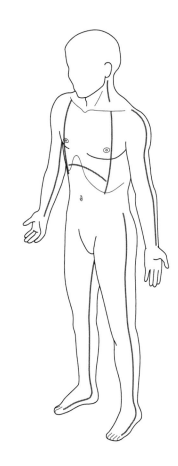

In what type of patient is silver sulfadiazine (Silvadene) contraindicated?

Those with glucose-6-phosphate dehydrogenase (G-6-PD) deficiency and allergy to sulfa drugs

Silver sulfadiazine is ineffective against which bacteria?

Gram-positive and *Pseudomonas*

What is the major side effect of silver nitrate?

Electrolyte wasting (salt, calcium, potassium; think of silver nitrate as 2 electrolytes, thus, electrolyte wasting is the side effect)

Define the following types of grafts.

Autograft

A skin graft from the same individual

Allograft

A skin graft from an individual of the same species (cadaver)

Homograft

Same as an allograft

Xenograft

A skin graft from a different species (porcine)

What are the signs of burn wound infection?

1. Peripheral wound edema
2. Conversion of second-degree burn to third-degree burn
3. Ecthyma gangrenosum
4. Hemorrhage of underlying tissue
5. Green fat
6. Black skin around wound
7. Rapid eschar separation
8. Focal areas on a burn wound that turn black, brown, or purple-red, or show generalized discoloration

Name the most common topical agent for an infected third-degree burn.

Mafenide

What topical agent has the greatest eschar penetration?

Mafenide (think: **M**afenide = **M**ost)

What is the most common viral infection of burn wounds?

Herpes (type I)

What tissue organism counts correlate with the absence of burn-wound invasive infection?

$< 10^5$ organisms per gram of burn-wound tissue

What percentage of patients with tissue counts $> 10^5$ organisms per gram of burn tissue will have an invasive burn-wound infection?

Only about 50%. Histology is necessary to diagnose an invasive infection.

What is the appropriate treatment of thrombophlebitis in burn patients?

Complete excision of the vein/pus (changing IV sites/central lines every 3 days helps prevent this complication)

What is the most common cause of death in burn injuries?

Smoke inhalation

What is the best clinical indication in burn patients of adequate fluid resuscitation?

Urine output

Which vitamin can decrease initial fluid requirements and wound edema in burns?

Vitamin C (ascorbic acid) in high IV dose

How do you estimate percentage of burn in children?

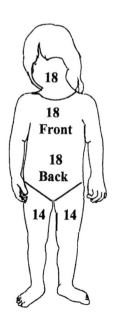

What is the hemoglobin CO_2 affinity vs oxygen?

CO_2 has 240 times greater affinity than oxygen.

What is the treatment for hydrofluoric acid burn?

Calcium gluconate $\rightarrow$ gel, subcutaneous, and rarely intra-arterially

37   Upper GI Bleeding

Which patients with GI tract bleeding can be worked up as outpatients?	Melena or occult bleeding in hemodynamically stable patients (those with hematochezia and hematemesis must be hospitalized)
What is the treatment for a bleeding gastric leiomyoma?	Wedge resection
What is a Cameron's ulcer?	Linear ulcer at level of diaphragm in patients with paraesophageal hiatal hernias (rarely, may cause massive upper GI bleeding)
What is the treatment of aortoenteric fistula?	Resection of graft and extra-anatomic bypass
What is the treatment of bleeding duodenal or jejunal diverticula?	Resection

ACUTE HEMORRHAGIC GASTRITIS

Describe the initial treatment.	Reduce acid production with H_2 blocker or proton pump inhibitor and treat for *Helicobacter pylori*
What are the options with uncontrolled refractory hemorrhage?	1. Vasopressin via left gastric artery 2. Last resort: gastric resection

HEMOSUCCUS PANCREATICUS

What is hemosuccus pancreaticus?	Blood from pancreatic duct into ampulla of Vater, then into duodenum
What are the signs?	Upper GI bleed via ampulla of Vater, upper abdominal pain, melena

What is the main risk factor?   Chronic pancreatitis

What are the anatomic causes?
1. Bleeding into a pseudocyst
2. Spleen artery pseudoaneurysm
3. Erosion into smaller pancreatic or splenic arterial branch

What is the treatment?   Often requires distal pancreatectomy and ligation of splenic artery, or angiogram embolization

BLEEDING DUODENAL ULCER

How do you suture ligate a bleeding duodenal ulcer?   By the "principle of 3-point vessel ligation" of the posterior ulcer exposed through a duodenotomy or as part of a pyloroplasty

What arteries are ligated?
1. Proximal gastroduodenal artery
2. Distal gastroduodenal artery
3. Transverse pancreatic artery

Illustrate the 3-point ligation for bleeding duodenal ulcer.

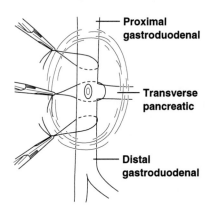

38

The Stomach

GASTRIC ULCERS (SEE ALSO DIAGRAMS IN CHAPTER 29)

Define.

Type I	Along a lesser curvature
Type II	In the body of the stomach, in combination with a duodenal ulcer (think: Type II = 2 ulcers)
Type III	Prepyloric ulcer (think: Type III = prepyloric)
Type IV	Next to the gastroesophageal (GE) junction (think: Four = next to the door—GE junction)

What are the most common operations for each of the following types of ulcers?

Type I	Distal gastrectomy with Billroth I (3% recurrence rate; 15% recurrence)
Type II	Antrectomy with truncal vagotomy (because acid secretion is elevated, as evidenced by the duodenal ulcer), truncal vagotomy and pyloroplasty, or truncal vagotomy and drainage
Type III	Antrectomy and vagotomy with incorporation of the ulcer in the specimen
Type IV	Excision of the ulcer or distal gastrectomy with vertical extension of the resection specimen to include the ulcer

Is it necessary to perform a vagotomy with a type I ulcer in a patient with no history of duodenal ulcers?	No
What is a Dieulafoy ulcer?	A gastric vascular malformation in which a small (2–4 mm) mucosal defect bleeds from a large submucosal artery, resulting in painless hematemesis
What is the appropriate treatment of a Dieulafoy ulcer?	Endoscopic coagulation or surgical resection

GASTRIC CANCER

When is a splenectomy indicated?	**Only** if the cancer is invading the spleen directly
When is a distal pancreatectomy indicated?	**Only** when invaded by cancer directly
Name the stages of gastric cancer by tumor (T), node (N), metastasis (M) [TNM] staging system.	
Stage Ia	T1 (to lamina propria/submucosa), N0, M0
Stage Ib	1. T1 with N1 (+ perigastric lymph nodes [LNs]) 2. T2 (muscularis propria/subserosa), N0, M0
Stage II	1. T2 (muscularis propria/subserosa), N1 (+ perigastric LN), M0 2. T1 (lamina propria/submucosa), N2 (+ LN > 3 cm from stomach/hepatic/splenic/celiac) 3. T3 (through serosa), N0, M0
Stage IIIa	1. T2, N2, M0 2. T3, N1, M0 3. T4 (invades surrounding tissues), N1, M0
Stage IIIb	1. T3, N2, M0 2. T4, N1, M0

Stage IV
    1. Distant METS (any T, any N, M1)
    2. T4, N2, M0

How are the lymph nodes designated?
    D1, D2, D3, D4

Define.

    D1
    6 nodes: left cardia, right cardia, lesser curve, greater curve, suprapyloric, infrapyloric

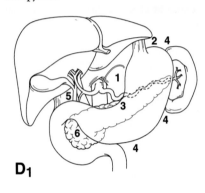

    D2
    Left gastric artery, common hepatic artery, celiac artery, splenic hilum, splenic artery

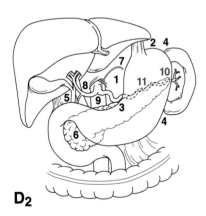

What percentage of patients have metastases at the time of diagnosis?
    75%

GASTRIC LYMPHOMA

At what age is the highest incidence noted?	Peaks at 60 to 70 years
What is the most common GI site?	Stomach (> 50% of GI lymphomas arise in this location; most common organ involved in extranodal non-Hodgkin lymphoma)
What are the associated symptoms?	Epigastric pain, anorexia, nausea and vomiting, weight loss
How is the diagnosis confirmed?	Endoscopy is the method of choice; biopsy with brushings provide diagnosis in more than 90% of cases.
What else should be done if biopsy for lymphoma is positive?	Evaluation for systemic involvement is necessary and includes CT of the chest and abdomen, bone marrow biopsy, and biopsy of enlarged peripheral lymph nodes.
Define the following stages of gastric lymphoma.	
Stage I	Confined to the stomach
Stage II	Spread to the perigastric nodes
Stage III	Spread to nodes other than perigastric
Stage IV	Spread to other abdominal organs
Describe the treatment of gastric lymphoma.	Controversial. Either: 1. Chemotherapy with radiation therapy or surgery for recurrent or refractory disease (M.D. Anderson) 2. Gastrectomy
What chemotherapy is used?	Doxorubicin and cyclophosphamide

GASTRIC SARCOMA

What is the incidence?	Mean age is 60 to 70 years old; incidence is the same in men and women.

What is the histology?	Most are leiomyosarcomas.
What are the associated symptoms?	Similar to those of adenocarcinoma; masses usually attain a large size before causing symptoms
Describe the appearance.	Grossly, they are firm gray-white masses that occasionally contain a pseudocapsule.
What determines the behavior of these tumors?	The number of mitoses per high-power field (hpf), with 5–10 mitotic figures/hpf demonstrating increased propensity for metastases
What is the most common route of metastasis?	Hematogenous (90%)
What is the appropriate treatment?	Surgical resection of the tumor with negative margins
What is the prognosis?	Low-grade: 75% 5-year survival rate High-grade: 33% 5-year survival rate

GASTRIC CARCINOID

What is a leading risk factor?	Pernicious anemia
What test confirms the diagnosis?	Esophagogastroduodenoscopy (EGD) with biopsy
What are the associated findings?	Yellow or pink submucosal gastric nodules
What is the appropriate treatment?	Resection for cure

39

Bariatric Surgery

What is the long limb gastric bypass?	Lengthening of the Roux-en-Y limb to add a malabsorptive component to the gastric bypass
Who is eligible for the long limb gastric bypass?	"Superobese"
What is the operative mortality of a gastric bypass?	0.5%–1%
What is the most feared operative complication after a gastric bypass?	Anastomotic leak!
Name the signs of an anastomotic leak.	**Tachycardia,** tachypnea; fever and increased WBC later. Peritonitis is often hard to detect in morbidly obese!
What is the treatment for an anastomotic leak?	OR STAT for repair, washout, ± drain placement
What complication may postoperative hiccups herald?	Roux limb obstruction at the anastomosis of the jejunojejunostomy (distended gastric pouch on abdominal x-ray) may lead to gastric pouch perforation!
What percentage of patients develop a marginal ulcer?	10%
Name the treatment for a gastrojejunostomy stenosis.	Balloon dilation
Name the most common cause of postoperative neuropathy after gastric bypass.	Thiamine deficiency

What percentage of patients will develop gallstones after a gastric bypass and weight loss?

33%

How is the postoperative complication of gallstones prevented?

1. Cholecystectomy, or
2. At least 6 months of oral ursodeoxycholic acid

What is the lap-band?

Laparoscopically placed **band** around stomach with a subcutaneous port to adjust constriction; results in smaller gastric reservoir

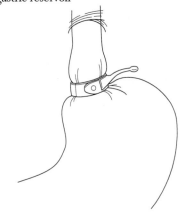

What is a jejunoileal bypass?

Surgery initially used for morbid obesity; bypasses the ileum with an end-to-end anastomosis between the proximal jejunum and distal ileum. No longer performed because of the large number of complications.

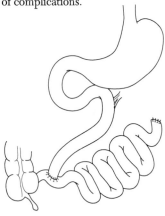

What complications are associated with the old jejunoileal bypass?

Cirrhosis (from protein calorie malnutrition, GI toxin absorption), bacterial overgrowth with resultant vitamin K deficiency, interstitial nephritis, iron deficiency anemia, bypass enteritis; also, hypocalcemia, resultant severe osteoporosis, and a rheumatoid-like arthritis

What is the "biliopancreatic bypass" operation?

Anastomose the proximal small bowel to the terminal ileum because the bile and pancreatic juices "bypass" the bowel (not usually performed in the United States)

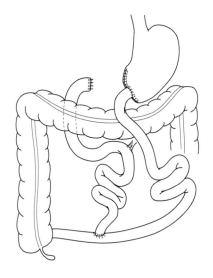

40   Ostomies

What is another name for continent ileostomy?

Kock pouch

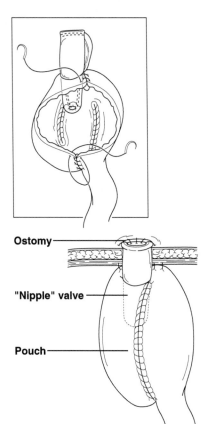

What is the usual sodium concentration in ileostomy effluent?

~115 mEq/L

In the immediate postoperative period, what IV fluids should be used to replace ileostomy output?

Normal saline or LR with 40 KCl/L at equal volumes (mL for mL)

Patients with ileostomies typically have what type of body fluid abnormality?

Mild dehydration with a chronic state of sodium and water depletion

Which type of stomas are candidates for the irrigation method of bowel control?

Descending colon and sigmoid colostomies

What does the eversion technique of Brook ileostomy help prevent?

Serositis, leading to obstruction and high-output ileostomy diarrhea with associated dehydration/electrolyte abnormalities; protects skin

What does placing the ostomy through the rectus muscle help to prevent?

Parastomal hernia
Prolapse

In general, ostomies should be placed through the anterior abdominal wall within a triangle composed of what landmarks?

Stoma triangle: umbilicus, pubis, and anterior superior iliac spine

Upon completion of an end ileostomy, how far beyond the skin should the "bud" protrude?

2–3 cm

Through which muscle should proper ileostomy formation always place the ostomy?

Rectus abdominis muscle

Where should a stoma be placed on a small lower abdominal fat fold?

At the apex (not above, not below fold)

In general, in a very obese patient with many skinfolds, where should a stoma be placed: upper or lower abdomen?

Upper abdomen, above the panniculus

What length of ileum should be brought out above skin to fashion an end ileostomy?	4–6 cm
When creating a stoma, how many "average"-size fingers should you be able to admit through fascia and skin?	2
What is the average incidence of small-bowel obstruction following loop ileostomies?	10%
Is the incidence of small-bowel obstruction with loop ileostomies higher or lower than for loop colostomies?	Higher
Is parastomal hernia more common in ileostomy or colostomy?	Colostomy
What is the most common dermatologic problem associated with stomas?	Chemical irritation from effluent
What is the most common organism associated with peristomal skin infection?	*Candida albicans*
Name the 5 most common colostomy complications.	Ischemia Retraction Stenosis Prolapse Peristomal hernia
What is diversion colitis?	Inflammation of the distally diverted portion of the colon
What is the cause of diversion colitis?	Thought to be secondary to a lack of trophic factors to mucosa, particularly short-chain fatty acids

What is the appropriate treatment of diversion colitis?	Reversal of the colostomy is curative (if feasible).
What are the indications for repair of parastomal hernias?	Repair/relocate for pain, obstruction, inability to fit appliance adequately, cosmetic reasons
What is the best surgical option for parastomal hernia?	Relocation of the stoma
What sodium and potassium abnormalities do patients with profuse ileostomy diarrhea usually have?	Hyponatremia and hypokalemia
What is the most common cause of colostomy stenosis?	Ischemia
What is the most common cause of pericolostomy abscess?	Perforation caused by an irrigating device
What is the most common technical error in stoma construction leading to peristomal hernia?	Stoma brought out laterally to the rectus
What is the most common complication following closure of a colostomy?	Wound infection
What is the most frequent cause of ileostomy fistulas?	Crohn's disease
What is the most common cause of arterial insufficiency in colostomy?	Excessive clearance of mesentery from the bowel
What is the appropriate treatment of mild colostomy strictures?	Dilation
How can the depth of ischemia/necrosis be assessed in an ileostomy?	By inserting a small test tube into the stoma and illuminating with a flashlight to assess mucosa down to and below the fascia

Why do patients with ileostomies have increased incidence of gallstones?

Ileal disease or resection interrupts the enterohepatic circulation by decreasing the availability of bile acids and favoring precipitations of cholesterol stones.

Which limb is usually involved in prolapse of a loop colostomy?

Distal

High ileostomy output can result in which type of acid-base disorder?

Metabolic acidosis, secondary to excessive bicarbonate loss from ileostomy

What is the most common type of urinary stone in ileostomy patients?

Uric acid stones (60%)

What medical condition can result in peristomal venous complexes?

Portal hypertension (basically peristomal caput medusae)

41

Small Intestine

SMALL BOWEL OBSTRUCTION

ILEUS

Describe ileus.	Paralytic ileus is a functional obstruction of the small bowel that occurs in most patients following abdominal surgery, and is caused by neural, humoral, and metabolic factors. It also occurs with inflammatory processes in the abdomen (e.g., pancreatitis, peritonitis), retroperitoneal hemorrhage, spine injury, electrolytes, and medication.
What are the associated signs of ileus?	Lack of bowel sounds, bowel distention, no flatus, no stool, +/−emesis
What are the other common causes of ileus?	Opiates, hypokalemia, hyponatremia
What is the order of return of motility following abdominal surgery?	1. Small intestine 2. Stomach 3. Colon
What is one theory regarding the physiologic mechanism of ileus?	Sympathetic hyperactivity, which slows GI propulsion and constricts sphincters
How is the diagnosis of ileus confirmed?	History and physical examination Abdominal plain film demonstrating air throughout the GI tract with or without air-fluid levels
What is the appropriate treatment of ileus?	Conservative: Nothing by mouth, nasogastric tube (NGT), IV fluids until patient passes flatus; electrolyte replacement as needed

ANTICOAGULANT-INDUCED OBSTRUCTION

What is anticoagulant-induced obstruction?	Patients taking warfarin may develop an intramural hematoma of the small bowel.
What is the most frequent site?	Proximal jejunum
What are the associated signs/laboratory findings?	Elevated prothrombin time (PT), ecchymoses, hematuria
What are the associated radiologic findings?	Affected segment appears narrow and rigid; "picket fence" appearance of mucosa
What is the appropriate initial treatment?	Discontinue the anticoagulant vitamin K Nasogastric suction/IV fluids

SMALL BOWEL OBSTRUCTION

How can you remember the 6 impending signs of bowel ischemia/necrosis with small bowel obstruction?	**FATAL:** **F**ever **A**cidosis **T**achycardia **A**bdominal pain **L**eukocytosis

SMALL BOWEL TUMORS

What is the differential diagnosis of benign tumors of the small intestine?	Leiomyoma, lipoma, lymphangioma, fibroma, adenoma, hemangioma
What is the most common benign tumor of the small intestine?	Leiomyoma (followed by lipoma and adenoma)
What is the differential diagnosis of malignant tumors of the small intestine?	Adenocarcinoma, carcinoid tumor, lymphoma
What is the most common malignant small bowel tumor?	Adenocarcinoma

What is the incidence of small bowel malignancies?	< 2% of all malignancies arise in the small bowel.
What 5 factors are important in preventing malignancies in the small bowel?	Fast transit time, thus limiting contact of carcinogens with mucosa Alkaline pH and decreased bacterial contamination High activity of benzopyrene hydroxylase, which detoxifies carcinogens Rapid turnover of mucosal cells Secretory IgA
What is the usual presentation?	Insidious onset, weight loss, anorexia, malabsorption with steatorrhea, dull aching pain, symptoms of obstruction, occult or massive bleeding
How are the tumors identified?	Upper gastrointestinal (UGI) series with enteroclysis Esophagogastroduodenoscopy (EGD) for duodenal lesions

ADENOCARCINOMA OF THE SMALL BOWEL

What is the incidence of adenocarcinoma?	Most common small bowel neoplasm; 30–50% of all small bowel cancers
What is the mean age?	Peaks at 60–70 years (parallels colonic adenocarcinoma)
What is the most common location of adenocarcinoma?	The duodenum, especially in the periampullary region, which accounts for two-thirds of all small bowel adenocarcinomas; occurs least frequently in the ileum
What are the signs of duodenal/ampullary adenocarcinoma?	Extrahepatic biliary obstruction
What is the usual presentation of adenocarcinoma?	Duodenal/periampullary—obstructive jaundice Jejunoileal—slow, progressive obstruction
What is the appropriate treatment of adenocarcinoma?	Surgical resection with removal of draining lymph nodes

What is the prognosis?	Usually poor, because patients present with advanced disease
	With lymph node metastases—5-year survival rate of 15%
	Without lymph node metastases—5-year survival rate of 50–70%
How does the prognosis of periampullary neoplasm compare with that of pancreatic cancer?	More frequently resectable for cure than pancreatic cancer; 5-year survival rate is 40%, compared with < 10% for pancreatic cancer.

LYMPHOMA OF THE SMALL BOWEL

What is the incidence of lymphoma?	10–15% of all small bowel malignancies. Primary involvement of the small bowel is the 2nd most common site after the stomach.
What is the mean age of occurrence?	Peaks at 50–60 years
What is the associated cell type?	Virtually all primary small bowel lymphomas are non-Hodgkin B-cell lymphomas
What is the most common location in the small bowel?	Ileum (remember Peyer's patches = lymphatic tissue)
What is the usual presentation?	Fatigue, malaise, weight loss, abdominal pain, bowel obstruction, fever and night sweats, malabsorption, guaiac-positive stool
How is the diagnosis made?	UGI series with enteroclysis (demonstrates submucosal nodules, ulcerations, or diffuse mucosal thickening)
	CT (demonstrates bulky nodes and bowel wall thickening)
What are the associated medical conditions?	Celiac disease, Crohn's disease, AIDS, systemic lupus erythematosus (SLE), Wegener's disease, X-linked agammaglobulinemia

What is the staging?	Follows Ann Arbor classification: Stage I—confined to the small bowel Stage II—with regional lymph nodes Stage III—with nonresectable lymph nodes beyond regional nodes Stage IV—metastases to other organs in and beyond the abdomen
What is the appropriate treatment?	Surgery; resection with primary anastomosis and removal of draining lymph nodes
What is the indication for postoperative chemotherapy?	Intermediate/high-grade lymphoma

ENTERIC INFECTIONS

Through what mechanisms do enteric infections act?	Osmotic Secretory (i.e., cholera) Inflammatory (i.e., *Shigella*)
Which diagnostic tests are indicated?	Stool smear, Wright's stain for WBCs, Hemoccult testing, stool culture, examination for ova and parasites
What are the sites of intestinal involvement?	Small intestine (cholera, *Escherichia coli*, *Giardia*, viruses) Ileum and colon (*Salmonella, Yersinia, Campylobacter*) Colon (*Shigella, E. coli* [invasive, hemorrhagic], *Amoeba, Giardia*)
What is the most common cause after drinking from a mountain stream?	*Giardia*
What causes food poisoning?	Preformed toxins elaborated by *Staphylococcus aureus, Clostridium perfringens,* or *Bacillus cereus*
What part of the history differentiates gastroenteritis?	Vomiting is **followed** by pain and diarrhea.

BLIND-LOOP SYNDROME

What is blind-loop syndrome?	Bacterial overgrowth in the small intestine. The organisms that tend to overgrow are not the normal flora of the small bowel, but are more representative of colonic flora (e.g., gram-negative bacteria [*E. coli*]). Often overgrowth of strictly anaerobic bacteria, such as *Clostridium* and *Bacteroides*.
What are the causes?	Anything that disrupts the normal flow of intestinal contents (i.e., causes stasis): strictures, Crohn's disease, postvagotomy, scleroderma, diverticula, decreased gastric acid secretion, and incompetent ileocecal valve
What are the associated signs and symptoms?	Diarrhea, steatorrhea, malnutrition, abdominal pain, hypocalcemia, B_{12} deficiency, and resultant megaloblastic anemia
What is the pathogenesis of B_{12} deficiency?	1. Bacterial utilization of B_{12} 2. Bacterial toxins inhibit the absorption of B_{12} across the small bowel mucosa
Which diagnostic tests are indicated?	Schilling test—demonstrates an intrinsic factor-resistant B_{12} malabsorption Hydrogen breath test—lactose is swallowed and hydrogen expiration is monitored; with bacterial overgrowth, there is increased H_2 production earlier than normal
What is the appropriate treatment?	Surgical correction of the underlying disorder, if feasible; otherwise, antibiotics to inhibit bacterial overgrowth
What are the other causes of B_{12} deficiency?	Gastrectomy (decreased secretion of intrinsic factor) and excision of terminal ileum (site of B_{12} absorption)

42

The Appendix

Who first described the pathogenesis of acute appendicitis?

Fitz in 1886 (Harvard pathologist)

What was the mortality for acute appendicitis in 1886?

45% died!

What is Dunphy's sign?

Exacerbation of abdominal pain with **coughing** (seen with peritonitis from appendicitis)

What is the "hamburger" sign?

Ask patients with suspected appendicitis if they would like a hamburger or favorite food; if they can eat, seriously question the diagnosis.

What often happens to the leukocytosis seen with acute appendicitis soon after appendiceal perforation?

WBC count falls!

What lab value (rarely used) is almost always elevated with acute appendicitis?

C-reactive protein

What percentage of the time will you see free air on abdominal x-rays with a perforated appendix?

Approximately 1% of the time

What kind of CT scan should be obtained for evaluation of acute appendicitis?

Spiral CT with rectal enema contrast

What are the CT findings with acute appendicitis?

1. Thickened appendix > 6 mm
2. Fat stranding
3. Cecal thickening
4. Appendicolith
5. No contrast in appendix (unopacified)
6. Arrowhead sign

What is the CT "arrowhead" sign of acute appendicitis?

Contrast in the **cecum** forms an "arrowhead" pointing to the occluded appendiceal orifice

Where is the appendix anatomically in the right lower quadrant with pregnancy by month 5?

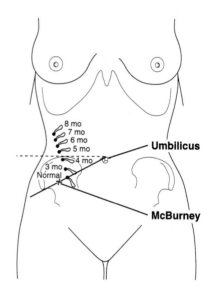

What is the fetal mortality with acute _non_perforated appendicitis in pregnancy?

< 10%

What is the fetal mortality with _perforated_ appendicitis in pregnancy?

33%

What is the incidence of wound infection after _non_perforated appendectomy?

Only about 3%!

What is pyelophlebitis?

Rare post-appendicitis complication marked by fever and jaundice due to septic clot in portal vein

While incidental appendectomy is controversial, in which group is it almost *never* indicated?

Elderly

What is the mortality for a perforated appendix in the elderly vs the young?

Young: < 1%
Elderly: 5%

What should you order if a patient's appendiceal specimen returns with a rare opportunistic pathogen?

HIV test for the patient

What percentage of all appendiceal specimens will reveal a tumor?

1%

What is "pseudomyxoma peritonei"?

Peritoneal cavity is filled with mucinous secretions and diffuse spread and implants of mucinous carcinomatous cells.

What appendiceal tumor can cause pseudomyxomatous peritonei?

Mucinous **cystadenocarcinoma** of the appendix after rupture of appendiceal mucocele

What is an appendiceal mucocele?

Blockage of the appendiceal lumen and accumulation of mucus forming a large mucous-filled mass of the appendix

What causes an appendiceal mucocele?

Benign cystadenoma or malignant cystadenocarcinoma

What is the treatment of pseudomyxoma peritonei?

1. Wide resection of primary (right hemicolectomy)
2. Wide débridement of all feasibly removed peritoneal implants

What is the treatment of appendiceal cystadenoma?

Appendectomy

What is the treatment of ruptured appendiceal cystadenoma with mucinous ascites?

Appendectomy alone (benign mucinous ascites has no cells)

43   Carcinoid Tumors

PATHOLOGY/HISTOLOGY

What are tachykinins?
A family of vasoactive peptide hormones with very short half-lives

What percentage of patients with carcinoid tumors have elevated serotonin levels?
Approximately 60%

What percentage of patients with serotonin overproduction are symptomatic?
Approximately 66%

Are elevated serotonin levels responsible for the carcinoid syndrome?
Not entirely. Excessive serotonin levels seem to be involved in diarrhea and valvular disease; however, the other classic symptoms seem to be due to other vasoactive/endocrine products.

What are the associated valvular lesions?
Most commonly tricuspid, regurgitation, and pulmonic stenosis (predominantly right-sided valvular lesions)

What causes the valvular lesions?
Subendocardial fibrosis, thought to be secondary to elevated serotonin levels

Why are the valvular lesions predominantly right sided?
The lungs (like the liver) act as a filter to deactivate the bulk of the humorally active substances and thus protect the left side of the heart.

Do desmoplastic (fibrotic) changes occur at other sites as well?
Yes; most commonly, the gut wall, mesenteric vessels, and retroperitoneum; less commonly, the penile fascia and joints

Can these fibrotic changes cause trouble?	Absolutely. The intense mesenteric and gut-wall fibrosis is the most common cause of bowel obstruction in carcinoid tumor patients; the mesenteric vascular fibrosis can lead to intestinal ischemia.
Which humoral product causes flushing?	Bradykinin is thought to be the most likely culprit.

CLINICAL MANIFESTATIONS

Is GI bleeding common with carcinoid tumors?	No. Carcinoids are submucosal and do not commonly bleed. However, bleeding is seen with rectal carcinoids.
What disease is associated with carcinoid tumors of the ampulla of Vater?	Neurofibromatosis
In patients with multiple endocrine neoplasia-I (MEN-I), what are the most frequent locations of carcinoid tumors?	Men—thymus Women—lung
Which primary site(s) are most commonly associated with carcinoid syndrome?	Two-thirds of all cases occur with ileal primaries.

TREATMENT

Where are appendiceal carcinoids located?	Tip—70% Body—20% Base—10%
What is the 5-year survival rate for appendiceal carcinoids?	99%
How common are metastases from appendiceal carcinoids?	Very rare, and almost always limited to the regional lymph nodes
What is the most common metachronous primary GI malignancy?	Colon adenocarcinoma
What is octreotide, and how does it work?	A synthetic somatostatin analog; thought to inhibit release of humoral products by the carcinoid

What are the side effects of octreotide?	Steatorrhea Cholelithiasis secondary to biliary stasis
How effective is octreotide?	Response rate of 60–80%, with excellent relief of diarrhea and flushing. However, tachyphylaxis occurs with time in most patients because of receptor down-regulation, with a median response time of 9 months.
How effective is alpha interferon (α-IFN)?	Response rate of 50–80% with symptom alleviation. Tachyphylaxis also occurs with α-IFN, most likely because of the development of antibodies.
In what cases should hepatic resection be attempted?	Only in low-risk patients in whom > 90% of a metastatic tumor mass can be extirpated safely
Can hepatic resection ever be considered curative?	Yes, if all primary abdominal disease and all metastatic disease is resected
Why is cholecystectomy indicated at the time of initial operation for carcinoid tumors?	Two reasons: 1. To prevent potential gallbladder ischemia, if future hepatic artery embolization is necessary 2. Due to increased risk of gallstones with octreotide
What is the blood supply for most carcinoid liver metastases?	Hepatic artery (not the portal vein)
What is the rationale for hepatic artery embolization?	The liver has dual blood supplies, and thus 2 oxygen sources. The hepatic artery branches supplying the tumor can be interrupted without causing excessive damage to the normal liver.
What are the potential side effects of embolization in carcinoid patients?	Increased release of humoral substances from the tumor. Infection of necrotic liver
What precautions must be taken prior to any tumor embolization, manipulation, or anesthesia induction?	Octreotide "blockade," to prevent excessive humoral product release from the tumor

What is the proper surgical therapy for bronchial carcinoid?

For typical carcinoids, local excision is adequate.

If carcinoid is atypical, the lesion should be treated as a bronchogenic carcinoma.

What is carcinoid crisis?

Severe cramping, abdominal pain, and diarrhea, with or without cardiac disturbances (hypotension and/or tachycardia) and wheezing

What causes carcinoid crisis?

Extremely high humoral product levels (especially serotonin, which in high levels can cause mesenteric vasoconstriction)

GI symptoms are caused by ischemia, not by mechanical obstruction.

Why should catecholamines be avoided in the treatment of carcinoid bronchospasm?

There is evidence that humoral product release by enterochromaffin cells may be controlled by adrenoreceptors, and thus catechols/agonists may actually worsen the bronchoconstriction by increasing the release of the causative factors!

What is the appropriate therapy for carcinoid crisis?

Octreotide; administer fluids to alleviate hypotension acutely; administer aprotinin for bronchospasm, if present

What is aprotinin?

An inhibitor of kallikrein

Can carcinoid tumors cause paraneoplastic syndromes?

Yes. Carcinoids are a common cause of ectopic cortisol secretion (Cushing's syndrome); acromegaly and hypercalcemia have also been reported.

What nutritional deficiency occasionally occurs secondary to carcinoid tumors?

Pellagra, because of excessive tryptophan consumption in making excess serotonin (tryptophan is a niacin precursor)

When is cytotoxic chemotherapy indicated?

In anaplastic variants of carcinoid, etoposide and cisplatin yield response rates of 67%; this therapy is not useful in other variants.

44   Fistulas

What is the most common cause of enterocutaneous fistulas?

Abdominal operations (anastomotic leak and inadvertent enterotomies)

Which *FRIEND* factor (*F*oreign body, *R*adiation, *I*nfection, *E*pitheliazation, *N*eoplasm, *D*istal obstruction) is the most common reason for keeping a fistula open?

Distal obstruction

What is the difference between external and internal fistulas?

External is cutaneous (e.g., colocutaneous)
Internal connects to internal hollow organs (e.g., colovesical)

Define the following.

    Simple fistula

One tract (complicated fistulas have multiple tracts)

    Low-output fistula

< 500 cc output per day

    High-output fistula

> 500 cc output per day

What is the most common cause of death with a fistula?

Infection

What are the medical therapy options for decreasing output from a proximal (e.g., gastric) fistula?

H_2 blocker (e.g., ranitidine) somatostatin

After a definitive surgical operation for an enterocutaneous fistula, what is the recurrence rate postoperatively?	10%
What length of enterocutaneous fistula is more likely to close?	> 2 cm long
What percentage of enterocutaneous fistulas close in 6 weeks?	Approximately 60% (think: 60% in 6)
Has octreotide (somatostatin) been shown to decrease enterocutaneous fistula output?	Yes, (50–85% decrease)
Has octreotide been shown to speed up the closure of enterocutaneous fistula?	No

45 Colon and Rectum

COLON ANATOMY AND PHYSIOLOGY

Where is the rectosigmoid junction consistently located?

15–18 cm from the anal verge

What is the arc of Riolan?

Proximal collateral in the colonic mesentery that links the superior mesenteric artery (SMA) and the inferior mesenteric artery (IMA)

Should a sigmoid colostomy be brought through the rectus or oblique muscles?

Rectus muscle (lower incidence of peristomal hernias)

Which procedure has the higher morbidity, takedown of an end colostomy or a loop colostomy?

End colostomy

Which ion is preferentially absorbed from the normal colonic lumen?

Na^+

Which ions are preferentially secreted by the normal colonic epithelium?

K^+, HCO_3^-

Where in the GI tract does the majority of H_2O absorption take place?

Ascending colon

By what mechanism does H_2O absorption occur?

Passive diffusion, which is linked to active Na^+ transport

What is the effect of bile acids on colonic epithelium?	They produce secretory diarrhea by inducing Na^+ and H_2O secretion.

COLON CANCER

What are the indications for colon resection after endoscopic malignant polypectomy?	1. Positive margin 2. Angiolymphatic invasion 3. Invasion of muscularis mucosa (Haggitt level 3) 4. Invasion of submucosa in sessile polyp (Haggitt level 4) 5. Poorly differentiated
Which is more accurate for assessing the distance of a rectal tumor from the anus: rigid or flexible sigmoidoscopy?	Rigid
What is the value of the Valsalva maneuver when performing a digital rectal exam?	A high rectal tumor may descend within reach of the examiner's finger
Which procedure should come first: colostomy maturation or abdominal closure?	Abdominal closure (decreased risk of infection)
Which chemotherapeutic agents are considered standard for:	
Stage III colon cancer?	5-fluorouracil (5-FU) and levamisole
Stage IV colon cancer?	5-FU and leucovorin
Why is radiotherapy (RT) not a standard adjuvant therapy for colon cancer?	Because of frequent complications of radiation enteritis and renal injury
What are the contraindications for hepatic resection of colon cancer liver metastases?	1. > 5 metastases 2. Other distant metastases 3. Positive portal/celiac lymph nodes

What margins do you need with resection of liver metastases?	1 cm
What percentage of patients survive 3 years after liver resection?	Approximately 33% are alive at 3 years.
What percentage of patients are alive 5 years after resection of a SOLITARY liver metastasis?	Up to 60% are alive at 5 years!
What do you do in the event of recurrence after successful resection for liver colorectal metastases?	Redo the resection with 1-cm margins.

COLON OBSTRUCTION

With colon obstruction, is perforation more likely with competent or incompetent ileocecal valve?	Competent; results in a closed loop obstruction through the one-way valve
What is the diagnostic workup for colon obstruction?	Abdominal x-ray (AXR), Gastrografin enema study
What are the major causes of colon obstruction?	Cancer (# 1 cause) Volvulus Diverticulitis Inflammatory bowel disease
What are the indications for a cecostomy with colon distention with colonic obstruction?	Unstable, very poor prognosis
What do you use for an open cecostomy tube?	Malencott or Foley catheter

OGILVIE'S SYNDROME

What is Ogilvie's syndrome?	Nonobstructive colon distention (pseudoobstruction)

Describe the workup.	AXR (to rule out free air/measure cecum) Gastrografin enema (to rule out obstruction) Electrolyte levels
At what cecal diameter is there danger of perforation?	> 12 cm at high risk of perforation
What is the treatment if no free air is seen?	Neostigmine IV (parasympathomimetic), or colonoscopic decompression
How does neostigmine work?	As a cholinesterase inhibitor
At what cecal diameter is treatment mandated?	> 12 cm, or if no improvement in 36 hours

ISCHEMIC COLITIS

What is ischemic colitis?	Low blood flow to colon
What are the signs and symptoms of ischemic colitis?	Abdominal pain, hematochezia, diarrhea
What is the diagnostic test?	CT scan
What is the role of angiography with colon ischemia?	No role!
What is the treatment?	NPO, IV fluids, broad-spectrum antibiotics
What are the indications for laparotomy and resection?	Peritonitis, free air, transmural necrosis
After resection, what procedure should be done?	Colostomy/mucus fistula is safest choice

RECTAL CANCER

Give the original Dukes' staging (simplified).	
A	Limited to the mucosa/submucosa
B	Invasion of muscularis propria
C	Positive regional lymph nodes
D	Dukes' did not describe a stage D!
For what tumor was the Dukes' classification originally described?	Rectal cancer (not colon cancer)
What is TRUS?	TransRectal UltraSound
What are the ultrasound rectal cancer stages for:	
uT1?	Tumor confined to mucosa/submucosa
uT2?	Invades muscularis propria
uT3?	Invades perirectal fat
uT4?	Invades adjacent organ
N0?	No lymph node enlargement seen
N1?	Lymph node enlargement
Which rectal tumors get preop chemotherapy and radiation therapy (neoadjuvant)?	All rectal tumors except uT4
What treatment is used for neoadjuvant rectal cancer?	5-FU and leucovorin 5000 cGy radiation therapy Followed postoperatively by chemotherapy and radiation therapy for 6 weeks
What is total mesorectal excision?	Total removal of the mesorectum with its lymph nodes

What is a coloanal anastomosis?

For distal rectal tumors: anastomose a colon J pouch to the anus

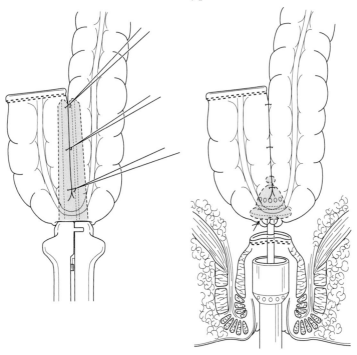

What are the criteria for transanal rectal cancer resection?

Small (< 4 cm), well or moderately differentiated, distal, less than a third of lumen circumference, no biopsy-proven lymphatic or vessel invasion, T1 (submucosa), no positive nodes

46 The Anus

ANAL CANCER

Define the anal verge, anal margin, and anal canal.

The anal verge separates the anal canal from the anal margin. The anal margin is 5 cm of perianal skin.

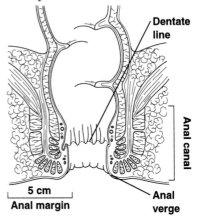

What are the risk factors for anal cancer?

Human papillomavirus (HPV), HIV, any immunosuppressive state, anal-receptive intercourse

What are the signs and symptoms of anal cancer?

Bleeding, pain, pruritus, tenesmus, change in bowel movement habits

Define tenesmus.

Feeling of need to have bowel movement with "ineffectual" painful **straining**

What is the diagnostic test for anal canal tumors?

EAUS = EndoAnal UltraSound

Describe the stages of anal cancer.

Stage I

Tumor < 2 cm , no nodes, no metastases (T1, N0, M0)

Stage II	Tumor > 2 cm, (T2, N0, M0)
Stage IIIA	1. Tumor > 2 cm with positive perirectal lymph nodes, no metastases (T1–3, N0, M0) 2. Tumor invades adjacent organ (T4, N0, M0)
Stage IIIB	1. Tumor invades adjacent organs and has positive perirectal nodes (T4, N1, M0) 2. Any tumor with positive inguinal or iliac nodes (any T, N2–3, M0)
Stage IV	Distant metastases (any T, any N, M1)
In general, to what lymph node basin does anal cancer *distal* to the dentate line (anal margin and distal anal canal) spread?	Inguinal nodes
In general, where do anal canal tumors *proximal* to the dentate line spread?	Inferior mesenteric lymph nodes, mesorectum, paravertebral lymph nodes (like rectal cancers)
What should be done if residual tumor remains in the anal canal after treatment according to NIGRO protocol?	Chemotherapy with different agent Radiation therapy
What should be done if disease recurs or residual tumor remains in the anal canal after 2 attempts of chemotherapy and radiation?	Abdominoperineal resection (APR)
What percentage of patients have a complete response to treatment with modified NIGRO protocol?	90%
After treatment with modified NIGRO protocol, what percentage of patients are alive at 5 years?	85%

What is the most common site of distant metastases with anal cancer?

Liver

ANORECTAL ABSCESS

Define the abscess.

1. Supralevator
2. Perianal
3. Intersphincteric
4. Ischiorectal

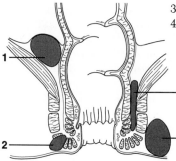

Where should a simple isolated supralevator abscess be drained?

Through the rectum

What test is very helpful when entertaining the thought of supralevator abscess?

CT scan

ANAL CONDYLOMA

What causes anal condyloma?

Human papillomavirus (HPV)

What is the incubation period for anal condyloma?

6 weeks until signs

What are the nonsurgical treatments for anal condyloma?

Aldara, 5-fluorouracil (5-FU) cream, intralesional interferon injection, podophyllin

What is Aldara?

Imiquimod—a cream that is an immunostimulant

What is the treatment of anal canal disease?

Surgical resection and intralesional interferon injections

What is the treatment of external perianal disease?	Surgical excision and/or topical medication

MISCELLANEOUS

What is the most common cause of anal stricture?	Hemorrhoidectomy
What is the most common cause of anal pruritus?	**Idiopathic;** other causes include tumors, infections, anorectal disorder, skin disorder (e.g., psoriasis), jaundice

47

Lower GI Bleeding

Define massive lower GI bleeding.

> 3 units of blood in 24 hours

Why is a nuclear-tagged RBC study not used with massive lower GI bleeding as the first-line test?

Because > 50% of patients will not be localized until after 6 hours!

What causes lower GI bleeding in patients acutely after abdominal aortic aneurysm (AAA) repair?

Left colon ischemia due to loss of inferior mesenteric artery (IMA)

What condition causes bright red blood per rectum and per mouth?

Duodeno-aortic fistula (large volume bleeding!)

The small bowel is the source of lower GI bleeding in what percentage of cases?

Approximately 4%

What is the most common cause of small bowel lower GI bleeding?

Angiodysplasia

How do you evaluate the small bowel for mass or mucosal abnormality?

Enteroclysis (not upper GI study), but this does not diagnose angiodysplasia!

What is the most common cause of lower GI bleeding in children and adolescents?

Meckel's diverticulum with ectopic gastric mucosa resulting in an ulcer

What percentage of significant bleeding originates in the upper vs lower GI tract?

85% are **upper** GI ("most common cause of massive blood per rectum is upper GI bleeding")

What is angiodysplasia?

A.K.A. arteriovenous malformation; dilated (ectatic) vessels in the submucosa. Breakdown of overlying mucosa results in bleeding.

What is the most common location of colon angiodysplasia?

Right sided

Why does right-sided angiodysplasia bleed more often than left sided?

Thought to be because the right colon wall has less muscle (i.e., it's thinner)

Give the differential diagnosis of lower GI bleeding in adolescents.

Meckel's diverticulum (ectopic gastric mucosa)
IBD
Polyps

What is one exam that many patients require prior to laparotomy for lower GI bleeding?

Esophagogastroduodenoscopy (EGD; to rule out UGI bleed)

How can you mark the spot of colon bleeding for localization at laparotomy?

Inject **India ink** via colonoscope!

How often is colonoscopic treatment of colonic angiodysplasia definitive?

Approximately 85% of the time

What percentage of patients with lower GI bleeding that spontaneously stops will rebleed?

Up to 25%!

What is the differential diagnosis of lower GI bleeding and pain?

IBD, ischemic bowel, ruptured abdominal aortic aneurysm (AAA) with occlusion of inferior mesenteric artery (IMA), Meckel's diverticulum with ulcer, intussusception

48

Inflammatory Bowel Disease: Crohn's Disease and Ulcerative Colitis

What is the treatment for short segment small bowel strictures in Crohn's disease?

Heineke-Mikulicz stricturoplasty

What is the surgical treatment of long segment small bowel stricture in Crohn's disease?

Isoperistaltic side to side stricturoplasty:
  Transect strictured bowel
  Overlap ends
  Anastomose side to side to enlarge lumen

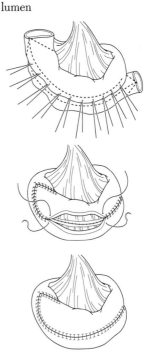

In general, should the small bowel ever be surgically bypassed in Crohn's disease?

No (increased risk of cancer, bleeding, perforation)

What is the one exception regarding bypass in Crohn's disease?

Duodenal involvement; "bypass" with gastrojejunostomy

When is colonic resection in Crohn's disease relatively contraindicated?

In a patient who has had many small bowel resections, the bowel becomes very important for water and electrolyte absorption! Consider "stricturoplasty" of large bowel.

What is a popular surgical anastomosis after total abdominal colectomy for ulcerative colitis?

Ileoanal anastomosis—create pouch of ileum and then anastomose to anus/rectum

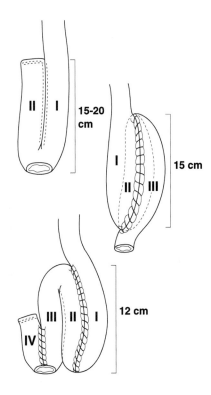

What is the function of the "pouches"?

Act as a reservoir for stool

What is a relative contraindication for ileoanal anastomosis?

Controversial, but most believe that an ileoanal anastomosis should not be performed with Crohn's disease

How many bowel movements per day do patients have after an ileoanal anastomosis?

Average 4–7

What is the treatment for colon to other organ fistulas in Crohn's disease?

Resect colon segment

What is the role of Infliximab in Crohn's disease?

Immunosuppressive; an antibody against tumor necrosis factor receptors, which results in lysis of inflammatory cells

What is the role of cyclosporine in inflammatory bowel disease (IBD)?

Usually as a last resort (in refractory cases)

What is olsalazine?

5-ASA dimer (cleaved by colonic bacteria)

49   Liver

ANATOMY

What fissure does the falciform ligament enter?	Umbilical fissure
What are the borders of the caudate lobe?	IVC, umbilical fissure, transverse hilar fissure
What are the 3 borders of the quadrate lobe?	Transverse hilar fissure Umbilical fissure Gallbladder fossa
Do the hepatic veins follow the segmental lobar anatomy of the liver?	No
Does the portal vein have valves?	No
What is the obliterated umbilical vein called?	Ligamentum teres
What percentage of left hepatic arteries are replaced entirely by a branch from the left gastric artery?	Approximately 10%
What percentage of left hepatic arteries are partially replaced by a branch of the left gastric artery?	Approximately 10%
What percentage of right hepatic arteries arise from the superior mesenteric artery?	Approximately 10% (Is there a pattern here?)

What percentage of right hepatic arteries pass anteriorly to the common hepatic bile duct?	Approximately 25%
What percentage of right hepatic arteries pass posteriorly to the portal vein?	Approximately 10%
What is the name of macrophages located in the liver?	Kupffer cells
What are the 3 components of a portal triad?	1. Arteriole (hepatic) 2. Portal venule 3. Bile duct

PHYSIOLOGY

What fraction of total liver blood flow comes from the portal vein?	Approximately two-thirds
What fraction of total liver blood flow comes from the hepatic artery?	Approximately one-third
What percentage of total cardiac output goes to the liver?	Approximately 20%
What protein is produced in the largest amount by the liver?	Albumin
What are the 9 hepatic acute-phase proteins?	Fibrinogen, haptoglobin, C-reactive protein, complement 3, ceruloplasmin, α-antitrypsin, α-antichymotrypsin, α-acid glycoprotein, amyloid A

HYDATID LIVER CYSTS

What is the appropriate treatment of cyst rupture and bile duct obstruction?	Endoscopic retrograde cholangiopancreatography (ERCP) with papillotomy

What are the 3 layers of a hydatid cyst?	Host pericyst Ectocyst (from parasite) Endocyst (from parasite)
Which layers must be removed in the OR?	The endocyst and the ectocyst, because both layers may contain live parasites
What is the recurrence rate of postoperative hydatid cysts?	Approximately 20%

TUMORS OF THE LIVER

CAVERNOUS HEMANGIOMA

What are the 2 types of hepatic hemangioma?	Capillary hemangioma Cavernous hemangioma
What is the significance of capillary liver hemangiomas?	Clinically insignificant
How common are cavernous hemangiomas?	Approximately 7% incidence (autopsy studies)
What percentage of cavernous hemangiomas are multiple?	Approximately 10%
What are the associated signs/symptoms?	Right upper quadrant pain/mass, shock, CHF
What are the possible complications?	Hemorrhage, CHF, coagulopathy
Which diagnostic tests are indicated?	CT with IV contrast
Should biopsy be performed?	No. There is a chance of severe hemorrhage with biopsy.
What is the appropriate treatment?	Observation; resection if the patient is symptomatic/hemorrhaging
What are the nonoperative treatment options?	Steroids, radiation

BILE DUCT ADENOMA

What is a bile duct adenoma?	Benign tumor < 1 cm composed of bile ducts and fibrous material
What is the incidence?	Nearly one-third of all people have these lesions!
What is the appropriate treatment?	Leave alone

HEPATOMA (HEPATOCELLULAR CARCINOMA)

What is the most common site of metastasis?	Lungs
What percentage of patients who receive a liver transplant for hepatoma will have a recurrence?	Approximately 50%
What options are available for treating a solitary, small hepatoma in a patient who is not an operative candidate?	Ethanol injection under US guidance Radiofrequency ablation
Which subtype has the best prognosis?	Fibrolamellar hepatoma (young adults); not associated with alpha-fetoprotein (AFP) elevations
Describe the staging of hepatoma.	
Stage I	Tumor < 2 cm (T1, N0, M0)
Stage II	T2, N0, M0: 1. Tumor < 2 cm with vascular invasion 2. Tumor > 2 cm without vascular invasion 3. Multiple tumors in one lobe < 2 cm without vascular invasion
Stage III	Positive nodes (T1–3, M0)
Stage IVA	T4, any N, M0: 1. Multiple tumors in > 1 lobe 2. Invasion of major venous structure

Stage IVB   Distant metastases with multiple tumors
                            in > 1 lobe or invasion of major venous
                            structure (T4, any N, M1)

**What are the standard liver
resections?**

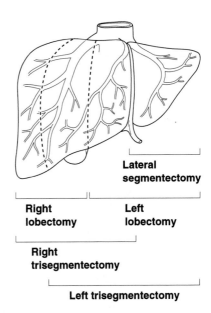

Lateral
segmentectomy

Right   Left
lobectomy   lobectomy

Right
trisegmentectomy

Left trisegmentectomy

**What 3 factors are most
related to mortality and
morbidity during and after
liver resection for
hepatoma?**

Blood loss, blood transfusion, and
operative time

BENIGN LIVER CYSTS

**What is the difference
between simple cyst and
cystadenoma or
cystadenocarcinoma?**

Simple cyst: No septa or associated mass,
    regular margins
Cystadenoma/cystadenocarcinoma:
    Septations, irregular margins,
    loculations

**What is the treatment of
cystadenomas?**

Complete resection due to risk of
transformation into a
cystadenocarcinoma

**What is the treatment of
asymptomatic simple liver
cysts?**

Observation

What is the surgical treatment for *symptomatic* simple liver cysts?	Unroofing/fenestration (in poor operative candidates, radiographically guided aspiration with alcohol injection is an option)

MISCELLANEOUS LIVER FACTS

What is Kasabach-Merritt syndrome?	Seen with liver hemangiomas: hemolytic anemia, platelet trapping, loss of fibrinogen
What 5-year survival rate is associated with colorectal carcinoma metastases to the liver without surgical resection?	0–7%
What 5-year survival rate is associated with colorectal liver metastases in patients who undergo resection?	Approximately 25–35% (with negative margins)
If a kidney from a patient with hepatorenal syndrome is transplanted into a patient with normal liver function, does the kidney recover function?	Yes
If a patient with hepatorenal syndrome receives a liver transplant, what happens to the kidneys?	They recover function.
From what source do metastatic tumors to the liver receive their blood supply?	The vast majority receive their blood from the hepatic artery.
What is the liver's "favorite" amino acid for gluconeogenesis (making glucose)?	Alanine
Which 2 serum tests are most sensitive for liver parenchyma damage?	Angiotensin sensitivity test (AST) and alanine aminotransferase (ALT)

What is the most sensitive and specific test for hepatocyte injury?	ALT
Which 3 tests are sensitive for bile duct damage or pathology?	1. Alkaline phosphatase 2. GGT 3. 5′ nucleotidase
What is the most common liver tumor?	Metastatic disease outnumbers primary tumors 20:1. The primary site is usually in the GI tract.
What hepatic defect is associated with Dubin-Johnson syndrome?	Faulty excretion of conjugated bilirubin from the liver (think: **D**ubin = **D**eparture defect)
What is Gilbert's syndrome?	Partial deficiency of glucuronyltransferase, leading to intermittent asymptomatic jaundice in the 2nd to 3rd decade of life
What is Crigler-Najjar syndrome?	Rare genetic absence of glucuronosyltransferase activity, causing unconjugated hyperbilirubinemia, jaundice, and death from kernicterus (usually within the 1st year)
What hepatic defect is associated with Crigler-Najjar syndrome?	Faulty conjugation of bilirubin (think: **C**rigler = **C**onjugation defect)
What hepatic defect is associated with Rotor's syndrome?	Faulty excretion of conjugated bilirubin due to a defect in the storage of bilirubin (think: **R**otor = **R**elease defect)
What do the Denver and LeVeen shunts do?	Drain ascitic fluid (fluid from ascites) from the peritoneal cavity into the central venous system
What dreaded complication is associated with the Denver and LeVeen shunts?	DIC (If refractory DIC occurs, the shunt must be emergently ligated!)
What type of amino acid should be limited in patients with liver failure?	The aromatic amino acids, because they are thought to be precursors of the false neurotransmitters involved with hepatic encephalopathy

Which amino acids are thought to be beneficial to patients with hepatic encephalopathy?

Branched amino acids (**L**eucine, **I**soleucine, **V**aline; think: **LIV** = **Liv**er)

What vitamin should every patient with liver failure and a coagulopathy receive?

Vitamin K (remember: 2, 7, 9, 10 are liver clotting factors)

Define the Pringle maneuver.

Compression of the hepatoduodenal ligament and its contents (i.e., hepatic artery and portal vein) to help control bleeding from the liver

What is the hepatorenal syndrome?

Renal failure of unknown cause in patients with liver failure (kidneys work fine when transplanted into a patient with a normal liver!)

50   Portal Hypertension

What level of portal pressure is associated with portal hypertension?	> 18 mm Hg
What is the most common cause of portal hypertension in the world?	Schistosomiasis
What are the 3 classes of portal hypertension?	Presinusoidal Sinusoidal Postsinusoidal
Give 2 examples of presinusoidal portal hypertension.	Schistosomiasis Portal vein thrombosis
Give an example of sinusoidal portal hypertension.	Cirrhosis
Give an example of postsinusoidal portal hypertension.	Budd-Chiari's syndrome (most common cause of portal hypertension with upper GI bleed in children)
What is a major cause of isolated gastric varices?	Splenic vein thrombosis secondary to pancreatitis
What is a common long-term medical treatment of portal hypertension?	Beta blocker (e.g., propranolol, nadolol)
If rebleeding takes place after multiple sclerotherapy episodes, what are the options?	TIPS, shunt procedure, or transplant

What does TIPS stand for?

Transjugular **I**ntrahepatic **P**ortacaval **s**hunt: a metallic shunt is placed from the hepatic vein to the right portal vein via a catheter introduced through the internal jugular vein

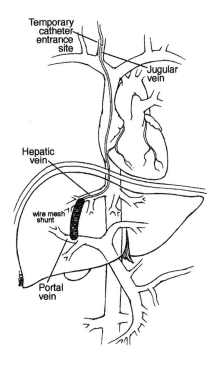

Which patients are good candidates for TIPS?

Those most likely to undergo liver transplantation subsequently
Poor operative candidates

Image the following shunts.

Mesocaval shunt "H" graft

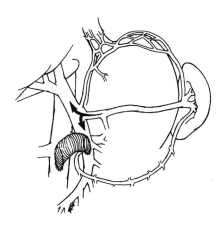

**End-to-side portacaval
shunt**

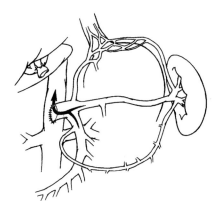

**Side-to-side portacaval
shunt**

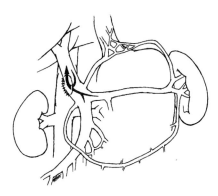

**Warren distal splenorenal
shunt**

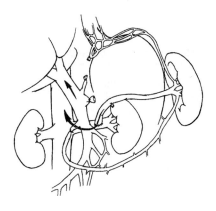

**Which vein must be tied off
with a distal splenorenal
shunt?**

The coronary vein

What is the advantage of a Warren distal splenorenal shunt?

Lower rate of encephalopathy

What are the relative contraindications for the Warren shunt?

Poorly controlled ascites (i.e., the Warren shunt often makes ascites)

What is a partial shunt?

Does not shunt all of the portal blood (i.e., decreases variceal bleeding but allows some liver blood flow to avoid encephalopathy) as illustrated:

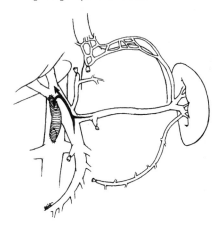

What is a Sugiura procedure?

Used rarely, the **esophagus** is **transected** and **reanastomosed,** with splenectomy and gastric devascularization.

PORTAL HYPERTENSION AND ASCITES

Why do patients with cirrhosis and portal hypertension have high aldosterone levels?

Low glomerular filtration rate (GFR) and low renal blood flow

Are sodium levels in the urine low or high?

Low

Why do patients with portal hypertension and ascites have a low GFR and decreased renal blood flow?

With portal hypertension, the splanchnic blood volume drastically increases with significant venous vasodilation, which leads to reduction in intravascular volume and results in decreased renal blood flow and decreased GFR.

What are the 2 most common electrolyte abnormalities in patients with cirrhosis and ascites?	Hyponatremia Hypokalemia
What is the best way to prevent hyponatremia in patients with cirrhosis and ascites?	Limit H_2O intake, because total body sodium is normal or elevated.
How does spironolactone work?	It is an aldosterone antagonist (results in sodium/H_2O loss and potassium retention).
What is a risk of spironolactone therapy in the patient with cirrhosis and mild renal dysfunction?	Hepatorenal syndrome

51 ___ Biliary Tract

BILIARY ANATOMY

What is the hepatocystic triangle?

1. Liver edge
2. Cystic duct
3. Common hepatic duct

What are Rokitansky-Aschoff sinuses?

Branching evaginations from the lumen into the mucosa and muscularis of the gallbladder

What causes these sinuses to form?

Increased intraluminal pressure in the gallbladder

Is the predominant blood supply to the bile ducts arterial or venous?

Arterial

Describe the anatomy of the arteries to the bile duct.

Two main vessels running axially (longitudinally) at approximately 3 o'clock and 9 o'clock
Arise mainly from retroduodenal artery below, and right hepatic artery above
Majority of the axial blood supply to the common bile duct is from below

What are the effects of vagal innervation on the gallbladder?

Excitatory (emptying)

What is the effect of sympathetic stimulation on the gallbladder?

Predominantly inhibitory motor effect on the gallbladder

BILE METABOLISM/PHYSIOLOGY

What are the main chemical components of bile?

Water, electrolytes, bile salts, cholesterol, lecithin, bile pigments (bilirubin)

What does bile do?	Emulsifies fats
What is the volume of bile secreted per day?	Approximately 600 mL
From what substance are bile acids formed?	Cholesterol
What is the source of this substance?	1. Cholesterol is synthesized de novo in the liver 2. Diet
What are the 2 primary bile acids?	Cholic acid and chenodeoxycholic acid
What are the 2 secondary bile acids?	Lithocholate and deoxycholate
What makes the secondary bile acids?	Bacterial action
What step do the primary bile acids undergo prior to secretion as bile salts?	They are conjugated in the liver with glycine or taurine.
What is a bile salt?	Conjugated bile acid at a neutral pH results in an ionic salt and thus a bile salt.
What is the enterohepatic circulation?	Secretion of bile salts into the gut, reabsorption, and return to the liver
In what part of the bowel are the bile salts reabsorbed?	In the terminal ileum, by active transport
What is the main bile pigment?	Bilirubin glucuronide
From what substance does it arise?	80–85% of bilirubin is derived from the catabolism of senescent red blood cells by the reticuloendothelial system (from heme).
Which enzymes participate in this conversion?	1. Heme oxygenase converts heme to biliverdin 2. Biliverdin reductase converts biliverdin to bilirubin

What is bilirubin conjugated to?	Glucuronic acid, by glucuronic transferase
What is the significance of urobilinogen in the urine?	Urobilinogen is produced in the terminal ileum from the breakdown of bilirubin glucuronide by bacterial action. Some of it is reabsorbed into the bloodstream. If urobilinogen is present in the urine (after being absorbed from the GI tract), then complete biliary obstruction must **not** be present.
What inhibits gallbladder emptying?	Somatostatin Sympathetic stimulation (Think: impossible to digest food and "flee" at the same time)
What are the effects of the female reproductive processes on gallbladder contraction?	Efficiency of gallbladder contraction is significantly reduced during the latter half of the menstrual cycle and in the last trimester of pregnancy.
At what level of serum total bilirubin is jaundice usually evident?	Usually, 2.5–3.0 mg/dL
Classically, at what anatomic site is jaundice first evident?	Under the tongue
What is the difference in jaundice associated with stone obstruction versus malignancy?	Stones "ball valve" and usually is < 6. Cancer can cause complete obstruction and is often > 6.
What is the approximate maximum bilirubin level?	When urinary daily losses of bilirubin match bilirubin production, jaundice stabilizes at a level of approximately 30 mg/dL.
What enzyme is found in the biliary endothelium?	Alkaline phosphatase (also found in bone!)

BILIARY IMAGING

How often can US diagnose ductal dilatation?	> 80% of the time
How often can US diagnose choledocholithiasis?	Only about one-third of the time!

How often can US diagnose the cause of biliary obstruction?	Only about 50% of the time
What is distal obstruction versus proximal biliary obstruction?	Proximal bile ducts are in or near the liver and distal is near the duodenum. (Bile flows proximal to distal—like arterial blood!)
What is the diagnostic test for biliary dyskinesia?	1. US (rule out stones) 2. Nuclear scan (HIDA) with cholecystokinin (CCK) and ejection fraction
What is the positive predictive value of a sonographic Murphy's sign and gallstones?	Approximately 90%

BILIARY DYSKINESIA

What is biliary dyskinesia?	Biliary colic due to gallbladder dysfunction—**not** stones
What are the signs of biliary dyskinesia?	Nuclear scan: EF < 35%, and/or reproducing of pain with injection of CCK
What are the indications for surgery?	EF < 35% Pain consistent with biliary colic
What is the treatment?	Laparoscopic cholecystectomy
What percentage of patients will be asymptomatic after surgery?	If EF < 35% and biliary colic pain was present preoperatively, approximately 90% will be asymptomatic.
What percentage of patients will have signs of chronic inflammation on pathology?	> 66%

GALLSTONES

How are gallstones classified?	Cholesterol stones (predominant in the United States) Pigment stones, brown or black (predominant in Asia)

What percentage of all gallstones do the following classes comprise?

    Cholesterol   Approximately 75%

    Black   Approximately 20%

    Brown   Approximately 5%

Which type of stone is most likely to be intrahepatic?

Approximately 95% of intrahepatic stones are pigment stones.

What are the 3 steps in the formation of cholesterol gallstones?

1. Cholesterol saturation
2. Nucleation
3. Stone growth

What is Admirand's triangle?

A tricoordinate phase diagram describing the concentrations of bile salts, cholesterol, and lecithin. Note the small area where cholesterol is entirely soluble!

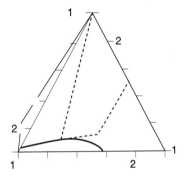

What substances are implicated in the nucleation of cholesterol gallstones?

Calcium, gallbladder mucus

Which tumor is associated with gallstone formation?

Somatostatinoma

What 6 factors predispose patients to pigment stone formation?

Hemolytic disorders
Cirrhosis
Biliary infections
Parasitic infection
Ileal resection
Long-term TPN

What is the mechanism of formation of pigment stones?

Unconjugated bilirubin precipitates to yield calcium bilirubinate and insoluble salts. Calcium bilirubinate is the main component in pigment stones.

What are the characteristics of "black" pigment stones?

Typically black and tarry
Frequently associated with hemolysis or cirrhosis
Almost always located in the gallbladder
Almost never associated with infection

What are the characteristics of "brown" pigment stones?

Earthy, brown, friable
Typically found in Asian patients
Frequently associated with infection
Primary common duct stones are almost invariably of this type

What is the mechanism of formation of "brown" pigment stones?

Stagnant bile with bacteria allows enzymatic hydrolysis of bilirubin glucuronide into free bilirubin and glucuronic acid. The free unconjugated bilirubin (insoluble) combines with calcium in the bile to produce a calcium bilirubinate matrix—the predominant component of most pigment stones.

Which enzyme is involved in this process?

Bacterial β-glucuronidase

Which bacteria commonly produce this enzyme?

Escherichia coli and *Klebsiella*

What is Mirizzi's syndrome?

Impaction of a large gallstone in the cystic duct, with extrinsic obstruction of the adjacent common hepatic duct

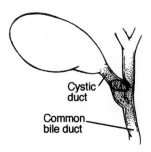

Cystic duct

Common bile duct

Which antibiotic is associated with cholestatic jaundice and gallbladder sludge?	Ceftriaxone

ENDOSCOPIC RETROGRADE CHOLANGIOPANCREATOGRAPHY (ERCP) EXTRACTION OF COMMON BILE DUCT (CBD) STONES

What morbidity rate is associated with endoscopic stone extraction?	Approximately 5–10%
What is the associated mortality rate?	Approximately 1%
What 4 specific complications are associated with this procedure?	GI hemorrhage Duodenal perforation Biliary sepsis Pancreatitis
Should you routinely check post-ERCP labs the following A.M. for amylase and lipase?	**No**! Unless the patient has abdominal pain, almost all patients will have a "chemical" pancreatitis after ERCP.

CBD EXPLORATION

What CBD size is a relative contraindication to CBD exploration?	< 6 mm
What maneuver must be performed before a CBD exploration?	Kocher maneuver
What type of suture must be used in suturing the CBD after T-tube placement?	**Absorbable**

What is the correct orientation for incisions on the CBD?

Longitudinal (parallel to the blood supply) between 2 stay sutures

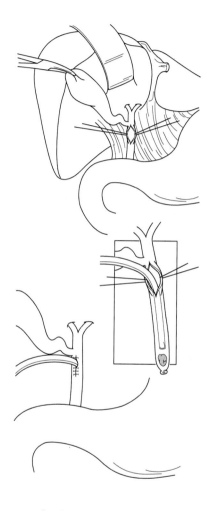

What backup procedure can be used in the rare instance that a stone is impacted in the distal common duct and cannot be removed with transductal manipulation?

A transduodenal sphincterotomy

BILIARY STRICTURES

What is the most common source of benign biliary strictures?	Iatrogenic
What procedures precede postoperative benign strictures?	> 90% result from cholecystectomies (an incidence of from 1/400 to 1/500 cases) Approximately 5% follow exploration of the biliary ducts Partial or subtotal gastrectomy Pancreatoduodenectomy Liver resection for trauma
What are some noniatrogenic conditions causing biliary stricture?	Mirizzi's syndrome Radiotherapy (rare) Idiopathic
Describe the Bismuth classification of benign biliary strictures.	
Grade I	Stricture of CHD > 2 cm from confluence of left and right hepatic ducts
Grade II	Stricture of CHD < 2 cm from confluence of left and right hepatic ducts
Grade III	Stricture at confluence of left and right hepatic ducts
Grade IV	Obliteration of all extrahepatic ducts by stricture
What is the success rate of biliary repair based on the Bismuth classification?	
Bismuth grade I or II strictures	75–90% long-term success rate for repair
Bismuth grade III lesions	Approximately 70% success rate
Bismuth grade IV lesions	50% of patients will have recurrent cholangitis on follow-up.

Is there benefit in the use of external percutaneous transhepatic biliary drainage before surgery in cases of biliary obstruction with jaundice?	Preoperative drainage has failed to show benefit.

ORIENTAL CHOLANGIOHEPATITIS

What is oriental cholangiohepatitis?	Recurrent cholangitis, in association with recurrent formation of primary common duct stones
With what other disorders is it associated?	Parasitic infection: *Clonorchis sinensis, Ascaris lumbricoides, Trichuris trichiura* (Parasites may cause stasis, damage to bile ducts.) Bacterial colonization with *E. coli* (produces β-glucuronidase, which causes deconjugation of bilirubin and subsequent production of pigment stones)
What is the endemic area?	Asia
What is the appropriate therapy?	Choledochoenterostomy and antiparasitic medications

CAROLI DISEASE

What is it?	A type V choledochal cyst; congenital dilatation of the intrahepatic biliary ducts
What are the 4 "C"s of Caroli disease?	Caroli Congenital Choledochal cyst Cholangitis
What is the clinical presentation?	Often presents as recurrent cholangitis
Is surgical therapy recommended under any conditions?	Hepatic lobectomy is the therapy of choice if only one lobe of the liver is involved.

PERIAMPULLARY TUMORS

What is the definition?	Malignant tumors arising adjacent to or from the ampulla of Vater
What are the 4 possible anatomic sites of origin?	Distal pancreatic duct (40–60%) Ampulla itself (20–40%) Distal bile duct (10%) Duodenum (10%)
What are the most common cell types?	Adenocarcinoma, but the cancer may arise from any cell type in the region
Why are these grouped, despite their variations in anatomy and histology?	Because they have the same mode of presentation (jaundice), and the same operation (pancreatoduodenectomy) is performed for curative intent
How do periampullary tumors usually present?	Jaundice is the most common sign (80–90% of patients); 75% of patients lose weight.
What is the tumor marker for periampullary tumors?	CA 19–9 has the best sensitivity and specificity (both close to 90%).
What is the operative mortality rate of pancreatoduodenectomy, past and present?	Operative mortality has decreased from 25% in older reports to 1–2% in most current series.

What is the survival rate after pancreatoduodenectomy performed "for cure"?	5-year survival rate depends on cell type:
	    Pancreatic (15–20%)
	    Distal bile duct (40%)
	    Duodenal (40%)
	    Ampullary (50–70%)

GALLBLADDER TUMORS

What is the incidence of gallbladder cancer in comparison with cancer of the common bile duct?	Gallbladder cancer is about 4 times as common.
What are the risk factors for gallbladder cancer?	**Gallstones,** porcelain gallbladder, gallbladder adenoma, infection by *Salmonella typhi* of bile ducts/gallbladder

What is the rate of incidental presentation of gallbladder cancer?	Approximately 1% of all laparoscopic cholecystectomy specimens
What proportion of all gallbladder cancer is discovered incidentally?	Approximately 20–30%
What are the symptoms of gallbladder cancer?	Pain, nausea/vomiting, weight loss, jaundice
How effective is US in diagnosing gallbladder cancer?	Approximately 75% of gallbladder cancers can be diagnosed by US, but approximately 50% of US diagnoses of gallbladder cancer are false positives.
What is the most common cell type?	Adenocarcinomas (85%). The remainder are undifferentiated or squamous carcinoma.

Describe the stages of gallbladder cancer.

Stage I	T1, N0, M0: invades mucosa, no nodes, no distant metastases
Stage II	T2, N0, M0: invades perimuscular connective tissue (below serosa)
Stage III	T3, N0, M0: through serosa, < 2 cm into liver parenchyma
Stage IVA	T4, N0–1, M0: Tumor > 2 cm into liver, or invades 2 adjacent organs
Stage IVB	1. Any T, any N, M1: Distant metastases 2. Any T, N2, M0: Positive nodes around pancreas/duodenum/superior mesenteric artery/celiac

Describe the treatment of gallbladder cancer by stage.

Stage I	Laparoscopic cholecystectomy
Stage II	Radical cholecystectomy, node dissection (N2)

Stage III	Radical cholecystectomy, node dissection (N2)
Stage IVA	Radical cholecystectomy and node dissection (N2 peripancreatic/duodenal, superior mesenteric artery/celiac)
Stage IVB	**Nonoperative**—palliative only
What is the rate of resectability at presentation?	Most patients present with advanced disease characterized by extensive local invasion and a low resectability rate(25%).
What is a radical cholecystectomy?	Resect gallbladder bed with gallbladder en bloc, with 2 cm liver margins around gallbladder
What is the prognosis?	5-year survival for stage I: approximately 50% 5-year survival for stage IVB: 0%
What is the appropriate management of porcelain gallbladder?	Resection upon identification, because 25–75% of patients develop malignancy

HEMOBILIA

What are the causes?	Trauma, other disease, accidental tumors, blunt or penetrating trauma, operative/interventional aneurysms, gallstones, and inflammation
What is the appropriate workup?	Arteriography, which is often therapeutic by means of embolization

PRIMARY BILIARY CIRRHOSIS

What is the etiology/ histology?	An autoimmune disease causing granulomatous destruction of the medium-sized intrahepatic bile ducts
What is the final common pathway?	The final event is an attack by cytotoxic T cells on biliary epithelium. Suppressor T cells are reduced in number and function.
What is the usual presentation/clinical course?	Ductal destruction leads to cholestasis, with subsequent cirrhosis, portal hypertension, and liver failure.

What are the associated signs/symptoms?

Fatigue and pruritus (usually occur early)

Jaundice (usually occurs later; does not always correlate with pruritus)

Xanthelasmas and xanthomas (appear as signs of chronic liver disease)

Evidence of an associated extrahepatic autoimmune disorder, such as Sjögren's syndrome or rheumatoid arthritis (incidence of up to 80%)

Is medical therapy effective?

No. A variety of immunosuppressive drugs and penicillamine have proved unsuccessful.

What is the appropriate surgical therapy?

Liver transplant. Primary biliary cirrhosis (PBC) is the most frequent indication for transplantation in the cholestatic group of patients.

52   Pancreas

ANATOMY

On what structure does the pancreatic head rest?	The IVC, renal vessels
On what structure does the uncinate process (a prolongation of the pancreatic head) rest?	The aorta
What lies behind the pancreatic neck?	The superior mesenteric vessels
How is blood supplied to the head of the pancreas from the celiac axis?	The gastroduodenal artery branches into the superior posterior and anterior pancreaticoduodenal arteries.
How is blood supplied to the pancreatic head from the SMA?	The SMA branches into the inferior posterior and anterior branches of the pancreaticoduodenal arteries.
Which arteries supply the body and tail of the pancreas?	The dorsal pancreatic artery from the splenic artery branches and joins a branch from the SMA to form the inferior pancreatic artery. Multiple branches from the splenic artery, along with the inferior pancreatic artery, supply the tail.
Into which veins do the pancreatic veins drain?	The splenic vein and the portal vein
Which nodal groups drain the pancreas?	From the head—nodes in the pancreaticoduodenal groove drain into subpyloric, portal, mesocolic, and aortocaval nodes From the body and tail—retroperitoneal nodes in the splenic hilum drain into the celiac, mesocolic, mesenteric, or aortocaval nodes

PHYSIOLOGY

What do the islets of Langerhans produce?	Insulin—β-cells Glucagon—α-cells Somatostatin—δ-cells Pancreatic polypeptide, gastrin, and vasoactive intestinal peptide (VIP)
What types of cells constitute the exocrine pancreas?	Acinar, centroacinar, intercalated ductal, and ductal cells
Describe the composition of pancreatic secretions.	
pH	pH = 8
Concentration of HCO$_3$	30–120 mEq/L
Cl	30–100 mEq/L
Enzymes	Inactive forms of peptidases: trypsin, chymotrypsin, elastase, kallikrein, carboxypeptidase A and B, phospholipase, lipase, colipase, carboxylesterase, amylase, ribonuclease, deoxyribonuclease
What stimulates exocrine secretion?	Vagal efferents and secretin stimulate HCO$_3$ secretion; cholecystokinin and acetylcholine stimulate enzyme secretion.
What other GI hormone is structurally similar to cholecystokinin?	Gastrin, which may explain why it is a weak stimulator of pancreatic enzyme secretion
How are the peptidases activated?	Intraluminally by enterokinase

PANCREATITIS

CHRONIC PANCREATITIS

What is a Duval procedure?	Resection of the tail of the pancreas, and then anastomosis of the pancreatic remnant and the limb of the Roux-en-Y

GALLSTONE PANCREATITIS

What is the most common cause of deadly severe pancreatitis?	**Gallstones**

What are the indications for preop endoscopic retrograde cholangiopancreatography (ERCP) in gallstone pancreatitis?	Cholangitis Severe refractory pancreatitis with choledocholithiasis

PANCREATIC FISTULAS

How are pancreatic pleural and peritoneal effusions managed?	Initially, nonoperatively: NPO, repeated evacuation percutaneously, and TPN
What defines a high-output pancreatic fistula?	> 200 cc/day
How should pancreatocutaneous fistulas be managed?	Initially, nonoperatively with TPN, electrolyte replacement, and skin care. Octreotide may help reduce output. Most fistulas will close spontaneously.
What is the operative management for refractory pancreatic fistula?	Refractory distal duct fistulas are best managed by distal pancreatectomy, proximal duct fistulas with pancreaticojejunostomy.
What side effect is associated with somatostatin?	Gallstones and gallbladder sludge

PANCREATIC NECROSIS

Should patients with necrotic pancreatitis receive prophylactic antibiotics?	Yes. Antibiotics decrease rate of conversion of pancreatic necrosis to infected pancreatic necrosis.
What has been shown to work as a prophylactic antibiotic?	Imipenem
What type of bacteria usually is found infecting necrotic pancreatic tissue?	Gram-negative organisms (e.g., *Escherichia coli, Pseudomonas*)
What is the indication for operative debridement?	Infected necrotic pancreatic tissue

PANCREATIC DIVISUM

How does pancreas divisum occur?	The primordial ductal systems do not fuse.

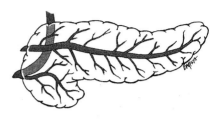

What percentage of the population has pancreatic divisum?	Approximately 6–10%
What percentage of patients undergoing ERCP for idiopathic pancreatitis has pancreatic divisum?	Up to 50%
How does a surgeon determine if the tumor has invaded the IVC?	Kocher maneuver; then, if hand cannot pass through plane between pancreas and IVC, consistent with invasion of IVC
How does the surgeon make sure that the pancreatic cancer has not invaded the superior mesenteric vein (SMV)?	Index finger to index finger dissection underneath pancreatic neck and above the SMV

OTHER PANCREATIC TUMORS

Name the various endocrine tumors of the pancreas.	Insulinoma, glucagonoma, vasoactive intestinal peptide tumors (VIPoma), somatostatinoma, gastrinoma; also, tumors secreting pancreatic polypeptide, calcitonin, and neurotensin
Which is the most common pancreatic endocrine tumor?	Insulinoma
How do insulinomas classically manifest?	Whipple's triad: fasting blood sugar < 50 mg, symptoms of hypoglycemia when fasting, symptomatic relief following glucose replacement

How is insulinoma diagnosed?

Monitored 72-hour fast with blood glucose and insulin levels, insulin/glucose ratio > 0.4, elevated C-protein and proinsulin

Should an imaging study be performed with a presumed pancreatic endocrine tumor?

Yes. CT with contrast often helps localize the tumor.

Where are insulinomas located?

Head (1/3)
Body (1/3)
Tail (1/3)

How should insulinomas be treated?

Resection: enucleation for small lesions, distal pancreatectomy for large lesions

What is the role of diazoxide for patients with unresectable disease?

It can attenuate hypoglycemia.

What is Zollinger-Ellison syndrome?

Peptic ulcers in unusual places, refractory hypersecretion of gastric acid, pancreatic endocrine tumor that secretes gastrin (gastrinoma)

Is a hereditary factor associated with Zollinger-Ellison syndrome?

Yes, in some cases. Most cases are sporadic, but some are associated with MEN I syndrome.

What is Verner-Morrison syndrome?

WDHA syndrome:
Watery **D**iarrhea
Hypokalemia
Achlorhydria, associated with VIPoma

Where are VIPomas located?

Typically in the body and tail

Should VIPomas be resected?

Yes, although more than half of patients have metastases at diagnosis

What action should be taken if no tumor is identified in a patient with WDHA syndrome?

Occasionally, diffuse islet-cell hyperplasia can cause WDHA. In this case, subtotal pancreatectomy is an option.

What condition would a patient with diabetes and a migratory rash be likely to develop?

Glucagonoma is the characteristic necrolytic migratory erythema associated with this tumor. These patients may also have anemia, glossitis, and weight loss.

How is it diagnosed?	Elevated serum glucagon level
Where are these tumors usually found?	Body and tail
How should they be treated?	Resection for cure is possible in only one-third of cases. Steroids, zinc, and octreotide have helped in treatment of the rash. Octreotide may also help control hyperglycemia.
What is a somatostatinoma, and what is the appropriate treatment?	A very rare tumor, usually of the head of the pancreas; may present with diabetes, steatorrhea, and gallstones. If possible, it should be treated by excision with cholecystectomy.
Why a cholecystectomy?	There is a high rate of gallstone formation with somatostatinoma.
Are nonfunctional islet-cell tumors malignant?	Yes, in 90% of cases; however, they usually run an indolent course.
What is the most common benign neoplasm in the pancreas?	Cystadenoma
What is the most common cystic lesion of the pancreas?	Pancreatic pseudocyst
What is the appropriate management of cystic lesions of the pancreas that are incidentally found?	Tissue diagnosis must be confirmed; it is impossible to distinguish malignancy radiographically. If the lesion is not associated with pancreatitis (i.e., not a pseudocyst), it should be resected.
How is pancreatic lymphoma diagnosed and treated?	Percutaneous radiographically guided needle biopsy with appropriate staging, followed by chemotherapy

53

The Breast

ANATOMY/HISTOLOGY

When raising a skin flap, between which layers should dissection be performed?

In the bloodless plane located just subdermally; the final thickness of the flap should be approximately 4 mm at the edge and < 6 mm at the base.

What structure is responsible for the mobility of the breast, and between what layers of fascia is it located?

Retromammary bursa, formed by the deep layer of superficial fascia and deep investing fascia of the pectorales major muscle

What 3 arteries supply blood to the breast?

1. Internal mammary artery (via perforators)
2. Intercostal arteries
3. Axillary artery (via the lateral thoracic and thoracoacromial arteries)

What 3 veins drain blood from the breast?

1. Axillary vein (main route of drainage)
2. Internal mammary vein
3. Intercostal veins

What plexus probably mediates much of breast cancer metastases to the skull, vertebral column, CNS, and pelvis?

Batson's vertebral plexus of veins: encircles the vertebrae from skull to sacrum and communicates with thoracic, abdominal, and pelvic viscera

What nerves provide sensory innervation to the breast?

Lateral and anterior cutaneous branches of **intercostal** nerves 2 through 6

How many lactiferous duct orifices are there on the nipple?

Approximately 15–20

At what stage of the menstrual cycle do breasts tend to be engorged and painful?	**Premenstrual** (i.e., late luteal) phase
Why is this clinically significant?	Breasts may be rather nodular, possibly causing concern for malignancy—least favorable time for a breast exam.

PHYSIOLOGY

PROLACTIN (PRL) SECRETION

What primarily controls the secretion of PRL?	Dopamine
What is the role of each of the following hormones in mammary development?	
Estrogen	Starts ductal development, up-regulates epithelial E and P receptors
Progesterone	Involved in epithelial cell differentiation and lobule development
PRL	Involved in the development of mammary epithelial and adipose tissue; up-regulates E receptors; synergizes with E in ductal development and with P in lobular development

BREAST DISCHARGE

What type of discharge suggests an underlying malignancy?	Unilateral, bloody (or heme-positive) discharge coming from one duct
What is the likelihood that such a discharge indicates an underlying carcinoma (in the absence of a palpable mass)?	Cancer is found in only about 5% of cases.
What is microdochectomy?	Surgical excision of breast duct and lobule after marking duct with dye injection

BREAST CANCER

What is the "triad of error" with breast cancer?	The **triad** of risk for missing a breast carcinoma diagnosis: 1. Young patient ($<$ 45 years of age) 2. Negative mammogram 3. Mass found by patient
What is relative risk?	Ratio of [risk of disease in the presence of some characteristic] to [risk in the absence of the characteristic]

What relative risk of breast cancer is associated with the following factors:

Family history of a mother < 60 years old with breast cancer	2
Family history of 2 first-degree relatives (i.e., mother, sister) with breast cancer	5
Age of menarche < 15 versus 16 years old	1.3
Nulliparous versus < 20 years old at first childbirth	2
Menopause past 55 years versus 45–54 years	1.5
Atypical hyperplasia versus never biopsied	4

MAMMOGRAMS

What type of mass is likely to be missed, and in what kind of breast?	Large, noncalcified lesions in radiographically dense breasts (common in premenopausal women)
What percentage of palpable masses are missed by mammography?	Approximately 5–15%

For the mammographic diagnosis of breast cancer, what is the:

Sensitivity? — > 90%

Specificity? — > 90%

Positive predictive value? — 10–40%

How many more cancers are likely to be detected if mammograms are "double-read" (read by 2 different radiologists)? — Approximately 15%

What percentage of breast cancers are detected by mammograms as a mass and/or cluster of calcifications? — Approximately 80%

Do breast cancers tend to be more or less radiodense than normal breast tissue? — Cancer is usually more radiodense.

How often does a radiolucent lesion turn out to be cancer? — Rarely

What mammographic quality of a lesion is most highly suggestive of breast cancer? — An irregular or spicular margin

How frequently will a mass with a sharp margin be cancer? — Approximately 5% of cases

What percentage of breast cancers have mammographically detected calcifications? — As many as 50%

Roughly what percentage of clustered microcalcifications in the absence of a mass will ultimately prove to be cancer? — Up to 33%

What is the mammographic technique of displacing a breast implant to visualize the breast tissue?	Eklund

What are the indications for open biopsy after a core or Mammotome biopsy?	1. Atypical hyperplasia 2. Radial scar 3. Pathology doesn't make sense based on mammographic finding

BREAST CANCER STAGING

What does an "x" indicate?	Parameter cannot be assessed
What does "0" indicate?	No evidence for that feature
What does "Tis" represent?	Carcinoma in situ or Paget disease of nipple with no other tumor
What are the key divisions in diameter that separate T1 through 3?	T1: < 2 cm T2: 2–5 cm T3: > 5 cm
Define T4.	Invading chest wall and/or skin (any size) or inflammatory carcinoma
Define N1 through N3.	N1: ipsilateral; positive axillary nodes N2: same as N1, but matted or fixed N3: ipsilateral; positive internal mammary nodes
Define M1.	Distant metastases or positive supraclavicular nodes

STAGES 0 THROUGH IV

What is stage IV?	M1 plus anything else
What is stage 0?	Tis/N0
What is stage I?	T1/N0
What is stage IIIB?	The worst T (T4) with any N, or the worst N (N3) with any T (Think: 3B = worst N or T. Now you can forget about T4 and N3!)
What primarily separates stages II and III?	Once you've gotten up to N2, or T3, N1, you are in stage III

What is the difference between IIA and IIB?	IIA: sum of T and N is less than or equal to 2 IIB: sum of T and N is 3 (think: IIB = 3; Remember, no N2s in this stage.)
What is stage IIIA?	N2 with any T, but add T3, N1
Which staging factor most reliably predicts long-term survival?	Number of pathologically positive nodes (physical examination is not reliable prognostically)

What is the approximate 5-year survival rate for each of the following numbers of pathologically positive axillary nodes:

None	80%
1–3	60%
> 3	30%
What is the most common distant site to which breast cancer metastasizes?	Bone metastases are present in approximately 50% of cases.
What are some other common sites to which breast cancer metastasizes?	Lung (20%), pleura (15%), soft tissues (10%), and liver (10%)

NODAL METASTASES

What is the general sequence in which levels I through III become positive?	I-II-III
Which level is an ominous sign if positive?	III

Define the following types of recurrence.

Local	Regrowth of malignancy in ipsilateral-lateral breast, skin, chest wall, underlying muscles, and other associated soft tissues
Regional	Regrowth of malignancy in regional nodes (i.e., internal mammary, axillary, supraclavicular, and/or Rotter's)

How should breast biopsy incisions be oriented for optimal cosmetic results?

Curvilinear; following Langer's lines

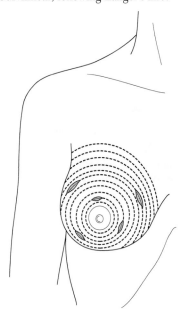

ESTROGEN RECEPTOR (ER) AND PROGESTERONE RECEPTOR (PR) LEVELS EXPRESSED IN BREAST CANCERS

Is ER/PR positivity generally more common for breast cancers in pre- or postmenopausal women?

Postmenopausal women

Roughly what percentage of breast cancers are positive for both ERs and PRs?

About half (45% in premenopausal women, 65% in postmenopausal women)

Roughly what percentage of breast cancers are negative for both ERs and PRs?

Approximately 10% (15% in premenopausal women, 5% in postmenopausal women)

Give the approximate response rate to endocrine therapy in patients with the following ER and PR status.

ER+ PR+

80%

ER+ PR−	35%
ER− PR+	45%
ER− PR−	10%

HER-2/*NEU* (*C-ERB* B2)

In what fraction of breast cancers is it amplified (and overexpressed)?	One-third
To what receptor is it homologous?	The epidermal growth factor (EGF) receptor
What is its purported prognostic significance in breast cancer?	Overexpression correlates with decreased disease-free survival.

CATHEPSIN D

What is it?	Lysosomal protease secreted by estrogen-stimulated breast tumor cells
What process is it thought to facilitate in the natural history of breast cancer?	Metastasis
What is its purported prognostic significance?	Higher levels correlate with decreased disease-free and overall survival.
What oncogene is amplified (in gene-copy #) in 20–30% of breast cancers?	Myc
Why is this fact important?	Portends a poor prognosis

TUMOR SUPPRESSOR GENES/PROTEINS

What tumor suppressor is (at least functionally) missing in about half of breast cancers?	p53
What does it normally do?	Prevents DNA replication if DNA damage is detected

Why is this function important?	It helps prevent widespread mutations/rearrangements of genomes and, hence, transformation to malignancy.

BRCA1/BRCA2

What are they?	Inherited genes associated with breast cancer. They are tumor suppressor gene mutations.
How are they inherited?	Autosomal dominant with varying degrees of penetrance
What percentage of all breast cancers are thought to be associated with these inherited genes?	Only 5%
Of all "inherited" breast cancers, what percentage are due to BRCA1 or BRCA2?	> 75%
What is the risk of developing breast cancer if the patient is a carrier of BRCA1?	> 50% (50–85%)
What is the risk of developing ovarian cancer if the patient is a carrier of BRCA1?	Approximately 33% (15–45%)
What are the options for breast and ovarian cancer prevention in women who carry BRCA?	1. Very aggressive screening 2. Bilateral prophylactic mastectomies and prophylactic oophorectomy

DUCTAL CARCINOMA IN SITU (DCIS)

What chemotherapy is now used for treatment of DCIS?	Tamoxifen, postoperatively, for cancer prophylaxis

54

Endocrine

ADRENALS

ANATOMY

What is the normal weight?	Approximately 4 g
What is the source of arterial supply?	Variable; usually from the inferior phrenic, renal arteries, and branches directly off the aorta
What is the venous drainage of the right adrenal gland?	IVC
What is the venous drainage of the left adrenal gland?	Left renal vein
What embryologic tissue gives rise to the adrenal cortex?	Mesoderm
What are the 3 histologic layers of the adrenal cortex?	1. Zona **g**lomerulosa (think "salt") 2. Zona **f**asciculata (think "sugar") 3. Zona **r**eticularis (think "sex") (Think: GFR = salt, sugar, sex)
What is produced in the zona glomerulosa?	Mineralocorticoids (e.g., aldosterone) = "salt"
What is produced in the zona fasciculata?	Glucocorticoids = "sugar"
What is produced in the zona reticularis?	Androgens and estrogens = "sex"
What embryonic tissue gives rise to the adrenal medulla?	Neural crest

What is produced in the adrenal medulla?	Catecholamines
What are the 2 most common sites for ectopic adrenal medullary tissue?	Sympathetic paraganglia along the aorta Mediastinum
What is the organ of Zuckerkandl?	Sympathetic paraganglia near the aortic bifurcation (common location for extra-adrenal pheochromocytoma)
What are the 3 most common sites for extra-adrenal cortical tissue?	Ovary, testes, and kidney

GLUCOCORTICOIDS

Where are they produced?	Zona fasciculata
How are they regulated?	Adrenocorticotropic hormone (ACTH), from pituitary corticotropin-releasing factor

MINERALOCORTICOIDS

Where are they produced?	Zona glomerulosa

PHEOCHROMOCYTOMA

Where are catecholamines produced?	In the adrenal medulla
What normally controls catecholamine synthesis and release?	Sympathetic innervation
What are the 4 adrenergic receptor subtypes?	α-1, α-2, β-1, and β-2
What does α-1 receptor mediate?	Vasoconstriction, pupillary dilation, intestinal relaxation, and uterine contraction
What does α-2 receptor mediate?	Vasoconstriction, feedback inhibition of NE release from sympathetic neurons; inhibits renin release and insulin release

What does β-1 receptor mediate?	Increases force and rate of cardiac muscle contraction Increases lipolysis Increases amylase production
What does β-2 receptor mediate?	Relaxes smooth muscle Increases glycogenolysis Increases insulin and glucagon secretion Increases renin secretion
Which familial syndromes are associated with pheochromocytoma?	Isolated familial pheochromocytoma MEN IIa MEN IIb Von Recklinghausen neurofibromatosis
Do patients with pheochromocytoma have nonepisodic hypertension?	Yes. Half of patients may have sustained hypertension only as a manifestation of pheochromocytoma.
What are the classic postoperative complications?	Persistent hypertension Hypotension Hypoglycemia Bronchospasm
Why does hypoglycemia occur?	Decreased circulating catecholamines; increased insulin release
Why does postoperative bronchospasm occur?	Decreased β-2 activation after removal of pheochromocytoma
What is the recurrence rate after resection?	Approximately 5–10% (monitor catecholamine levels annually for the first 5 years)
What percentage of patients with von Hippel-Lindau syndrome have a pheochromocytoma?	50%!
What is the most likely tumor site in a patient with palpitation, headache, and diaphoresis with urination?	Bladder pheochromocytoma
What risk is associated with angiography to localize a pheochromocytoma?	May precipitate a hypertensive crisis

CUSHING'S SYNDROME

What findings on HIGH-dose dexamethasone test are associated with the following conditions?

Healthy patient	**Decreased** urinary 17-hydroxycorticosteroid (OHCS)/serum cortisol level less than half the previous baseline levels
Cushing's disease (pituitary cause)	**Decreased** urinary 17-OHCS/serum cortisol to about half the previous baseline levels
Ectopic ACTH-producing tumor	**No effect** in more than 70% of cases (no response to cortisol; autonomous ACTH production)
Adrenal tumor	**No effect** (autonomous cortisol production)

What findings on corticotropin-releasing hormone (CRH)-stimulation test are associated with the following conditions?

Healthy patient	**Mild increase** in ACTH/cortisol
Cushing's disease (pituitary cause)	**Great increase** in ACTH/cortisol
Ectopic ACTH-producing tumor	**No effect** (ACTH is already high)
Adrenal tumor	**No effect** (cortisol production does not respond to ACTH)

What type of "sampling" may distinguish a pituitary versus an ectopic source of ACTH?	Inferior petrosal sinus sampling

What is mitotane?	Medication that selectively **kills the cells that produce cortisol** (kills zona fasciculata and zona reticularis); used in inoperable cases of adrenal carcinoma (think: **MIT**otane = un**MIT**igated murder of cortisol-producing cells)

ADRENOCORTICAL INSUFFICIENCY

What eponym refers to this disorder?	Addison's disease
What is the most common cause?	Iatrogenic suppression of ACTH secretion by exogenous steroids
What other causes are possible?	Autoimmune disease Histoplasmosis Bilateral adrenal hemorrhage Bilateral adrenal TB Adrenal fungal infection
What is Waterhouse-Friderichsen syndrome?	Acute hemorrhagic adrenal necrosis caused by bacteremia, usually *Meningococcus*
What is Addisonian crisis?	Acute adrenocortical insufficiency (medical emergency)
What type of patient is most likely to develop this condition?	Patients with chronic insufficiency who are subjected to stress (e.g., surgery)
Describe the pathophysiology.	In response to stress, inadequate mineralocorticoids and glucocorticoids result in an inability to retain Na^+, secrete K^+, and maintain adequate intravascular volume. Hypovolemia and electrolyte imbalance are exacerbated by vomiting.
What are the associated signs/symptoms of adrenocortical insufficiency?	Weakness, fatigue, weight loss, nausea, vomiting, hypotension, abdominal pain, fever, diarrhea; progresses rapidly to lethargy, weakness, and cardiovascular collapse
What are the associated laboratory findings?	**Hyponatremia, hyperkalemia,** hypoglycemia, acidosis, elevated BUN, decreased chloride, depressed plasma cortisol

What is the appropriate initial treatment?	1 L NS plus 200 mg hydrocortisone over 30 minutes Followed by NS plus 100 mg hydrocortisone/L, with glucose, replace electrolytes Identify and treat underlying causes (e.g., infection, trauma)
What preventative measures should be taken in patients with known adrenal insufficiency undergoing surgery?	Stress-dose steroids: 100 mg cortisol IM or IV on the day of surgery and then every 8 hours Taper as tolerated postoperatively to maintenance dose

NEUROENDOCRINE GI TUMORS

What are the cells of origin?	APUD cells (**A**mine **P**recursor, **U**ptake, and **D**ecarboxylation); tumor = **apud**oma
What is the etiology?	Sporadic Familial (MEN I) Approximately 5% of insulinomas are associated with MEN. Approximately 30% of gastrinomas are associated with MEN.
What is the overall incidence?	< 10 cases per million per year
What is the average age at diagnosis?	Fourth decade
What is the most common source of symptoms?	Usually caused by a single secreted hormone. A mass effect is rare.
Are multiple hormones secreted from a single tumor?	Rarely
What is the appropriate treatment?	Surgical removal
How does octreotide work?	As a somatostatin analog. It inhibits hormone release.
What is the major complication of octreotide?	Gallstones, in 25–30% of cases

What is the best way of preventing complications?	Cholecystectomy at the time of surgery for those undergoing chronic octreotide treatment

GLUCAGONOMA

From which islet cells do these tumors arise?	α-cells
What percentage of all islet cell tumors do they comprise?	Approximately 1%
What is the clinical triad for diagnosing glucagonoma?	1. Necrolytic migratory dermatitis 2. Diabetes mellitus 3. Weight loss
What laboratory test confirms the diagnosis?	Elevated plasma glucagon > 150 pg/mL (many patients will be > 1000 pg/mL)
What is the rate of malignancy?	Two-thirds of cases
What is the most common location?	Pancreas
Which test is used for localization?	CT
What is the appropriate treatment?	Surgical. Removal of tumor should include a rim of normal tissue or distal pancreatectomy, if located in tail of pancreas.
What other treatments may be beneficial?	Chemotherapy or octreotide
What is the appropriate treatment for metastases?	Surgical removal, if possible
What are the most common metastatic sites?	Liver and nodes
What is the prognosis?	Only one-third of patients are cured; recurrence is common. Aggressive therapy may be indicated because the tumor is slow growing. Overall, the 5-year survival rate is 50%.

INSULINOMA

What percentage of islet cell tumors do they comprise?	Approximately 25%. Almost all are small, single adenomas.
From what islet cell do these tumors arise?	β-cells
How can insulinoma be distinguished from factitious hyperinsulinemia?	Insulinoma—C-peptide:insulin = 1:1 Factitious disease—C-peptide:insulin < 1:1
What is the normal insulin:glucose ratio?	Less than or equal to 0.25; useful for detecting abnormal insulin secretion in the setting of normal insulin levels
What is the rate of malignancy?	Approximately 10%
How is malignancy determined?	Only by evidence of local invasion or metastases to nodes or liver
What tests provide localization prior to surgery?	CT and MRI (poor tests) Endoscopic ultrasound Angiography Venous sampling Octreotide indium scan
What is the appropriate treatment?	Surgery, ranging from enucleation to subtotal pancreatectomy, depending on location
What is the appropriate medical treatment?	Possibly diazoxide, octreotide, or 5-fluorouracil (5-FU) and streptozotocin
What is the prognosis?	Up to 95% cure rate

NONFUNCTIONING ISLET CELL TUMOR

What is it?	An islet cell tumor that does not cause a syndrome related to excess hormone secretion
What percentage of all islet tumors do they comprise?	Up to 30% (second to insulinomas among **apud**omas)

What is the average age at onset?	Sixth decade (as opposed to fourth decade for other islet cell tumors)
What are the associated histologic findings?	Islet cell type staining for neuronal-specific enolase or chromograffin
What are the associated signs/symptoms?	Vague epigastric or back pain, usually from mass effect, or possibly jaundice
What is the rate of malignancy?	Almost 100%
What is the usual size of tumors?	Large (approximately 10 cm)
Are metastases common?	Yes, to liver, nodes, peritoneum, bones, and lung
How is the diagnosis made?	History, normal serum hormone levels, and histologic findings
What tests provide localization?	Ultrasound, CT, MRI
What is the most common location?	Pancreas
What is the appropriate treatment?	Surgical resection, depending on location (e.g., subtotal or total resection of pancreas)
What is the appropriate nonsurgical treatment?	Possibly 5-FU and streptozotocin
What is the prognosis?	Variable, but 10-year survival rate may be as high as 50%

VIPOMAS

What does VIP stand for?	**V**asoactive **i**ntestinal **p**olypeptide
What is a VIPoma?	A tumor arising from VIP-secreting cells of the GI tract
What are the other names for this condition?	Verner-Morrison syndrome WDHA syndrome (see Chapter 52)

What percentage of all islet cell tumors does it comprise?	< 2% (rare)
What are the associated signs/symptoms?	Severe secretory diarrhea, leading to dehydration, hypokalemia, and acidosis, achlorhydria
What are the associated laboratory findings?	Usually VIP will be increased Electrolyte abnormalities, especially hypokalemia and acidosis
What other hormones may be elevated?	Pancreatic polypeptide Neurotensin Prostaglandin (PGE_2)
What tests provide localization?	Ultrasound, CT (often tumor is 3 cm or larger), angiography (second line)
Where is it usually found?	Pancreas (approximately 90% of cases)
What is the rate of malignancy?	Approximately 50%
What is the appropriate treatment?	Enucleation or surgical resection, depending on location

SOMATOSTATINOMAS

What percentage of all islet cell tumors do they comprise?	< 1%
Where are they usually found?	In the pancreas—50% Outside of the pancreas (e.g., duodenum, ampulla of Vater)—50%
Is metastasis common?	Yes, usually to the liver and nodes
What is the usual number and size of primary tumors?	Single and large (approximately 5 cm)
Is there a relationship between somatostatinomas and MEN I syndrome?	Yes. Approximately 50% of patients with somatostatinomas have MEN I.

What are the associated clinical symptoms?	Usually none, but there is an associated inhibitory syndrome triad: Mild diabetes mellitus Cholelithiasis Diarrhea
How is the diagnosis made?	Markedly elevated somatostatin level
What is the normal somatostatin level?	Less than 100 pg/mL
Is localization necessary prior to surgery?	Yes. CT, ultrasound, or angiography is sufficient, because this type of tumor is often large.
What is the appropriate treatment?	Resection
What is the appropriate management of unresectable disease?	Debulking
What is the appropriate medical therapy?	Possibly streptozotocin and 5-FU
Is cure possible?	Yes, for localized disease Poor prognosis for advanced disease (15% 5-year survival rate)

55

Thyroid Gland

ANATOMY

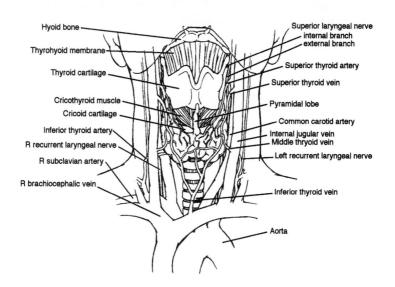

Hyoid bone

Thyrohyoid membrane

Thyroid cartilage

Cricothyroid muscle

Cricoid cartilage

Inferior thyroid artery

R recurrent laryngeal nerve

R subclavian artery

R brachiocephalic vein

Superior laryngeal nerve
internal branch
external branch

Superior thyroid artery

Superior thyroid vein

Pyramidal lobe

Common carotid artery

Internal jugular vein
Middle thyroid vein

Left recurrent laryngeal nerve

Inferior thyroid vein

Aorta

What is a nonrecurrent laryngeal nerve?	Variant in which the laryngeal nerve passes from the vagus directly into the larynx at the level of inferior horn of thyroid cartilage
How common are nonrecurrent laryngeal nerves?	1/200 cases
On what side is a nonrecurrent laryngeal nerve likely to be found?	Almost always on the right (can be seen with an aberrant right subclavian artery)
What is the function of the superior laryngeal nerve?	Motor to the cricothyroid and sensory to the supraglottic pharynx

What structure is closely associated with the superior thyroid nerve?

Superior thyroid artery

To avoid damaging the superior laryngeal nerve, where should the superior thyroid artery be ligated?

The point at which the superior thyroid artery enters the thyroid gland

Describe the relationship of the posterior recurrent laryngeal nerve to the inferior thyroid artery.

Variable. Nerve is inferior to the thyroid artery between the branches of the artery (7%); the nerve is superficial to the artery (20%).

What is the incidence of lingual thyroid?

1/3000

What is the usual presentation?

Dysphagia or problems speaking because of goiter enlargement

PHYSIOLOGY

Outline the basic steps in thyroid hormone synthesis and release.

1. Iodine uptake by synthesis in the GI tract and conversion to I^-; I^- concentrated by thyroid
2. Peroxidases couple I^- to tyrosine residues on thyroglobulin, forming mono- and di-iodotyrosine (MIT and DIT)

3. Coupling of MIT and DIT forms T_3; DIT and DIT form T_4 (still attached to thyroglobulin)
4. Upon secretion, lysosomal enzymes cleave T_3 and T_4 from thyroglobulin

What is T$_3$?	3,5,3' Tri-iodothyronine
What is T$_4$?	Thyroxine $= 3,5,3',5'$-tetra-iodothyronine
What is Wolff-Chaikoff-White block?	The phenomenon in which iodine binding by thyroid and production of T$_3$ and T$_4$ are inhibited as plasma iodine levels accumulate beyond a critical level ($\sim$25 mic/100 mL)
Clinically, why is this relevant?	Iodine is the most effective means to rapidly decrease thyroid hormone levels (Lugol's solution, Na ipodate).
What is Lugol's solution?	Potassium iodide
Where is T$_4$ produced?	Thyroid gland (only source)
What do the parafollicular cells of the thyroid secrete?	Calcitonin, in response to increased serum Ca^{2+}
What does calcitonin do?	Inhibits osteoclast activity
What do osteoclasts do?	Resorb bone
What do osteoblasts do?	Form bone
What is reverse T$_3$ (rT$_3$)?	More inactive form of T$_3$ produced by the same enzyme that converts T$_4$ to T$_3$
When is rT$_3$ elevated?	Severe illness (e.g., sick euthyroid states; See Chapter 62)

THYROID FUNCTION TESTS

What does serum T$_4$ measure?	Total serum T$_4$
What does free thyroxine (FT$_4$) measure?	Circulating, unbound T$_4$
In what situations is FT$_4$ useful?	It is the test of choice for following thyroid after treatment of hyperthyroidism.
What does resin T$_3$ uptake (RT$_3$U) measure?	Relative levels of thyroid-binding globulin (TBG)

What does an elevated RT$_3$U indicate?

Hyperthyroid or decreased TBG

What does a decreased RT$_3$U indicate?

Hypothyroid or increased TBG

What are the differential diagnoses for increased ^{123}I uptake by the thyroid?

Graves' disease, toxic nodular goiter, early Hashimoto's nephrotic syndrome, pregnancy, iodine-deficient diet

What are the differential diagnoses for decreased ^{123}I uptake?

Subacute thyroiditis, thyroid gland damage (from surgery, radiation, thyroiditis), circulating iodine contrast dyes, ectopic thyroid, hypopituitarism, severe Graves' disease

What test is the single most sensitive and specific indicator of thyroid function?

Thyroid-stimulating hormone (TSH)

THYROIDITIS

ACUTE THYROIDITIS

What is it?

Inflammation of the thyroid gland, usually caused by bacterial infection (most uncommon form of thyroiditis)

What is the etiology?

Suppurative infection, usually arising from contiguous structures of thyroid; may be caused by hematogenous seeding local trauma (rare)

What is the most common cause of recurrent cases?

Piriform sinus fistula

Is the condition associated with hyperthyroidism?

No. Usually thyroid function tests (TFTs) are normal.

What are the associated signs/symptoms?

Sudden onset, diffuse, painful enlargement of thyroid with fever, chills, and dysphagia

What is the most common infection prior to acute thyroiditis?

Almost always follows upper respiratory infection in children and adolescents

What are the associated diagnostic findings?

Normal TFTs, normal radioiodine uptake. Ultrasound may show abscess.

What are the most common causative organisms?	*Streptococcus, Staphylococcus, Pneumococcus*
What is the appropriate treatment?	Surgical drainage and antibiotics Fistulectomy, if indicated Recovery usually occurs in 48–72 hours

SUBACUTE THYROIDITIS

What is another name for this disorder?	De Quervain thyroiditis
What is the etiology?	Viral
Who is most likely to develop this condition?	Adults 30–50 years of age; women 5 times more likely than men
What are the associated signs/symptoms?	Diffuse enlargement, sore throat
Hyperthyroid or hypothyroid?	Both—transient hyperthyroid, followed by euthyroid, then hypothyroid
What are the associated laboratory findings?	Elevated erythrocyte sedimentation rate (ESR) and serum γ-globulin; normal or elevated thyroid hormones; low radioiodine uptake
What is the appropriate treatment?	Self limiting within 2 to 6 months Nonsteroidal anti-inflammatory drugs (NSAIDs), β-blockade (antithyroid drugs not effective in treating hyperthyroid phase)

CHRONIC THYROIDITIS

What is another name for this disorder?	Hashimoto's thyroiditis
What is the incidence?	Common (1.5/1000); most common cause of goitrous hypothyroidism in adults
Who is most likely to develop this condition?	Women 10 times more likely than men; peak age 30–50 years
What is the etiology?	Autoimmune

What are the associated signs/symptoms?	Painless, diffusely enlarged gland, sometimes with nodularity; hypothyroidism
What are the associated diagnostic findings?	Increased serum antimicrosomal and thyroglobulin antibody; T_3 and T_4 may be within normal limits; decreased radioiodine uptake
What is the appropriate treatment?	Long-term thyroid hormone replacement

FIBROUS THYROIDITIS

What is another name for this disorder?	Riedel's thyroiditis
What is the incidence?	Very rare
What is the pathophysiology?	Thyroid replaced by fibrous tissue; unknown etiology
What are the associated signs/symptoms?	Stony hard gland, with or without invasion into adjacent structures; pressure symptoms, hypothyroidism (differential diagnosis is malignancy)
What is the appropriate treatment?	Surgery, if pressure symptoms require relief Subtotal thyroidectomy may be required, although surgery may be difficult because of extensive fibrosis

THYROID NODULE

WORKUP OF THYROID NODULE

What does initial workup involve?	History and physical examination, thyroid panel, calcitonin (if medullary cancer is suspected), fine needle aspiration (FNA)
How accurate is FNA?	Approximately 70–97% (varies with the experience of the surgeon and cytopathologist)
What is the false-positive rate associated with FNA?	Approximately 6%

What is the false-negative rate associated with FNA?	Approximately 5%
What percentage of FNAs are positive?	Approximately 10%
What percentage of FNAs are negative?	Approximately 70%
What proportion of FNAs are indeterminate?	Approximately 20%
Of the indeterminate lesions, what percentage turn out to be malignant?	Approximately 20%

NODULE SUPPRESSION THERAPY

What is it?	Attempt to shrink thyroid nodules by thyroid hormone replacement (thyroxine) to suppress TSH
What percentage of benign nodules will shrink with suppressive therapy?	20%
Why is suppression therapy controversial?	Even if nodule shrinks, cannot be 100% sure it is not cancer; up to 50% of benign nodules shrink spontaneously at some subsequent point!

RECURRENT LARYNGEAL NERVE INJURY

What action should be taken preoperatively?	Assess nerve function and document any abnormalities
What is the risk of damage to the recurrent laryngeal nerve during thyroidectomy?	< 5%
What preventative steps should be taken?	Identify the nerve intraoperatively
What are the points at which risk of injury to the recurrent laryngeal nerve is greatest?	Dissection around the ligament of Berry Ligation of the inferior thyroid artery Dissection around the thoracic inlet

How can recurrent laryngeal nerve injury be diagnosed?

Postoperative laryngoscopy

What findings are associated with unilateral injury?

Cord on the affected side is in the paramedian position.

What findings are associated with bilateral injury?

Both cords are in the midline position (airway compromise with stridor).

In cases of temporary paralysis, when should function be expected to return?

Within 6–8 weeks

If the nerve is obviously injured intraoperatively, should repair be attempted?

Controversial. Repair is associated with less cord atrophy, but more cord adductor spasm because of random reinnervation.

POSTOPERATIVE HYPOPARATHYROIDISM

What are the associated risk factors?

Magnitude of surgery (i.e., risk of total thyroidectomy is greater than that of isthmectomy)
Previous thyroid surgery
Surgery for large thyroid cancer with lymphadenectomy

What is the incidence?

Between 0.6% and 17% (depending on the experience of the surgeon)

What is the most common cause?

Devascularization of the parathyroid gland

What is the major source of blood supply to the parathyroids?

Inferior thyroid artery (80%)

How can postoperative hypoparathyroidism be prevented?

Avoid ligating the inferior thyroid artery at the main trunk. Ligate branches close to the thyroid gland.

What is the treatment for mild asymptomatic hypocalcemia?

1. Calcium carbonate PO
2. Vitamin D (1,25 dihydroxyvitamin D_3)

What is the treatment for hypocalcemia tetany?

IV calcium gluconate or IV calcium chloride

56

Parathyroid

Who discovered parathyroid glands, and how?	Legend has it that Sir Richard Owen discovered parathyroid glands while performing an autopsy on a rhinoceros!

PHYSIOLOGY

What is the significance of the calcium-phosphate product?	If the product is > 40, there is a chance of salt precipitation in tissues.
How much calcium is ionized?	Approximately 50%
What is the normal parathyroid hormone (PTH) level?	Approximately 20 mEq/mL or less
What PTH levels are associated with hyperparathyroidism?	Approximately 60 mEq/mL or more
How does PTH work?	Increases bone resorption of calcium and phosphate Increases renal resorption of calcium Increases renal secretion of phosphate Stimulates vitamin D formation
What stimulates PTH secretion?	Decreasing calcium
How does vitamin D work?	Increases intestinal calcium and phosphate absorption
How does calcitonin work?	Inhibits bone resorption and probably increases urinary excretion of calcium

How does mithramycin work?	Inactivates osteoclasts, inhibits RNA synthesis
Where is calcium absorbed?	Duodenum and proximal jejunum

PERSISTENT AND RECURRENT POSTOPERATIVE HYPERPARATHYROIDISM (THE "MISSED" GLAND)

What percentage of parathyroidectomies will result in postoperative "missed gland" with postoperative hyperparathyroidism?	Approximately 5%
What are the potential sites of an ectopic parathyroid gland?	

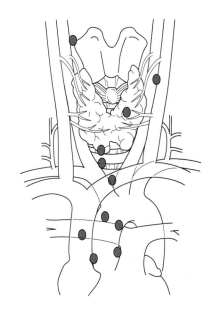

Define.

Persistent hyperparathyroidism	Postoperative hyperparathyroidism < 6 months after the operation
Recurrent hyperparathyroidism	Postoperative hyperparathyroidism > 6 months after the operation

What is the differential diagnosis of postoperative hyperparathyroidism?	1. Missed parathyroid gland at first operation 2. 5 glands 3. Metastatic spread of parathyroid cancer 4. Residual parathyroid cancer 5. **Ectopic** gland 6. PTH secreted by another carcinoma (e.g., lung carcinoma) 7. Hyperplasia of autotransplanted parathyroid tissue
Are any preoperative localization tests needed?	Common sense would dictate preoperative localization for any reoperation.
What are the best studies for localizing neck parathyroid?	**Sestamibi scan** (technetium Tc 99m Sestamibi) Ultrasound Venous sampling for PTH
What are the best studies for localizing an ectopic gland in the mediastinum?	Sestamibi CT MRI Venous sampling Angiogram

HYPERCALCEMIC CRISIS

What are the symptoms of hypercalcemic crisis?	Polyuria, dehydration (leading to increased calcium), muscle weakness, nausea, vomiting, lethargy, coma
What is the appropriate treatment of hypercalcemic crisis?	Fluids Furosemide (if hydrated) Calcitonin Mithramycin Biphosphonates

PARATHYROID AUTOTRANSPLANTATION

What site is used for autotransplanting a parathyroid?	1. Parathyroid pathology = nondominant forearm 2. No parathyroid pathology (e.g., inadvertent parathyroid injury during thyroidectomy) = sternocleidomastoid muscle

How is parathyroid transplanted into the forearm?

Slice into small pieces (approximately 1 × 1 × 3 mm), implant approximately 20 pieces into several sites in nondominant forearm muscle, then mark with Prolene

Why mark autotransplanted parathyroid gland?

Prolene stitch allows for identification if parathyroid tissue need to be removed later.

When does the transplanted tissue resume endocrine function?

About 3 weeks

57   Spleen

What is the largest single mass of lymphatic tissue in the body?

The spleen

By which ligament is the spleen attached to the stomach?

The gastrolienal ligament

What important structures are contained in the gastrolienal ligament?

The short gastric vessels and the left gastroepiploic vessel

Which ligament attaches the spleen to the kidney?

The lienorenal ligament

Which organ is in close proximity to the spleen?

The tail of the pancreas (which is prone to injury during splenectomy). The tail is classically said to "tickle" the spleen.

What portion of the circulating platelets are usually within the spleen?

Approximately one-third

What are Howell-Jolly bodies?

Nuclear remnants of RBCs, usually removed by the spleen

Why is the absence of Howell-Jolly bodies on a patient's blood smear important following splenectomy?

May signify the presence of unresected accessory splenic tissue

When is the best time to vaccinate after a trauma splenectomy?

At 14 days postoperatively is the optimal timing (but not always possible because many patients do not return for follow-up!)

| How do you differentiate between normal postsplenectomy leukocytosis and leukocytosis due to postoperative infection? | The following, if present, are highly associated with postoperative infection: 1. WBC > 15,000 2. Platelet count to WBC ratio of < 20 |

DISEASES OF THE SPLEEN

IMMUNE THROMBOCYTOPENIC PURPURA (ITP)

What is the etiology of ITP?	Circulating immunoglobulin (Ig)G is directed against platelet-associated antigen, resulting in destruction of platelets by the reticuloendothelial system.
What are the associated signs/symptoms?	Persistently low platelet count, easy bruising, petechiae, mucosal bleeding, menorrhagia, increased megakaryocyte counts on bone marrow aspirate
Is ITP more common in men or women?	Women (particularly young women)
What is the appropriate treatment?	Prednisone Platelet transfusions may be necessary for bleeding complications Plasmapheresis
What is the indication for splenectomy in ITP?	When patients are refractory to medical management
What percentage of patients eventually require splenectomy?	Approximately 75%
What is the prognosis after splenectomy?	In approximately 80% of patients, platelet counts return to normal by the 6th postoperative week. Another 15% improve sufficiently to no longer require steroids.
What condition may cause thrombocytopenia to recur after splenectomy for ITP?	The presence of an accessory spleen that was not resected during the initial splenectomy

THROMBOTIC THROMBOCYTOPENIC PURPURA (TTP)

What pentad of clinical manifestations is associated with TTP?	1. Thrombocytopenia 2. Fever 3. Neurologic changes 4. Renal failure 5. Microangiopathic hemolytic anemia
What is the etiology of TTP?	Unknown
Who is the typical patient with TTP?	A woman 30–40 years of age
What are the histologic findings associated with TTP?	Capillary and arteriole occlusion by aggregates of fibrin and platelets
What is the current medical treatment of TTP?	Antiplatelet agents, fresh frozen plasma, and corticosteroids
What is the indication for splenectomy in the setting of TTP?	Failure to respond to medical treatment
What percentage of patients will respond to medical treatment?	Approximately 80%

FELTY'S SYNDROME

What are the clinical manifestations?	Triad of "**SRG**": **S**plenomegaly **R**heumatoid arthritis **G**ranulocytopenia (Think: Felty SRG = "Felt a Surge")
What is the underlying cause?	Formation of antibodies against granulocytes

HEREDITARY SPHEROCYTOSIS

What is the etiology?	A genetic defect results in an abnormal **RBC membrane,** which leads to increased trapping and destruction of RBCs by the spleen.
What is the associated molecular deficit?	Defect of the membrane skeletal protein spectrin

What are the associated signs/symptoms?	Anemia, fatigue, jaundice, pigmented gallstones, and splenomegaly
What is the appropriate treatment?	Splenectomy

SPLENIC VEIN THROMBOSIS

What is the most common etiology?	Pancreatitis
What are the associated signs?	Isolated **gastric** varices, episodes of upper GI bleeding
How is the diagnosis made?	Celiac angiography or ultrasound
Is splenic vein thrombosis an indication for splenectomy?	Yes

SPLEEN TUMORS

What is the most common primary tumor of the spleen?	Benign hemangioma
What is the most common primary lymphoid tumor of the spleen?	Lymphoma (note: tumors may diffusely involve the spleen and present as splenomegaly rather than as mass lesions)
What are the types of splenic cysts?	Post-traumatic Parasitic (usually *Echinococcus*) Primary cyst (epithelial lined)
What are the indications for excision of a "true" splenic cyst?	A cyst > 10 cm in diameter should be removed because the risk of rupture and subsequent hemorrhage is greatly increased.

58

Surgically Correctable Hypertension

What causes surgically correctable hypertension?

Neuroblastoma
Pheochromocytoma
Renal artery stenosis
Coarctation of the aorta
Hyperparathyroidism
Conn's syndrome
Cushing's syndrome
Increased intracranial pressure
Cancer
Renal parenchymal disease

What percentage of hypertensive patients has one of these conditions?

Between 5% and 10%

Who should be evaluated for one of these conditions?

Young patients with hypertension
Patients with no family history of hypertension
Patients with diastolic blood pressure > 110 mm Hg that cannot be controlled medically

What is the appropriate initial evaluation?

History and physical examination
Serum electrolytes
Serum BUN and creatinine
Chest x-ray

NEUROBLASTOMA

What is it?

Embryonal tumor of neural crest origin; seen in children

What causes hypertension (HTN) in neuroblastoma?

Increased catecholamines

PHEOCHROMOCYTOMA

What is it?	Tumor of the adrenal medulla and similar tissues (e.g., sympathetic ganglion) that produces catecholamines (epinephrine, norepinephrine, dopamine)
What causes HTN in pheochromocytoma?	Increased catecholamines

RENAL ARTERY STENOSIS

What is it?	Narrowing of the renal artery, resulting in decreased perfusion of the juxtaglomerular apparatus and subsequent activation of the aldosterone-renin-angiotensin system
What are the signs/ symptoms?	Most patients asymptomatic Some may have headache, diastolic HTN, flank bruits (present in 50% of cases), and decreased renal function Note: Approximately 7% of patients with essential HTN also have flank bruits

COARCTATION OF THE AORTA

What is it?	Congenital abnormality consisting of narrowing of thoracic aorta, with or without intraluminal "shelf" (infolding of the media), usually found near the ductus/ligamentum arteriosum
What causes HTN in coarctation?	Increased resistance to flow to the distal body and, thus, increased flow to the upper body

HYPERPARATHYROIDISM (INCREASED PARATHYROID HORMONE [PTH])

Define increased PTH.	Increased secretion of PTH
What percentage of patients with hyperparathyroidism have HTN?	Approximately 10%
What causes HTN in hyperparathyroidism?	Hypercalcemia

CONN'S SYNDROME

What is it?	Hyperaldosteronism. Aldosterone is abnormally secreted by an adrenal adenoma/carcinoma/hyperplasia or by an ovarian tumor.
What are the 2 classic signs of Conn's syndrome?	HTN and hypokalemia
What causes HTN in Conn's syndrome?	Hypervolemia

CUSHING'S SYNDROME

What is it?	Excessive cortisol production
What percentage of patients with Cushing's syndrome have HTN?	> 75%!
What causes HTN in Cushing's syndrome?	Hypervolemia

INCREASED INTRACRANIAL PRESSURE (ICP)

What causes HTN in increased ICP?	The Cushing's response (reflex), consisting of HTN and bradycardia

CANCER

What causes HTN in cancer?	Paraneoplastic syndromes

RENAL PARENCHYMAL DISEASE

What causes HTN in renal parenchymal disease?	Hypervolemia Increased renin (which increases angiotensin [vasoconstriction] and aldosterone [hypervolemia])

59

Soft Tissue Sarcomas and Lymphomas

NON-HODGKIN'S LYMPHOMA (NHL)

What is NHL?	A lymphoma other than Hodgkin's disease. NHL has an established cellular origin (usually monoclonal B cells, but may also originate in T cells) based on the stages of lymphocyte differentiation.
How is NHL classified?	Nodular (low grade) versus diffuse (high grade). The Working Classification groups NHL according to natural history and therapeutic response.
Which is worse, high grade or low grade?	High grade
How does the presentation differ compared with that of Hodgkin's disease?	Patients with NHL are usually older (often debilitated), but less often have B symptoms. NHL often presents with peripheral nodal (especially epitrochlear) or extranodal disease. It may present as a retroperitoneal or mesenteric mass or as hepatomegaly and/or splenomegaly.
How does NHL spread?	Via the bloodstream, thereby involving noncontiguous areas
What are some of the more dramatic presentations of NHL?	Superior vena cava syndrome Acute spinal cord compression syndrome Ureteral obstruction Meningeal involvement
How is the diagnosis made?	Biopsy
What are the most common malignancies requiring abdominal surgery in patients with AIDS?	NHL Kaposi's sarcoma (KS)

When is splenectomy indicated in NHL?	Symptomatic splenomegaly Pancytopenia, secondary to hypersplenism Recurrent splenic infarcts
Define hypersplenism.	Hyperfunctioning spleen Documented loss of blood elements (WBCs, hematocrit, platelets) Splenomegaly Bone marrow

GASTRIC LYMPHOMA

What is the most common site of extranodal NHL?	The stomach
What are the signs/ symptoms of gastric lymphoma?	Abdominal pain and weight loss (80%) B signs (40%) Nausea, vomiting, malaise (possibly) Upper GI bleeding (rare)
What are the major differential diagnoses?	Gastric adenocarcinoma Ménétrier's disease Zollinger-Ellison syndrome Hypertrophic gastritis
Which diagnostic tests are indicated?	Upper GI endoscopy with biopsy is the method of choice. Grossly, lesions are superficial, well-demarcated, stellate ulcers that involve a large area of the stomach.
What signs appear on upper GI series?	May show a mass, ulcers, enlarged mucosal folds, and/or decreased gastric mobility
What is the appropriate treatment of disease confined to the stomach?	**Controversial:** 1. Surgical resection ± postoperative radiation therapy and chemotherapy, OR 2. Chemotherapy and radiation therapy alone

SOFT TISSUE SARCOMA (STS)

What type of tumor is associated with polyvinyl chloride and arsenic exposure?	Hepatic angiosarcoma

Where is polyvinyl chloride found?	In plastics industry
What is Stewart-Treves syndrome?	An angiosarcoma that develops in an extremity with lymphedema, classically following radical mastectomy and axillary lymph node dissection for breast cancer
What is the importance of surgical clips after sarcoma resection?	The sites of highest risk of recurrence should be marked with radiopaque clips for radiation therapy.

PULMONARY METASTASES

What is the appropriate treatment?	Isolated pulmonary metastases may be resected. Aggressive resection improves survival.
What factors are associated with an improved prognosis?	Slower doubling time Unilateral disease On CT, 3 nodules or less

MALIGNANT FIBROUS HISTIOCYTOMA (MFH)

What is MFH?	A sarcoma that originates from fibroblastic cells (histiocytes)
Where does it present?	Most commonly in the deep soft tissues of the extremities and in the abdominal/retroperitoneal areas
How common is it?	Accounts for approximately 20% of all cases of adult STS Pleomorphic MFH is the most common postradiation sarcoma.
What is the rate of local recurrence?	Approximately 25%
What are the 2 routes of metastases?	Via blood (most cases), most commonly to the lung (90% of cases) Via lymphatics (rare)
What is the appropriate treatment?	Radical surgery plus adjunctive radiation therapy or chemotherapy

LIPOSARCOMA

What is it?	A sarcoma originating from adipose cells
What is the usual presentation?	More common in men than in women Often develops singularly in the thigh or retroperitoneum, but may be multicentric Rarely found in subcutaneous tissue
What is unique about this type of sarcoma?	Common adult STS (23%) Largest sarcoma (on average) Most common retroperitoneal sarcoma
Describe the various types.	Well-differentiated—does not metastasize; extensive local recurrence; 10-year survival rate 40–60%; may dedifferentiate Myxoid Pleomorphic/round cell—metastasizes early; poor prognosis ($<$ 20% 5-year survival rate)
What is the appropriate treatment?	Surgery plus radiation therapy

RHABDOMYOSARCOMA (RMS)

What is RMS?	A sarcoma that originates from skeletal muscle cells
How common is it?	Embryonal RMS is the most common soft tissue sarcoma in infants and children.
What are the 3 various types of RMS?	1. Embryonal 2. Alveolar 3. Pleomorphic
Describe embryonal RMS.	One of the "malignant small blue cell" tumors of children; occurs in first 2 decades of life; presents in head, neck, or genitourinary regions
Describe alveolar RMS.	Seen in teenagers/young adults
Describe pleomorphic RMS.	Rare; seen in adults

Name the other "malignant small blue cell" tumors.	Lymphoma, Ewing's sarcoma, and neuroblastoma
What is sarcoma botryoides?	An embryonal RMS consisting of **grape-like masses** that involve the mucosal surface or tubular viscera
What percentage of patients with RMS have lymph node metastases?	Approximately 10%
What percentage of patients with RMS have distant metastatic disease at diagnosis?	Approximately 30%
What is the appropriate treatment of localized (stage I) RMS?	Complete surgical resection plus adjuvant chemotherapy
What is the appropriate treatment of advanced (stage II or higher) RMS?	Combined modality therapy: surgical resection, radiation therapy, and chemotherapy. If the tumor is considered initially unresectable, primary chemotherapy, or primary chemotherapy with radiation therapy may be administered, followed by surgery and adjuvant chemotherapy.
What is the 5-year survival rate for embryonal RMS?	80–90%
What is the 5-year survival rate for alveolar RMS?	Approximately 50%

FIBROSARCOMA

What is it?	A sarcoma originating from intermuscular or intramuscular fibrous tissues, fascial tendons, and aponeuroses
How common is it?	Second most common sarcoma in children; less common in adults
What type of patient is at greatest risk?	African American men

What is the usual presentation?	Occurs most frequently in the deep soft tissues of the extremities
What is the 5-year survival rate?	Approximately 50%
What is the appropriate treatment?	Wide excision plus radiation therapy

DESMOID TUMORS

What are they?	Benign fibrous tumors occurring in fascial tissues; may occur in areas of previous scarring
What is the most common location?	The anterior abdominal wall
Is this type of tumor likely to metastasize?	No. Desmoid tumors are nonencapsulated and spread by local invasion.
What are the possible complications?	Pain, intestinal/ureteral obstruction, fistulas
What is the appropriate treatment?	Wide surgical excision ± chemotherapy and radiation therapy
What is the appropriate drug treatment?	1. Tamoxifen 2. The nonsteroidal anti-inflammatory drug sulindac
What is the prognosis?	Local recurrence highly likely (19–77% with adequate margins; 90% with minimal margins)
With what syndrome are desmoid tumors associated?	Gardner's syndrome

KAPOSI'S SARCOMA (KS)

What is KS?	A vascular sarcoma involving endothelial cell proliferation with reactive lymphoreticular elements
How does KS usually present?	Begins as blue to purple patches, which become plaques and nodules

Describe the various types.

Classic—affects patients of Mediterranean and European-Jewish ancestry

African—affects young black men in the sub-Sahara

Iatrogenic/immunosuppressed—affects renal transplant recipients

Epidemic—affects HIV-positive individuals (AIDS)

How do the classic and epidemic forms differ in presentation?

Classic: affects elderly males on their lower extremities, with only occasional visceral involvement

Epidemic: preferential distribution in head, neck, and trunk, with oral/perioral mucosal involvement in 55% of cases

How do the classic and epidemic forms differ in prognosis?

Classic: slowly progressive; 10- to 15-year survival rate is average

Epidemic: rarely the cause of death in HIV-positive persons; its treatment is palliative

What is the appropriate treatment of localized lesions?

Local radiation therapy or intralesional vinblastine

What is the appropriate treatment of disseminated KS?

Chemotherapy plus immunotherapy

How often does GI involvement occur in epidemic KS?

Approximately 40% of cases

What are the associated signs/symptoms of GI involvement?

Abdominal pain, massive hemorrhage, perforation, malabsorption, protein-losing enteropathy, bowel obstruction, obstructive jaundice, tenesmus, ulcerative colitis-like syndrome, or dysphagia

What is the most common tumor associated with AIDS?

KS

60

Skin Lesions

What are the most common cancers in the United States?	Nonmelanoma skin cancers
What percentage of all cancers are they?	33%
What are the 3 types of basal cell carcinoma (BCC)?	1. Nodular 2. Morpheaform 3. Superficial
What is the most common type of BCC?	Nodular (> 75%) Superficial (10%) Morpheaform (2%)
What does a morpheaform BCC look like?	Plaque, often resembling a stellate scar
Did a dermatologist invent Mohs' surgery?	**No.** Frederic Mohs is a **general surgeon.**
What is the treatment of Kaposi's sarcoma skin lesions?	Nonsurgical; observe if asymptomatic, or use cryotherapy, radiation therapy, or chemotherapy
What is a Merkel cell carcinoma?	Highly aggressive skin lesion that is highly metastatic
What does a Merkel cell carcinoma look like?	Red/purple nodule with telangiectasia
What other cancer must be ruled out with a Merkel cell carcinoma?	Oat cell carcinoma of the lung, as skin metastases look just like Merkel cell carcinoma microscopically

61 Melanoma

From what embryologic tissue do melanocytes arise?

Neural crest cells

Where do melanocytes reside in normal skin?

In the basal layer of the epidermis

What is an amelanotic melanoma?

Melanoma that is not pigmented. Occurs when malignant transformation of the melanocyte results in loss of pigment production.

Patients present with nonpigmented melanomas, which may go unnoticed and untreated for an extended period of time.

What is local recurrence?

A tumor that is < 5 cm from the primary site

What is the incidence of local recurrence in treated melanoma?

Approximately 15%

What is regional recurrence?

Typically, lymph node metastases, which are the most common manifestation of recurrent melanoma

What are the most common sites of distant metastases in melanoma?

The lungs and liver

What percentage of melanomas are ocular lesions?

2–5%

Where in the eye does ocular melanoma occur?

In the uveal tract (iris, ciliary body, and chorioid), conjunctiva, or retina

What is the most common site of metastasis from an ocular-tract lesion?

The liver (the uveal tract lacks lymphatic drainage)

Are visceral primaries common among melanoma patients?

No. They account for < 0.1% of all melanomas.

What percentage of melanomas present as metastases from unknown primaries?

Approximately 5%

How do most unknown primaries present?

With lymph node metastases

What is the appropriate management of such lesions?

Rule out cutaneous, ocular, or mucous membrane primary lesions. Then, treat metastases, usually by resection.

True or false: survival rate after melanoma that occurs during pregnancy is worse than that of nonpregnant patients with melanoma?

False. Recent reports have indicated that although patients who present with melanoma during pregnancy may have a predilection to develop lymph node metastases, survival is comparable to that of matched controls.

What mortality rate is associated with pulmonary metastases?

Pulmonary metastases are associated with a 70% mortality rate within 1 year and a 4% 5-year survival rate.

How should isolated pulmonary metastases be managed?

Isolated pulmonary metastases should be resected.

How are GI metastases generally discovered?

Usually, they cause bleeding, intussusception, or small bowel obstruction.

What percentage of melanomas < 1.0 mm ("thin") have positive nodal metastases?

10%

What percentage of melanomas 1–4 mm ("intermediate") have positive lymph node metastases?

25%

Has routine sentinel node biopsy in patients with melanoma been shown to improve survival?

No (studies pending)

When performing lymphoscintigraphy, what gamma counts are considered classic for a melanoma sentinel node?

Gamma counts 10 times more than background counts

Should you do a FROZEN section of the sentinel node?

No

What margins do you need for local recurrences?

1 cm

What is "in transit disease"?

Skin or subcutaneous metastases in between primary and regional nodal basin

What percentage of patients will develop "in transit disease"?

2%

What is the treatment of "in transit disease"?

Resection with 1-cm margins

62

Surgical Intensive Care

INTENSIVE CARE UNIT (ICU) FORMULAS

Define.

Vo_2	Oxygen consumption
Do_2	Oxygen delivery
Co	Cardiac output
Cao_2	Arterial oxygen content
CVo_2	Venous oxygen content
PAP	Pulmonary artery pressure
PCWP	Pulmonary capillary wedge pressure

What is the formula for oxygen delivery (Do_2)?	$Co \times Cao_2 \times 10$
What are normal values for Do_2?	600–1000 mL/min
What is the formula for oxygen consumption (Vo_2)?	$Co \times (Cao_2 - CVo_2) \times 10$
What are normal values for Vo_2?	110–150 mL/min/M^2
What is the formula for pulmonary vascular resistance (PVR)?	$80 \times (PAP - PCWP)/Co$
What are normal values for PVR?	100–200 dynes/sec/cm^{-5}

What is the formula for alveolar-arterial (A-a) oxygen gradient?	Alveolar O_2 − arterial $O_2 = P(A\text{-}a)O_2$
What are the normal values for alveolar-arterial oxygen gradient?	FIO_2 21% $= 4 - 25$ FIO_2 100% $= 10 - 60$
Define compliance.	Change in volume divided by change in pressure ($\Delta V/\Delta P$)
Define CPP (cerebral perfusion pressure)?	MAP − ICP
What is the normal value for CPP?	> 70 mm Hg

END POINTS OF RESUSCITATION

Why are end points of resuscitation so important?	Underresuscitation leads to poor outcomes: death, multiple organ failure (MOF), systemic inflammatory response syndrome (SIRS)
What is the substrate for lactate?	Pyruvate (anaerobic pathway: lactate is made from pyruvate by lactate dehydrogenase)
Describe the fate of lactate.	Converted into glucose in liver (or kidney) via Cori cycle
What is base deficit?	Indirect measurement of acidosis on arterial blood gas (ABG)
What is the weakness of base deficit as an end point of resuscitation?	Nonspecific; elevated with any form of metabolic acidosis, but correlates well in patients who do not have any other medical problems and are not elderly
What is the best currently available end point of resuscitation?	Lactate

RESPIRATORY SYSTEM

Define the spirometry waves:	1. TV-Tidal volume 2. ERV-Expiratory reserve volume 3. RV-Residual volume 4. IRV-Inspiratory reserve volume (Think top to bottom: "IRV watches TV with ERV in the RV")

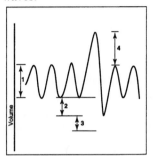

What is the normal I:E ratio?

Inspiration to expiration time. Normal is 1:2.

What is "reverse" I:E ratio?

Inspiration to expiration time of $> 1.1:1$

What is *static* lung compliance?

Compliance of lung parenchyma ONLY = Tidal volume divided by plateau pressure (minus any positive end-expiratory pressure [PEEP]; remember, compliance = $\blacktriangle V/\blacktriangle P$)

What is *dynamic* lung compliance?

Compliance of lung parenchyma AND airways = Tidal volume divided by peak inspiratory pressure (minus any PEEP)

What is the Tobin index?

RR divided by VT in liters; if > 105, unlikely to have a successful extubation

What is auto PEEP?

Alveolar pressure accumulating after incomplete exhalation (think of blowing up a balloon, and then letting the balloon deflate **incompletely** before re-blowing up the balloon)

What is the treatment for auto PEEP?

Decrease RR, decrease tidal volume, increase expiratory time: $\uparrow$ E time

ACUTE RESPIRATORY DISTRESS SYNDROME (ARDS)

Why was the name changed from adult to acute (respiratory distress syndrome)?

Children get the syndrome as well.

How is the diagnosis of ARDS made?	Capillary wedge pressure < 18, chest x-ray with bilateral infiltrates, ratio $PaO_2:FIO_2 < 200$
What is the difference between acute lung injury and ARDS?	Acute lung—$PaO_2:FIO_2$ ratio < 300 (and > 200). ARDS < 200.
How do you remember the ratio of ARDS?	$PaO_2:FIO_2$ or "PF"—think "**P**u**F**f"
What 2 barriers constitute the "alveolar-capillary" barrier?	1. Microvascular **endo**thelium 2. Alveolar **epi**thelium
What is the pathogenesis of the early acute phase of ARDS?	Breakdown of the alveolar capillary barrier and accumulation of transudate fluid (protein filled) in the alveolar air sac
What happens as the alveolar epithelial cells die?	No surfactant production; less removal of alveolar fluid; hyaline membranes replace the epithelial cells
What is the "fibrotic lung injury"?	Later stage of ARDS; deposition of cells, collagen, and fibronectin, resulting in "fibrosis" of lung
What is the treatment for ARDS?	Fix underlying cause, then support with ventilator: low tidal volume (< 6 mL/kg), plateau pressure < 35, PEEP prn

CRITICAL CARE MEDICATIONS

ACETAZOLAMIDE (DIAMOX)

What is it?	Diuretic with ability to remove bicarbonate in urine; use in metabolic alkalosis

AMINOPHYLLINE

What is it?	Bronchodilator
How does it work?	Increases cyclic adenosine monophosphate (cAMP), resulting in increased catechols

MILRINONE

What is the site of action?	Phosphodiesterase III inhibitor (PDE III); decreases breakdown of cAMP and therefore increases intracellular cAMP and intracellular calcium
How does it act?	Increases inotropy, decreases afterload (SVR), little or no increase in chronotropy with no net increase in myocardial oxygen consumption (MVO_2)
What is the usual dosage?	Load—50–75 mcg/kg over 10 minutes Maintenance—0.375 to 0.7 μg/kg/min
What should you do if milrinone loses its inotropic effect?	Add low dose epi/norepinephrine to increased cAMP intracellularly.

ISOPROTERENOL

What is the site of action?	$+++$ (β_1 and β_2 agonist)
How does it act?	Increases inotropy, increases chronotropy ($+$ vasodilation of skeletal and mesenteric vascular beds)

ESMOLOL

What is the site of action?	β-Adrenergic antagonist with very short half-life ($\approx$9 min), which necessitates intravenous infusion, but allows it to be easily titrated and turned off
In what cases is it indicated?	Control of ventricular response rate in patients with atrial fibrillation and rapid ventricular response, or with other supraventricular tachyarrhythmias; control of blood pressure (often in conjunction with sodium nitroprusside [SNP]) in patients with hypertensive emergency or with aortic dissection/traumatic aortic injury

LANDMARK ICU PAPERS

How long should you give IV dilantin for seizure prophylaxis in brain-injured patients?	7 days (Temkin, et al, NEJM 1990; 323:497–502)

What should the glucose level be in ICU patients?

80–110. Very tight control has been shown to decrease mortality. (Van den Berghe, et al: N Engl J Med 2001; 345:1359–1367)

What should the tidal volume and plateau pressures be in patients with ARDS?

Tidal volume 4–6 mL/kg and plateau pressures < 35 have been shown to decrease mortality. (ARDS Network. N Engl J Med 2000; 342:1301–1308)

What works better for prophylaxis against upper GI bleeding in ventilated patients: Zantac or sucralfate?

Zantac has a lower rate of GI bleeding and no difference in pneumonia. (Cook et al, N Engl J Med 1998; 338:791–797)

Does empiric administration of very powerful broad spectrum antibiotics for 72 hours while awaiting culture results lead to emergence of resistant bacteria?

No. Imipenem and gentamicin given for 72 hours in a trauma ICU while awaiting culture results did not lead to resistant bacteria. (Namias et al: J Trauma 45; (5):887–891)

When should ICU patients who do not have cardiac disease be transfused?

Hemoglobin < 7, unless acute MI or unstable angina (Herbert et al: N Engl J Med 1999; 340:409–417)

Who needs prophylaxis for upper GI bleeding in the ICU?

All patients intubated > 48 hours, all coagulopathic patients, burn patients, brain-injured patients, and all patients with recent history of peptic ulcer disease (Cook, et al: N Engl J Med 1994; 330:377–381)

What works best to avoid decrease in renal function due to radiocontrast agents?

Saline alone works better than saline with Lasix or mannitol. (Solomon, et al: N Engl J Med 1994; 331:1416–1420) Acetylcysteine PO the day before and the day of contrast administration also has been shown to protect renal function. (Tepel, et al: N Engl J Med 2000; 343:180–184)

What medication has been shown to decrease postoperative MI and death due to CAD?

Atenolol—beta-blockers (Mangano et al: NEJM 1996; 335:1713–1721)

What medication has been shown to improve outcome after spinal cord injury due to blunt trauma (controversial!)?	Steroids (methylprednisolone) 30 mg/kg, then 5.4 mg/kg/h × 23 hours (Bracken, et al: JAMA 1997; May 28; 277(20); 1597–1604)
What medication has been shown to decrease mortality in patients with severe sepsis?	Activated protein C (Bernard et al, NEJM 2001; 344:699–709)

MISCELLANEOUS

What is the most common symptom of pulmonary artery rupture from a Swann-Ganz catheter?	Hemoptysis
What is the treatment for Swann-Ganz pulmonary artery injury?	1. Deflation of balloon 2. Withdrawal of catheter 3. Ipsilateral side down (lateral decubitus) 4. Increased PEEP 5. Thoracic surgery consult
Does "renal dose" dopamine prevent or help treat renal failure?	**No**
What is the first step if the ventilator alarms are going off and difficulty with ventilation is apparent?	Take the patient off the ventilator, and hand bag him/her. Remove the ventilator from the equation!
Is there an increased rate of ICU pneumonia with H_2 blockers vs sucralfate?	No. Larger studies reveal no difference (smaller studies did show H_2 blockers as a risk factor due to bacterial overgrowth in stomach with H_2 blocker acid neutralization).
Can you add PEEP to bag ventilation?	**Yes**. Add PEEP valve to bag.
What percentage of ICU fevers represent true infection?	36%

What is a "differential blood culture" in patients with a central line?

Draw blood cultures from **central line** and **peripheral** vein. If ratio of catheter colony-forming units (CFUs) to peripheral vein CFUs is > 8, the diagnosis of catheter infection has a sensitivity of 93% and specificity of 100%.

How does Lasix affect fractional excretion of sodium (FENa)?

Because of salt wasting, it may falsely elevate FENa; thus, prerenal azotemia can be missed.

What can be done instead of FENa in the patient who has had Lasix?

FeUrea (use urea instead of sodium)

What ICU IV medication bag must be covered with aluminum foil because it will be broken down by light?

SNP

What is the physiologic effect of increasing dead-space ventilation?

Progressive hypoxemia and hypercapnia

What causes increased shunt fraction?

Underventilation (pneumonia, pulmonary edema, respiratory distress syndrome, mucus plugging) or overperfusion (loss of pulmonary vascular autoregulation as in massive pulmonary embolus), SNP, atelectasis

What is the physiologic effect of increasing shunt fraction?

Initially, progressive hypoxemia, followed by late hypercapnia

What mechanical situations cause a decrease in respiratory compliance?

Pneumothorax, atelectasis, pneumonia, pulmonary edema, alveolar air trapping, ARDS

What is the maximum O_2 that can be given via a nasal cannula?

Never more than 4 liters per minute— any more and you get no increase in O_2 but more uncomfortable and more nasal drying

How much diaphragm atrophy do you get after 7 days of complete ventilator support?

Loss of up to 50% diaphragm muscle mass!

What do you do if you have a patient with a left bundle branch block and absolute need for a Swann-Ganz catheter?

External pacer then float!

What percent of patients with a pulmonary embolus will not have a clinically documented decrease in O_2 saturation?

10%

What side down will increase O_2 saturation in a patient with a unilateral pulmonary contusion?

Good lung down! Will increase blood flow to the good lung and increase O_2 saturation!

What are the factors that effect SvO_2 (mixed venous saturations)?

Think of "**COSH**": **C**ardiac output, **O**xygen consumption, **S**aO_2, **H**gB concentration.

What percent of patients with tracheostomies will aspirate if fed orally?

Up to 50%! (Always get a swallowing study prior to feeding patients with tracheostomies!)

What is a contraindication for administering Haldol?

Prolonged QT internal—may result in *torsades de pointes!*

How can you calculate how much potassium is in potassium phosphate?

Number of millimeters of potassium phosphate times 1.47 = mEq potassium [Example: 13.6 mm of potassium phosphate = 20 mEq of K^+ (13.6 × 1.47 = 19.99)]

How can you detect hypovolemia on an A line tracing?

Cycling—the waveform moves up and down with respiration

Why give a patient with liver and kidney failure Nimbex (cisatricurium)?

Nimbex is metabolized by Hoffman degradation; it breaks down in the blood rather than by kidney or liver metabolism.

What is the half life of Amidarone?

52 days!

What is the equivalent dosing ratio of Bumex to Lasix?

1 mg of Bumex equals about 20 mg of Lasix

What is a common cause of ICU refractory hypertension?	Fluid overload
Which ICU benzodiazepine has the quickest period of time until peak effect?	Valium—about one minute until peak effect. Versed has 5 minutes and Ativan about 30 minutes until peak effect.
What is a Passy-Muir trach plug?	A speaking valve. It is a one-way valve (air comes in and none goes out) and therefore the trach balloon must be DOWN!
What should you do if milrinone stops working?	Add low dose Epi or NE increase cAMP
What is the antidote for cyanide SNP toxicity?	Sodium thiosulfate
What is the antidote for nitroglycerin toxicity?	Methylene blue
What is the tobramycin/ gentamicin "rule of sevens"?	1. Initial q 24 hr dosing **7** mg/kg 2. Check level at **7** hours post infusion 3. Level at 7 hours should be less than 7 mg/dl
Give the rough formula for pressure support.	$(PIP - peep) \times \frac{1}{2}$
Renal dose dopamine is one of two renal artery dilators. What is the other?	Fenoldopam—a DA1 dilator
With neck flexion, how far can an endotracheal tube travel in the trachea?	Up to 4 cm!
What is sick euthyroid syndrome?	**Normal** thyroid-stimulating hormone (TSH) but decreased thyroxine (T_4), decreased free triiodothyronine (T_3) with an increase in reverse T_3. This syndrome is seen in critically ill patients with previous normal thyroid function.
HCT of PRBCs?	60–70%
What percent of normal levels of clotting factors does a patient need for maximal clotting function?	Only 30%

How do you transfuse 1% of clotting factors?	1 cc/kg = 1% of clotting factors
What's the most common sign of pulmonary artery rupture due to Swann-Ganz catheter?	Hemoptysis
How should you treat a pulmonary artery rupture from a Swann-Ganz balloon?	1. Deflate and pull balloon back 2. Ipsilateral side down (lateral decubitus position) 3. Increase PEEP 4. STAT page thoracic surgery
What is the differential diagnosis for cause of increased trach secretions?	Bacterial infection, viral infection, fungal infection, or fluid overload
Has renal dose dopamine been shown to help prevent or treat renal failure?	No
What might be going on if the BUN rises disproportionately compared to creatinine?	GI bleed
What ICU endocrine disorder presents with hypothermia and bradycardia?	Hypothyroidism
What ICU endocrine disorder presents with fever and tachycardia?	Adrenal insufficiency

63

Vascular Surgery

ARTERIAL OCCLUSIVE DISEASE OF THE LOWER EXTREMITY

What named collateral path provides arterial flow to the lower extremity in the setting of complete aortoiliac occlusion?

Collaterals of **Winslow,** which connect the subclavian arteries with the external iliac arteries through the internal mammary and inferior epigastric arteries

What are the 5-year patency rates for:

Aortobifemoral bypass?

85–90%. (Rates are reduced by 15–20% if there is concurrent distal occlusive disease because patent outflow is crucial for long-term graft patency.)

Axillobifemoral bypass?

70–75%

Femorofemoral bypass?

80–85%

Percutaneous iliac artery angioplasty?

80–90%

What is the usual route by which blood reaches the foot in cases of superficial femoral artery occlusion?

The profunda femoris artery collateralizes through the genicular artery to the popliteal artery.

TIBIOPERONEAL OCCLUSIVE DISEASE

What patients are at increased risk for tibioperoneal occlusive disease?

Patients with diabetes or Buerger's disease

Why are these lesions more limb-threatening than more proximal disease?

Less abundant collateral pathways

What are the indications for surgery?

Limb salvage and ischemic ulcers only. (Because of the difficulty of successful bypass, the threshold for surgery in the patient with tibioperoneal occlusion is elevated.)

What are the surgical options?

Femorotibial or femoropopliteal bypass
Multiple short distal-distal grafts for multisegmental occlusions

What are the conduit options if insufficient vein is available for femorodistal bypass?

Composite graft: Proximal segment of polytetrafluoroethylene (PTFE) and distal segment of saphenous vein
Venovenous grafts: Anastomosis of short segments of available veins
Avoid using prosthetic grafts below the knee!

How is a patient with preoperative forefoot necrosis with infection managed?

Débridement and drainage ± limited amputation and IV antibiotics. Once infection clears, distal bypass is performed.

How is a patient with preoperative heel or posterior arch necrosis managed?

Extension of necrosis proximal to the forefoot rarely permits successful distal bypass. A below-the-knee amputation (BKA) is usually indicated.

What is the 5-year patency rate for femorodistal bypass?

50%

Name the labeled arteries on the anterior view of the lower extremity.

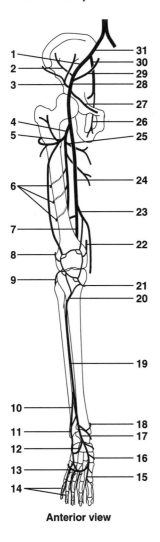

Anterior view

1. **External iliac artery**
2. Deep circumflex iliac artery
3. Superficial circumflex iliac artery
4. Profunda femoris artery
5. Lateral circumflex femoral artery
6. Perforating arteries
7. **Popliteal artery**
8. Superior lateral genicular artery
9. Inferior lateral genicular artery
10. Perforating branch of peroneal (fibular) artery
11. Lateral malleolar artery
12. Lateral tarsal artery
13. Arcuate artery
14. Dorsal digital artery
15. Deep plantar branch
16. Medial tarsal artery
17. **Dorsalis pedis artery**
18. Medial malleolar artery
19. **Anterior tibial artery**
20. Anterior tibial recurrent artery
21. Inferior medial genicular artery
22. Superior medial genicular artery
23. Descending genicular artery
24. **Superficial femoral artery**
25. Medial circumflex femoral artery
26. Obturator artery
27. External pudendal artery
28. **Common femoral artery**
29. Inferior epigastric artery
30. **Internal iliac artery**
31. **Common iliac artery**

Name the labeled arteries on the posterior view of the lower extremity.

1. Superior gluteal artery
2. Inferior gluteal artery
3. Medial circumflex femoral artery
4. **Profunda femoris artery**
5. **Superficial femoral artery**
6. **Popliteal artery**
7. Genicular arteries (originate from the popliteal artery)
8. **Posterior tibial artery**
9. Medial plantar artery
10. Deep branch of dorsalis pedis artery
11. Plantar arch
12. Lateral plantar artery
13. **Peroneal (fibular) artery**
14. **Anterior tibial artery**

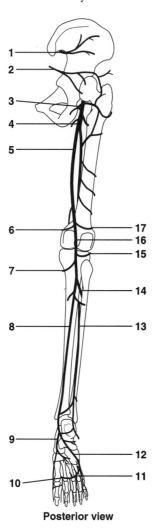

Posterior view

ARTERIAL OCCLUSIVE DISEASE OF THE UPPER EXTREMITY

Arterial occlusive disease of the upper extremity accounts for what percentage of cases of extremity ischemia?	5%
What are the etiologies?	Diverse; including atherosclerosis, embolism, trauma, thoracic outlet syndrome, arteritis (e.g., Buerger's and Takayasu's diseases), and vasospastic disorders (e.g., Raynaud's syndrome)
Why are proximal occlusions usually asymptomatic?	Extensive arterial collaterals around the shoulder girdle
What clinical test is performed to evaluate the patency of ulnar and radial arteries?	Allen's test
How are atherosclerotic lesions of the upper extremity different from those of the lower extremity?	Significantly increased incidence of atheroembolization
What is the most common site of stenosis?	Subclavian artery (75% occur on the left)
What are the treatment options?	Endarterectomy, bypass procedure, or, occasionally, percutaneous balloon angioplasty
What is the procedure of choice for subclavian artery stenosis in a patient without carotid occlusive disease?	Common carotid to subclavian artery bypass with a PTFE conduit. To avoid the use of prosthetic material, transect the subclavian artery and transpose the distal end to perform an end-to-side anastomosis.

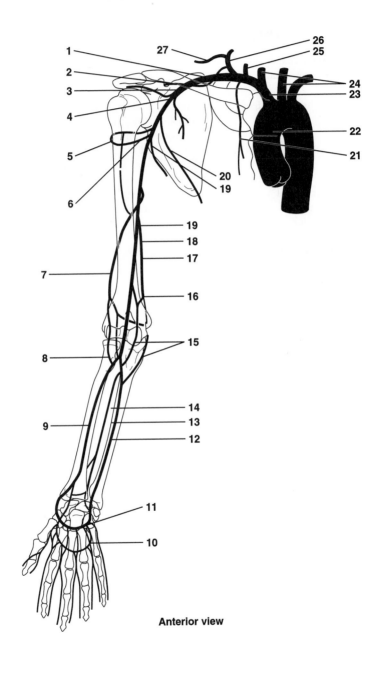

Anterior view

**Name the labeled arteries
of the upper extremity.
(See previous page.)**

1. **Subclavian artery**
2. Suprascapular artery
3. **Axillary artery**
4. Thoracoacromial artery
5. Posterior circumflex humeral artery
6. Anterior circumflex humeral artery
7. Profunda brachii artery
8. Radial recurrent artery
9. **Radial artery**
10. **Superficial palmar arch**
11. **Deep palmar arch**
12. Anterior interosseous artery
13. **Ulnar artery**
14. Common interosseous artery
15. Anterior and posterior ulnar
    recurrent arteries
16. Inferior ulnar collateral artery
17. Superior ulnar collateral artery
18. **Brachial artery**
19. Subscapular artery
20. Lateral thoracic artery
21. Internal mammary artery
22. **Aorta**
23. **Brachiocephalic trunk**
24. **Common carotid arteries**
25. **Vertebral artery**
26. Thyrocervical trunk
27. Transverse cervical artery

AMPUTATIONS

Define the following terms.

Syme's amputation   Amputation of the foot

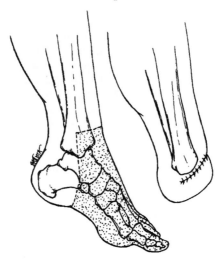

Ray amputation   Removal of the metatarsal head and digit of foot

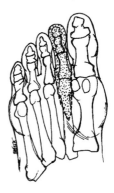

Transmetatarsal amputation

Foot amputation at the level of the metatarsals

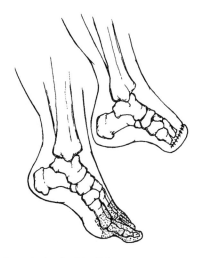

Hip disarticulation

Amputation by hip dislocation

What are 4 indications for amputation?

1. Gross overwhelming infection/ gangrene (refractory)
2. Rest pain or ulcers/infection without any graftable distal arteries
3. Malignant tumors
4. Trauma

What percentage of patients with claudication will receive an amputation in 5 years?

Only approximately 5%

Which type of amputation has the highest healing rate of all the lower extremity amputations?

Above the knee amputation (AKA)

What is the significance of a nonhealing AKA?

Bodes poorly; associated with a high mortality rate

What is the best amputation for a grossly infected limb?

Guillotine amputation with formal closure after infection clears

What is the best graft material after an infection clears?

Saphenous vein graft

Which flap—anterior or posterior—has the best blood supply for a BKA?

The posterior flap has more collaterals than the anterior flap because of the closer proximity to the popliteal artery

Should dog ears be removed from the skin closure during a BKA/AKA?

No (controversial)

What is the best type of suture for apposing the muscle fascia layer of a BKA or an AKA?

Absorbable (e.g., Vicryl)

Should electrocautery be used extensively during an amputation?

No. It is associated with a large necrotic tissue load and may cause infection/ischemia.

What are the 6 principles of operative technique for amputations?

1. Remove bone.
2. Avoid tension on closure.
3. Administer antibiotics.
4. Avoid hematoma.
5. Handle tissue with care.
6. Do not separate skin from underlying fascia.

What is the rate of operative mortality for an AKA or a BKA?

Approximately 10%

What is the most common cause of operative mortality in this group?

Heart attack/arrhythmia (accounts for 50%)

What is the mortality rate 3 years after an AKA or BKA?

Approximately 50%

Will a toe amputation heal in a patient with dry gangrene?

Usually not; therefore, do not perform an amputation until revascularization is completed.

What percentage of patients with an AKA will walk independently?

Only about one-third

What percentage of patients with a BKA will walk independently?

About two-thirds

In a BKA, how long should the fibula be in relation to the tibia?

Approximately 1 cm proximal to the tibia stump

What can help prevent post-BKA knee flexion contracture?

A knee immobilizer (or cast)

What bedside sign is used by many experienced surgeons to determine the level of amputation?

Warm skin

What is the best predictor of failure of a BKA to heal?

Absence of popliteal arterial pulsation on palpation or Doppler; < 70 mm Hg pressure

What toe pressure is thought to correlate with the failure of a transmetatarsal or toe amputation to heal?

Systolic toe pressures < 45 mm Hg (presence of a palpable pedal pulse correlates closely with the healing of a transmetatarsal amputation)

What systolic popliteal pressure is associated with healing of the stump?

> 70 mm Hg by Doppler

What percentage of all BKAs will heal?

Approximately 80%

What are the mortality rates for hip disarticulation, AKA, and BKA?

Hip disarticulation: 80%
AKA: 15%
BKA: 5%

What are the independent (prosthetic) ambulation rates after:

BKA?

66–80%

AKA?

35–50%

Bilateral BKA?

45%

Bilateral AKA?

10%

What is the overall survival rate at 1, 3, and 5 years after lower extremity amputation?	1 year: 75% 3 years: 50% 5 years: 35% Because of associated atherosclerotic lesions elsewhere (e.g., heart)
By how much do energy requirements increase with walking:	
BKA?	50%
AKA?	100%
What is a Gritti-Stokes amputation?	Amputation through the knee joint
Who benefits from a Gritti-Stokes?	Wheelchair-bound patients
Define.	
Lisfranc's amputation	Amputation through the distal tarsal bones
Chopart's amputation	Amputation through the tarsal navicular and calcaneocuboid joints (proximal to tarsal bones)
Pirogoff's amputation	Resect foot and pin heel Calcaneal remnant to tibia/fibula

EXTRACRANIAL CEREBROVASCULAR DISEASE

CAROTID VS. VERTEBROBASILAR DISEASE

How do the plaques in carotid disease differ from those in vertebrobasilar disease?	Carotid: High incidence of ulcerated plaques Vertebral: Usually a smooth intimal surface
Which type is usually associated with unilateral versus bilateral neurologic deficits?	Carotid: Usually unilateral Vertebral: Often bilateral
Where is the bruit auscultated in each type?	Carotid: Anterior border of the sternocleidomastoid muscle near the angle of the mandible Vertebral: Supraclavicular fossa

In which situation are "drop attacks" common?

Vertebrobasilar disease. The patient suddenly falls to the ground because of bilateral lower extremity motor deficit (± loss of consciousness with rapid recovery).

Name the labeled structures of a right carotid endarterectomy (CEA).

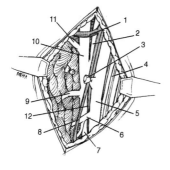

1. Hypoglossal nerve (CN XII)
2. Internal carotid artery
3. Ligated facial vein
4. Sternocleidomastoid muscle
5. Internal jugular vein
6. Superior thyroid vein
7. Common carotid artery
8. Ansa cervicalis
9. Superior thyroid artery
10. External carotid artery
11. Lingual artery
12. Vagus nerve

ANATOMY OF THE VISCERAL BRANCHES OF THE AORTA

MESENTERIC ARTERIES

What are the 3 main mesenteric arteries and the territory of bowel that each supplies?

Celiac artery: Stomach to ampulla of Vater (middle of the second portion of the duodenum)
Superior mesenteric artery (SMA): To the splenic flexure of the colon
Inferior mesenteric artery (IMA): To the rectum

What is the key "watershed" area?

Splenic flexure of the colon (often has a break in the continuity of the marginal artery of Drummond)

What are the branches of the celiac artery?

Left gastric artery
Splenic artery
Hepatic artery

What are the first 2 branches of the SMA?

Inferior pancreaticoduodenal (PD) artery
Middle colic artery

What are the branches of the IMA?

Left colic artery
Sigmoid arteries
Superior hemorrhoidal artery

What is the major arterial collateral path between the celiac artery and the SMA?	Celiac artery → Hepatic artery → Gastroduodenal artery → Superior PD artery → Inferior PD artery → SMA
What is the major arterial collateral path between the SMA and the IMA?	Arch of Riolan: SMA → Middle colic artery (left branch) → Left colic artery (ascending branch) → IMA
What is the "meandering mesenteric artery"?	The tortuous, enlarged, and dilated arch of Riolan that results with increased blood flow through this collateral

RENAL ARTERIES

Renal arteries are located at what lumbar level?	L1 to L2
Is the right renal artery anterior or posterior to the IVC?	Posterior
How is the right renal artery exposed intraoperatively?	Cattel and Kocher maneuvers (medial mobilization of the hepatic flexure of the colon and the third portion of the duodenum) ± retraction of the IVC for exposure of the most proximal portion of the renal artery
What is the most common anatomic "anomaly" of the renal artery?	Accessory renal arteries (seen in 20–25% of the population)

VISCERAL ISCHEMIC SYNDROMES

ACUTE MESENTERIC ISCHEMIA

What are the etiologies?	Embolus Thrombosis Nonocclusive etiologies (i.e., vasospasm associated with low cardiac output, venous thrombosis)
What is the most common surgically treatable cause?	Arterial embolism
What is the most common site of embolism?	Proximal SMA (at the SMA origin or at the takeoff of the middle colic artery)

Why do emboli tend to enter this vessel?

The SMA is large, and its takeoff from the aorta is at an acute angle versus the more perpendicular celiac, IMA, and renal origins.

What are the symptoms?

Early: Severe abdominal pain with fairly benign abdominal findings. Pain is classically "out of proportion to the signs" on physical exam.

Later: Fever, tachycardia, hypotension, vomiting, diarrhea (often heme positive), abdominal distension, peritonitis

What is the general presentation of embolus versus thrombosis?

Embolus: Acute, rapidly progressive symptoms

Thrombosis: More insidious. Patients usually have a history consistent with chronic mesenteric ischemia.

What are the laboratory findings?

Severe leukocytosis (often > 20,000 if infarcted)

Metabolic acidosis (later in the course)

Elevated amylase and lactate values (nonspecific, but helpful)

Which patients often do not have leukocytosis?

Elderly patients

What are the abdominal x-ray findings?

Distended loops of bowel, air-fluid levels, and edematous bowel wall. In the setting of infarction, gas may be seen in the bowel wall or portal venous tree.

What is the diagnostic study of choice?

Angiogram. (Duplex ultrasound is gaining popularity.)

Which view is most helpful, and why?

The lateral view because it facilitates visualization of the classic atherosclerotic ostial lesions

What are the classic angiographic findings for embolus, thrombosis, and nonocclusive etiologies?

Embolus: Abrupt occlusion with a "meniscus sign," usually 5–8 cm from the origin of the SMA

Thrombosis: Occlusion of the origin itself or a very proximal region of the mesenteric arteries

Nonocclusive: Smooth, gradual tapering of more distal branches (because of vasospasm)

When is bowel nonviability determined?	After the revascularization procedure
How is bowel viability assessed intraoperatively?	Gross examination: Palpable pulses, pink color, visible peristalsis Wood's lamp inspection after IV fluorescein Doppler ultrasound of the mesenteric artery adjacent to the bowel in question
When is the decision made to perform a second-look laparotomy?	At the time of the original surgery!
What do the terms "antegrade" and "retrograde" refer to in describing aortovisceral bypass?	The site of aortic anastomosis with respect to the origin of the mesenteric vessel being bypassed (i.e., antegrade is proximal to the origin, retrograde is distal)
Which site is usually preferred, and why?	Antegrade, because it offers better long-term patency, but retrograde is a faster/easier procedure.
What is the mortality rate for acute mesenteric ischemia?	55–85%
What factor accounts for much of this high mortality rate?	Delayed diagnosis

ANEURYSMS

ABDOMINAL AORTIC ANEURYSM (AAA)

What is the characteristic gross appearance of inflammatory AAAs?	Dense, white, fibrotic inflammatory reaction that covers the aorta and adjacent abdominal structures (e.g., duodenum, ureters)
What are the most common etiologies of mycotic AAAs?	*Staphylococcus epidermidis* and *Staphylococcus aureus* *Salmonella* ("Mycotic" does not imply fungal causes in AAAs.)

What is the presentation of inflammatory AAA?

Chronic abdominal pain
Weight loss
Increased erythrocyte sedimentation rate

What are examples of the structural anomalies that can be seen on CT scan?

Retroaortic left renal vein. There is a risk of injury to this vein with aortic cross-clamp.
Horseshoe kidney

What is the classic finding of ruptured AAA on physical exam INSPECTION?

Ecchymosis in the inguinal and groin region (tracking of blood around the abdominal wall from the retroperitoneum)

What complication is common in inflammatory AAAs?

Ureteral obstruction. Inflammatory reaction results in fibrotic attachments with ureters, IVC, etc.

What surgical procedure is used?

"Resection," which is a misnomer because the AAA is usually merely filleted open. Aortic continuity is restored with a prosthetic tube or bifurcation graft (aortoaortic, aortoiliac, or aortofemoral bypass).

What is the graft material of choice?

Dacron (woven or knitted, $\pm$ collagen impregnation)
Second choice: PTFE

What are the 2 surgical approaches?

Transabdominal approach through a midline laparotomy incision
Retroperitoneal approach through a left flank incision

How do you get to the aorta via the retroperitoneal approach?

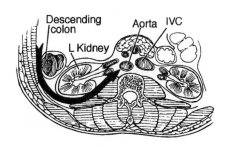

In a patient with a ruptured AAA, what is the first step after midline laparotomy?

Immediate compression of the supraceliac aorta against the vertebral bodies **through the lesser sac**

What are the next steps?	The left crus of the diaphragm is divided, the supraceliac aorta is clamped, the neck of the AAA (usually infrarenal) is exposed and clamped, the supraceliac clamp is removed, and the graft is placed.
What frequently obstructs access to the neck of the AAA in the transabdominal approach?	Left renal vein
What is the presentation of aortocaval fistula?	High-output CHF, hypotension, cyanosis, venous distension of the lower extremities, abdominal bruit, and palpable abdominal thrill
What is the treatment?	The fistula is closed: achieve proximal and distal control of the aorta and IVC; make an incision in the aortic graft; repair the fistula from within graft with large suture bites; and close the aortic graft.
What is excluded in the setting of pseudoaneurysm?	Graft infection

PERIPHERAL ARTERY ANEURYSM

What is the most common etiology of true peripheral aneurysm?	Atherosclerosis
What are the most common etiologies of false peripheral aneurysm?	Vascular bypass procedures Trauma
What are the most common locations of true aneurysms?	Popliteal artery (70%) Femoral artery (15–20%)
What diagnostic study is performed in patients with true peripheral artery aneurysms, and why?	Complete arteriogram of the abdominal aorta and its branches to the lower extremity. Between 75% and 85% of these patients have an additional aneurysm elsewhere.
What is the most common complication of true aneurysms?	Distal arterial occlusion caused by emboli from a mural thrombus within the aneurysm. Rupture is rare.

What percentage of true aneurysms are bilateral?	60–75%
What are the indications for surgery?	Symptoms caused by embolic events or local compression Aneurysm > 2 cm
What is the surgical procedure?	Excision or exclusion (proximal and distal ligation) of the aneurysm (to prevent further embolic events) plus a bypass procedure

VISCERAL ARTERY ANEURYSM

What is the etiology?	Medial degeneration of the arterial wall
What are the most common locations?	Splenic artery (60%) Hepatic artery (20%)
What is the presentation?	Vague upper quadrant or epigastric pain is occasionally present, but most patients are asymptomatic.
What is the most common complication?	Rupture
What is the incidence of splenic artery and hepatic artery aneurysm rupture?	Splenic artery: 2% Hepatic artery: 20%
What is the classic sequence of events in splenic artery aneurysm rupture?	"Double rupture": Herald bleed into the lesser omental sac (± transient hypotension); then rupture into the peritoneal cavity (± exsanguination)
What factor significantly increases the risk of rupture in patients with splenic artery aneurysm?	Pregnancy
What is the mortality rate if rupture occurs in the pregnant patient?	> 70%
What are the indications for treatment?	Symptomatic patient Aneurysm > 2 cm Splenic artery aneurysm in a patient who is pregnant or who plans to become pregnant

What surgical procedure is performed?

Excision or exclusion of aneurysm ± bypass procedure
Splenectomy is sometimes performed.
For intrahepatic aneurysms, hepatic resection may be indicated.

NONATHEROSCLEROTIC VASCULAR DISEASE

What feature common to these disorders may facilitate their diagnosis?

Symptoms of limb ischemia in a preatherosclerotic age-group of patients

THROMBOANGIITIS OBLITERANS (TAO; BUERGER'S DISEASE)

What is the target patient population?

Young men (20–35 years old) who are heavy tobacco abusers

What are the classic histologic findings?

Nonnecrotizing, segmental panarteritis with fibrous obliteration of the arterial lumen on healing; intraluminal thrombosis

How does TAO differ from atherosclerotic disease?

Involves all 3 layers of artery

Involves more peripheral vessels (small and medium arteries)

As many as 40% of patients have symptomatic upper extremity involvement

What is the etiology?

Uncertain, but believed to be autoimmune (possible association with human leukocyte antigens [HLAs] A9 and B5)

What are the symptoms?

Excruciating rest pain
Tender, bilateral digital ulceration and gangrene
Occasionally, claudication (but much less frequently than with atherosclerotic occlusive disease)

What are the classic arteriographic findings?

Uninvolved large vessels with abrupt occlusion in medium and small arteries; "corkscrew" or "tree root" appearance (thought to be caused by dilated vasa vasorum collaterals around the occlusion)

What treatment is most effective?

Abstinence from tobacco (disease usually goes into remission)

What is the surgical treatment?	Sympathectomy (for vasodilation; yields transient improvement in symptoms) Digital amputation for gangrene
Why is surgical bypass rarely possible?	Diffuse distal disease (i.e., no target for bypass)

POPLITEAL ENTRAPMENT SYNDROMES

What is the target patient population?	Young men (< 40 years old)
What is the etiology?	Congenital anomaly in the development of the popliteal artery or neighboring muscles, resulting in arterial compression
What structure is most often responsible for compression?	Medial head of the gastrocnemius muscle (> 80%)
Is involvement usually unilateral or bilateral?	Unilateral (75%)
What is the most common symptom?	Intermittent claudication of the leg or foot. Rest pain or gangrene is rare.
What is the classic finding on physical examination?	Loss of pedal pulses with ankle flexion or knee extension (contraction of the gastrocnemius muscle)
What diagnostic study is performed?	Arteriogram taken with the leg in various positions to show intermittent occlusion
What is the treatment?	Myotomy to divide the entrapping muscle ± Femorodistal popliteal bypass (frequently necessary because of popliteal stenosis or aneurysm)
What disorder mimics popliteal entrapment syndrome?	Adventitial cystic degeneration of popliteal artery (enlarging, **subadventitial** mucin-containing cysts causing obstruction)
How is this disorder distinguished from popliteal entrapment?	Arteriogram of adventitial cystic degeneration shows the pathognomonic "scimitar sign" (external compression of popliteal lumen by expanding cysts).

TAKAYASU'S ARTERITIS

What is the target patient population?	Young women (< 30 years old), often with Asian ancestry
What vessels are most commonly involved?	Thoracic aorta ± arch vessels (types I–IV) Abdominal aorta (types II and III) Occasionally, the pulmonary arteries (type IV)
What are the early symptoms?	Fever, arthralgia, myalgia, anorexia
What is the medical treatment?	High-dose steroids
What is the surgical treatment?	Bypass procedures for stenoses. (Endarterectomy fails in this disorder.)
What is the relative contraindication to surgery?	Active arteritis. The vascular inflammation must be reduced with steroids before a bypass procedure is attempted.
What are the complications?	Stroke Hypertension (usually caused by renal artery stenosis) CHF

VENOUS AND LYMPHATIC DISEASE

VENOUS ANATOMY AND PHYSIOLOGY

What is the basic gross anatomy of the venous circulation?	The superficial venous system is connected to the deep venous system by perforating veins that pass through the fascial layer of the extremity. The perforating veins have valves that are oriented to permit flow to pass only from the superficial to the deep system (except in the foot, where the reverse is true).
What are the 2 main superficial veins of the lower extremity and the deep veins they feed?	Greater saphenous vein: Empties into common femoral vein Lesser saphenous vein: Empties into popliteal vein

What is the main mechanism by which blood is returned to the heart?	Pumping action of the muscles of the leg, especially the calf muscles. Venous pressure normally decreases to less than half its resting level with exercise.
What are the sinusoids?	Thin-walled venous cavities within the muscles of the lower extremity. They play an essential role in the musculovenous pump.

DIAGNOSIS OF VENOUS INSUFFICIENCY

What 3 basic lesions lead to venous hypertension in the lower extremity?	Valvular incompetence Ineffective musculovenous pump Venous obstruction
What 2 clinical tests are used to evaluate the venous system of the lower extremity?	Trendelenburg test Perthes test
Describe how each test is performed.	1. Trendelenburg test: The leg is raised to drain the venous system, and a venous tourniquet is applied over the saphenofemoral junction. The patient then stands. 2. Perthes test: A venous tourniquet is applied proximal to varicoses or suspected incompetent perforators. Then the patient ambulates.
What is the purpose of each test?	Trendelenburg test: To exclude saphenofemoral and perforator valvular incompetence Perthes test: To exclude perforator valvular incompetence and deep venous occlusion
In the Trendelenburg test, what do the following observations suggest?	
Slow filling of varicosities before the tourniquet is released	Competent perforators (if filling is rapid, incompetent)

Rapid filling of varicosities when the tourniquet is released	Incompetent saphenofemoral valve
In the Perthes test, what do the following observations suggest?	
Increase in varicosities with exercise	DVT
Decrease in varicosities with exercise	Normal deep venous system and competent perforators
What is the diagnostic study of choice for venous disease, and why?	Duplex ultrasound: Shows the 2 basic pathologic venous lesions (valvular incompetence and venous occlusion)

LOWER EXTREMITY VARICOSITIES

What is the claim to fame of lower extremity varicosities?	Most common lower extremity vascular disorder, affecting 10–20% of population
What are the "types" and their main etiologies?	Primary varicosities: Genetic predisposition (exact mechanism is uncertain) Secondary varicosities: DVT, resulting in shunting of blood through incompetent perforators to the superficial system
What are the symptoms?	Fatigue, heaviness, or aching of the limb, especially when standing erect
What is the conservative therapy?	Elastic support stockings; elevation of the affected extremity when sitting
What are the indications for surgery?	Cosmetic Symptomatic (e.g., aching) Occasionally, complications of chronic venous insufficiency (e.g., recurrent superficial thrombophlebitis, ulcer)
What is the most frequently performed procedure?	Simple sclerotherapy (injection of a sclerosing agent into the varicose veins)

What agent is used?	Sodium tetradecyl sulfate
What is the contraindication to this therapy?	Incompetent saphenofemoral or saphenopopliteal valves
What is the procedure of choice if simple sclerotherapy is contraindicated?	Proximal ligation and division of the greater saphenous vein at the saphenofemoral junction Sclerotherapy or vein stripping (either of these ablation techniques is satisfactory)
What is the contraindication to proximal ligation or vein stripping?	DVT, which results in venous drainage, primarily through the superficial system
What are the other surgical options?	Procedures typically used for chronic venous insufficiency (e.g., subfascial ligation of perforators, valve transplant). Rarely indicated for simple varicose veins.

CHRONIC VENOUS INSUFFICIENCY

What are the etiologies?	Valvular venous incompetence (90%) Venous obstruction (10%) secondary to postphlebitic syndrome
What is the primary physiologic derangement?	Chronic venous hypertension
What is the result?	Local hypertension reduces capillary perfusion and causes interstitial accumulation of hemosiderin and fibrin (through dilated endothelial pores). Oxygen transport to tissue is reduced.
What are the clinical manifestations of reduced tissue oxygenation?	Poor healing of cutaneous traumatic lesions, eventually followed by spontaneous breakdown of the skin
What are the classic cutaneous changes of chronic venous insufficiency?	Brawny edema, hyperpigmentation, stasis dermatitis Liposclerosis (thick, hardened subcutaneous tissue because of fibrin deposits) Venous ulceration

What is the classic location of venous ulcers?

Superior and posterior to medial malleolus, the site of 5–6 perforators from the greater saphenous vein of the superficial venous system to the deep posterior tibial vein

Are these ulcers painful or painless?

Usually painless (unless infected)

What are the most common organisms associated with infected venous ulcers?

Staphylococcus aureus
Streptococcus faecalis
Klebsiella

What is Marjolin's ulcer?

Malignant transformation of a chronic venous ulcer

What is the conservative management of chronic venous insufficiency?

Meticulous skin care, limb elevation, elastic compression stockings, and hydrophobic dressing

What additional therapy is useful in the management of venous ulcer?

Unna boot (gauze with calamine, zinc oxide, and gelatin firmly wrapped around the foot or lower leg, and changed every week for 6–12 weeks)

When is this therapeutic adjunct contraindicated?

Patients with concurrent arterial occlusive disease

How successful is conservative therapy?

90–95%

What are the indications for surgery?

Persistent venous ulcer in:
1. Relatively young, active patients. Repetitive calf muscle contraction usually prevents healing with conservative therapy alone.
2. Compliant patients despite aggressive conservative management

What are the surgical options for incompetent valves?

1. Subfascial ligation of incompetent perforators (Linton procedure)
2. Correction of incompetence of deep venous valves by suture plication of the cusps (valvuloplasty)
3. Venous segment transposition, valve transplant, or valve banding

What is the procedure for venous obstruction?	Saphenous vein venous bypass procedure
What is the surgical management of venous ulcers?	Excision or débridement, followed by coverage with split-thickness skin graft

UPPER EXTREMITY DEEP VENOUS THROMBOSIS

What are the most common etiologies?	Effort-induced thrombosis (Paget-von Schrötter syndrome) Subclavian thrombosis caused by a central IV catheter
What is the usual presentation?	Edema, mild cyanosis, pain, and heavy sensation of the arm
Why is massive thrombosis rare?	Extensive venous collaterals around the shoulder girdle
What is the incidence of pulmonary embolus?	10–15% (higher than previously believed)
What is the treatment of effort-induced thrombosis?	Regional thrombolytic (urokinase) therapy; correction of thoracic outlet obstruction (if present)
What is the treatment of catheter-related thrombosis?	The catheter is removed if possible, and systemic heparinization is followed by 1–2 months of Coumadin therapy.
Why are these etiologies managed differently?	Effort-induced thrombi occur in young, healthy individuals who are at low risk for hemorrhage. In an ill or elderly patient with a central venous catheter, thrombolytic therapy is more likely to cause bleeding.
What is the prognosis?	Only 15–30% of patients have complete resolution of symptoms.

VASCULAR ACCESS FOR HEMODIALYSIS

What is the minimum flow rate required to drive the hemodialysis process?	150 mL/min

ACCESS FOR CHRONIC HEMODIALYSIS

What are the 2 general types of chronic access procedures?

1. Autogenous fistula: Direct anastomosis of artery to vein
2. Interposition AV fistula: Interposition of a prosthetic graft between artery and vein

Which specific type is the preferred first operation, and why?

Brescia-Cimino (aka "Cimino") autogenous fistula: Radial artery to cephalic vein. Autogenous fistulas are associated with improved long-term patency and reduced risk of infection; further, the Brescia-Cimino fistula requires minimal, superficial dissection.

What percentage of patients are candidates for an autogenous fistula?

15–20%. These patients, who often have a long history of illness, have few patent upper extremity veins.

What is the prosthetic material of choice for interposition AV fistula?

PTFE

What is the most common site used?

Forearm of the nondominant hand: PTFE loop between the radial (or brachial) artery and the antebrachial region vein (e.g., cephalic, basilic)

Compare, and explain the rationales for, the postoperative waiting periods required before the use of autogenous and interposition AV fistulas.

Autogenous: 3–6 weeks, to allow fistula to mature. The vein must hypertrophy and "arterialize" to permit repeated punctures with the large hemodialysis needle.

Interposition: 2 weeks. The prosthetic material will be the site of needle puncture, but a fibrous scar must develop around the graft so that hematomas will not develop at the puncture sites. (Hematomas predispose patients to infection.)

What is the most common cause of failure of an AV fistula?

Thrombosis as a result of poor **venous outflow** (acutely because of technical error, chronically because of neointimal hyperplasia)

What are the treatment options for thrombosis?	Thrombectomy (first-line procedure) Percutaneous balloon angioplasty Thrombolytic (urokinase) therapy Operative revision of fistula (e.g., patch angioplasty, new venous anastomosis)
In a patient who has distal extremity pain, what must be ruled out?	Arterial steal syndrome (ischemia distal to a fistula caused by retrograde flow through the distal artery)
What is the treatment?	Acutely, pressure is applied to the fistula to restore antegrade flow to the limb. Banding or ligation of the fistula or revision of arterial anastomosis is then performed.
What are the other complications of AV fistula?	Venous aneurysmal dilation caused by needle puncture Limb edema caused by venous hypertension distal to the fistula Pseudoaneurysm at the anastomosis or needle puncture site Infection Rarely, high-output cardiac failure caused by AV shunting
What are the 1-year and 5-year patency rates between autogenous and interposition AV fistulas?	1 year: Autogenous 65–80%; interposition: 75–80% 5 year: Autogenous 65–80%; interposition: 40–50%

OTHER VASCULAR TOPICS

CAROTID BODY TUMOR

What is it?	Tumor in the carotid body (bifurcation of common carotid artery)
What is the origin?	Afferent ganglion of the glossopharyngeal nerve
What are the gross characteristics?	Well encapsulated and tightly adherent to the adventitial surface of the carotid arteries
What is the presentation?	Asymptomatic mass at the angle of the jaw

What is the classic finding on physical exam?

Mass that is mobile in the horizontal axis (anteriorly and posteriorly), but fixed in the vertical axis

What is the classic radiographic finding?

Splaying of the bifurcation of the carotid artery. The carotid body rests in the crotch of the bifurcation.

What is the treatment?

Preoperative embolization to reduce blood loss at the time of surgery (very vascular tumors); usually reserved for masses > 3 cm

Excision of tumor ± carotid reconstruction

What is the incidence of metastasis?

5%

Section III

Subspecialty Surgery

64

Pediatric Surgery

What are the caloric and requirements by age for the following patients (per kg/day)?

Premature infants	80 kcal, 1–3 g
Children < 1 year old?	100 kcal, 3 g
Children 1–7 years old	85 kcal, 2 g
Children 7–12 years old	70 kcal, 2 g
Youths 12–18 years old	40 kcal, 1.5 g

What is the unique IV fluid route in children < 6 years of age?

Intraosseus

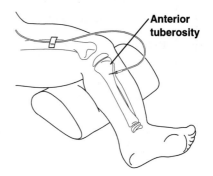

Anterior tuberosity

Define the *extracorporeal membrane oxygenation* (ECMO) circuit.

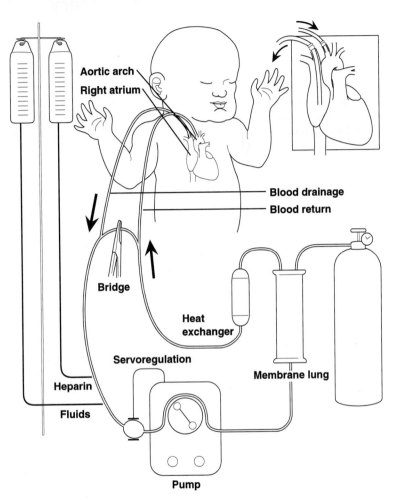

Aortic arch
Right atrium
Blood drainage
Blood return
Bridge
Heat exchanger
Servoregulation
Membrane lung
Heparin
Fluids
Pump

Define the Kasai procedure for biliary atresia.

Roux-en-Y to fibrous cord representing the atretic bile duct

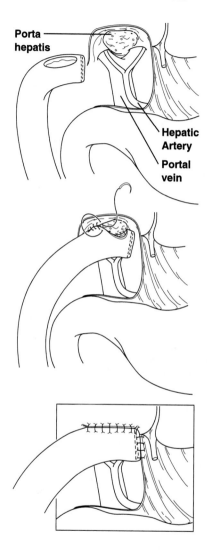

Porta hepatis

Hepatic Artery

Portal vein

FOREIGN BODIES: TRACHEA

What age group is affected most often?	2–4 years of age
What is the usual presentation?	1. Cough, wheezing, dyspnea, inspiratory and expiratory stridor, and/or fever 2. Unilateral diminished breath sounds or wheezing
A tracheal foreign body is often confused with what other diagnosis?	Severe asthma
How is the diagnosis made?	Neck and chest plain x-ray may show a radiopaque foreign body, a hyperinflated lobe or segment, or an atelectatic lobe or segment.
What are the indications for intervention?	Highly suggestive signs and symptoms with confirmatory x-rays or a suspicious history in a toddler
What is the usual treatment?	Rigid bronchoscopy with forceps retrieval of foreign body

FOREIGN BODIES: ESOPHAGUS

What are the common esophageal levels of lodgment?	Sites of esophageal narrowing: 1. Cricopharyngeal muscle 2. Arch of the aorta (level of carina) 3. Gastroesophageal junction
What is the usual presentation?	Drooling, dysphagia, and pain
What is the life-threatening sequela of a long-standing untreated esophageal foreign body?	Mediastinitis after erosion through the esophageal wall
How is the diagnosis made?	Plain x-ray showing radiopaque objects
What is the usual treatment?	1. At the level of the cricopharyngeus and carina: Rigid or flexible esophagoscopy with mechanical retrieval by forceps

2. At the gastroesophageal junction:
   Observation
   Most surgeons discourage the use of a
   Fogarty balloon catheter to retrieve
   esophageal foreign bodies.

**What are the risks of
treatment?**

1. Esophageal perforation
2. Aspiration, which is prevented by
   placing the patient in the prone
   position

EVENTRATION OF THE DIAPHRAGM

What is it?

Lack of a normal muscular component of
the diaphragm; results in an intact yet
elevated diaphragm

**What are the 2 types and
the etiology of each?**

1. Congenital: Embryologic muscular
   defect
2. Acquired: Usually caused by phrenic
   nerve injury

**What is the usual
presentation?**

Varies from asymptomatic to respiratory
distress, especially in infants, elevated
diaphragm (usually left)

**What diagnostic study is
performed?**

Fluoroscopy, which shows paradoxic
motion of the diaphragm

What is the usual treatment?

1. Asymptomatic patient: None
2. Symptomatic patient: Plication and
   stabilization of the diaphragm in the
   expiratory position

CONGENITAL PULMONARY CYSTIC DISEASES

What are the 4 types?

1. Cystic adenomatoid malformation
   (CAM)
2. Pulmonary sequestration
3. Bronchogenic cyst
4. Congenital lobar overinflation

Describe each type.

   CAM

Cystic and solid masses of immature lung
tissue that communicate with the normal
airway

Pulmonary sequestration	Collection of abnormal lung tissue with systemic venous drainage
Bronchogenic cyst	Extrapulmonary cysts, formed from immature bronchial tissue separated from the lung during early embryonic development, lined with ciliated columnar epithelium, and surrounded by a fibrous wall that contains cartilage
Congenital lobar overinflation	Normal lung tissue with abnormally formed bronchus that causes air trapping and overinflation

What is the usual presentation?

1. Respiratory distress caused by compression of a normal lung in the newborn
2. Recurrent infections in the older child
3. Bronchogenic cysts and extrapulmonary sequestrations are usually asymptomatic.

What diagnostic studies are performed?

1. Chest CT scan (study of choice)
2. Ultrasound
3. Esophagoscopy for patients with dysphagia
4. MRI and aortography, which can show systemic vasculature in sequestration

What is the usual treatment?

1. Bronchogenic cysts are excised.
2. Lobectomy is the treatment of choice for other congenital cystic diseases of the lung. It is well tolerated in infants, the complication rate is lower than that for segmental resections, and the lung parenchyma is still growing in small children, with resultant formation of new alveoli.

IMPERFORATE ANUS

Why is hyperchloremic acidosis associated with imperforate anus?

Colon absorbs Cl⁻ from urine from a bladder/urethra fistula.

CHOLEDOCHAL CYST

What are the anatomic variants of choledochal cyst?

Type I—Dilation of the common bile duct
Type II—Lateral saccular cystic dilation
Type III—Choledochocele represented by an intraduodenal cyst
Type IV—Multiple extrahepatic cysts, intrahepatic cysts, or both
Type V—Single or multiple intrahepatic cysts

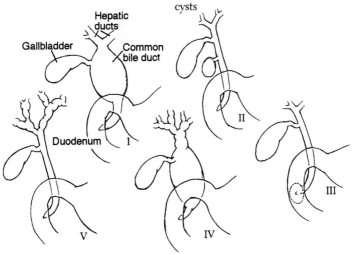

DUODENAL OBSTRUCTION IN THE NEWBORN

What are the causes of duodenal obstruction in the newborn?

1. Duodenal stenosis
2. Duodenal atresia
3. Duodenal web
4. Annular pancreas

What is an annular pancreas?

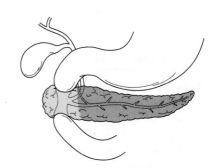

What are the usual locations?	90% occur distal to ampulla of Vater; 10% occur proximal to ampulla
What is the usual presentation?	1. Feeding intolerance and bilious vomiting in the first 24–48 hours of life 2. Distended stomach with an otherwise scaphoid abdomen
Are associated anomalies common?	Yes
What is the most common anomaly?	20–40% also have trisomy 21 (Down's syndrome); congenital heart defects are also seen.
What is the classic finding on x-ray?	Plain x-rays may show a "double bubble" (air-distended (1) stomach and (2) duodenum).
What additional study may be performed, and why?	Upper GI series, if the diagnosis is in doubt or malrotation is suspected
Why is surgery performed promptly?	Lethal malrotation is often included in the differential diagnosis.
What is the usual surgical treatment?	1. Duodenostomy (primary or bypass) 2. Duodenojejunostomy, if distal duodenal obstruction is present
What procedure is usually performed for duodenal webs?	Web resection with longitudinal duodenotomy

ENTERIC DUPLICATIONS

What is it?	An "extra" short parallel GI tract tissue forming a mesenteric cyst or cyst within bowel wall
What is the most common site of duplication?	Small bowel
What is the treatment?	Surgical resection

What percentage of duplications communicate with bowel lumen?	20%

INTESTINAL ATRESIA

What is intestinal atresia?	Intestinal obstruction from stenosis or atresia of the jejunum, ileum, or colon; thought to be caused by a vascular accident in utero or by intrauterine volvulus, hernia, intussusception, or malrotation
What are the types?	Type I: Intraluminal diaphragm or web Type II: Fibrous cord connecting 2 blind ends, with the mesentery intact Type IIIa: Discontinuous bowel with a V-shaped mesenteric defect (most common type) Type IIIb: Apple-peel deformity Type IV: Multiple atretic segments separated by relatively normal bowel
What is the usual presentation?	1. Antenatal polyhydramnios 2. Bilious vomiting 3. Abdominal distension 4. Failure to pass meconium
What contrast study is performed to aid diagnosis?	Contrast enema. Upper GI is often unnecessary and may complicate surgery.
What type of bowel biopsy may be performed during the evaluation?	Suction rectal biopsy
Why is this biopsy performed?	To rule out Hirschsprung's disease
What is the usual surgical treatment?	Resection of the affected bowel with primary anastomosis
What technical points should be considered for an optimal surgical result?	1. Preservation of bowel length, regardless of the number of anastomoses needed 2. Tapering of the dilated proximal end, to reduce the size discrepancy 3. Preservation of the ileocecal valve

GASTROINTESTINAL HEMANGIOMAS

What is the most common complication?	Bleeding (characteristically chronic and intermittent)
What 4 syndromes are associated with GI hemangiomas?	1. Osler-Weber-Rendu syndrome 2. Klippel-Trenaunay syndrome 3. Turner's syndrome 4. von Hippel-Lindau syndrome
What radiologic studies are usually performed?	1. Barium enema or enteroclysis to show mucosal filling defects or pseudopolyps 2. Selective angiography to show large aberrant vessels, dilated small vessels, rapid venous filling, or vascular tufts
What is the usual surgical treatment?	Careful cautery, laser, or ligature ablation of lesions. If multiple lesions are present, conserve bowel length by careful harvesting and segmental resection of clustered lesions.

PEDIATRIC HEPATOBILIARY AND PANCREATIC DISORDERS

HEPATIC NEOPLASMS

HEMANGIOMA

What is the usual location of hemangiomas?	Multicentric origin; therefore, often confused with metastases
What is the claim to fame of hemangiomas?	Most common benign liver tumor ($> 50\%$)
What is the most common symptom?	Upper abdominal discomfort
What diagnostic studies are performed?	Doppler ultrasound, dynamic CT, MRI, angiography, and tagged RBC scan (technetium-99m, ^{99m}Tc)
What are the associated complications?	1. Intraperitoneal bleeding 2. Chronic or subacute heart failure secondary to AV shunting through tumor vasculature 3. Thrombocytopenia and angiopathic anemia secondary to platelet or RBC trapping in tumor vasculature

| What is the usual treatment? | 1. Can be watched if the tumor is small (< 4 cm) and asymptomatic |
| | 2. Surgical resection or embolization (interventional radiology) if complications (see above) occur |

HEPATIC HAMARTOMAS

| What is a hepatic hamartoma? | Benign tumor secondary to new growth of **normal** epithelial tissues in the liver |

Hepatoblastoma

| Is hepatoblastoma benign or malignant? | Malignant |

| What is the average age at diagnosis? | 1 year |

| What laboratory value is frequently elevated? | α-Fetoprotein (> 90%) |

Hepatoblastoma is associated with what:

| Orthopedic abnormalities, and why? | Multiple pathologic fractures caused by abnormal calcium metabolism |

| Genitourinary abnormalities, and why? | Isosexual precocity, with genital enlargement and pubic hair secondary to human chorionic gonadotropin (hCG) production (10% of males) |

| What is the usual treatment? | Surgical resection and chemotherapy (doxorubicin, cisplatin) |

HEPATOCELLULAR CARCINOMA

| How is hepatocellular carcinoma histologically distinguished from the adult form? | Histologically indistinguishable: Invasive, multicentric, and frequently bile-stained (unlike hepatoblastoma) |

| What are the usual sites of metastatic spread? | Metastases to regional nodes, lung, and bone are common at diagnosis. |

| What is the average age at diagnosis? | 9–10 years |

What is the usual clinical presentation?	Abdominal pain, anorexia, and weight loss are common. Jaundice is seen in 20% of patients.
What laboratory values are frequently elevated?	1. α-Fetoprotein (in 50%); levels are lower than in hepatoblastoma 2. Liver enzymes and alkaline phosphatase
What is the usual treatment?	Same as hepatoblastoma (combination of surgical resection and chemotherapy), but chemotherapy is not as effective

RHABDOMYOSARCOMA

What is it?	Striated muscle sarcoma
Define the stages of rhabdomyosarcoma.	
Stage I	Localized, completely excised tumor
Stage II	Microscopic residual disease
Stage III	Gross residual disease
Stage IV	Distant metastases
What is the 3-year survival rate at each stage?	
Stage I	Approximately 80%
Stage II	Approximately 70%
Stage III	Approximately 50%
Stage IV	Approximately 25% (55% at 5 years)

PANCREAS DIVISUM

What is pancreas divisum?	Anatomic variant that occurs when the dorsal and ventral duct structures of the pancreas do not fuse during embryologic development

What is the main pancreatic duct?	Duct of Wirsung
What duct persists in pancreas divisum?	Duct of Santorini
What is the incidence?	10% of the population
What is the diagnostic study of choice?	Endoscopic retrograde cholangiopancreatography (ERCP)
What is the most common complication?	Repeated bouts of pancreatitis
What is the most common indication for surgery?	Documented recurrent acute pancreatitis
What is the procedure of choice?	Open dorsal duct sphincteroplasty
What procedure is performed in a patient with chronic pancreatitis and a dilated dorsal duct?	Anterior longitudinal pancreaticojejunostomy with a Roux-en-Y loop

PEDIATRIC GENITOURINARY DISORDERS

HORSESHOE KIDNEY

What is a horseshoe kidney?	Renal fusion anomaly in which the lower poles of 2 distinct renal masses are joined by renal parenchyma or fibrous tissue (isthmus of kidney)
What is the claim to fame of horseshoe kidney?	Most common renal fusion anomaly
What is the incidence?	Approximately 1:1000
What causes most complications?	Collecting system anomalies that result in hydronephrosis, infection, and renal stones
Affected individuals are at increased risk for what tumors?	Hydronephromas, Wilms' tumor, and collecting system and parenchymal tumors

INFANTILE POLYCYSTIC KIDNEY DISEASE

What is the claim to fame of infantile polycystic kidney disease?	Although rare, it is the most common genetically determined cystic disease of the kidney in childhood.
What is the route of genetic transmission?	Autosomal recessive
What is the finding on physical exam?	Palpable, often visible, massively enlarged hard flank masses at birth
What is included in the differential diagnosis?	1. Hydronephrosis 2. Renal neoplasm 3. Renal vein thrombosis
What diagnostic tests are performed?	1. Excretory urography: Radial streams of contrast material from the medulla to the surface of the cortex, with alternating radiolucent and radiodense areas (sun ray effect) 2. Ultrasound: Hyperechogenic masses and disseminated small cysts
What other organ is also diseased in these patients?	Liver: Proliferation and dilation of the bile ducts, with varying amounts of periportal fibrosis and, occasionally, portal hypertension
What is the prognosis for these patients?	Poor. Death usually occurs in the first several months of life.

URETEROPELVIC JUNCTION (UPJ) OBSTRUCTION

What is UPJ obstruction?	Fibrosis or interruption of smooth muscle continuity across the UPJ, interrupting the orderly transmission of peristaltic waves
What are the associated complications?	1. Hydronephrosis 2. Urinary tract infection (UTI) 3. If uncorrected, renal failure
What diagnostic studies are performed?	1. Ultrasound: Renal pelvic dilation 2. Renal scintigraphy if ultrasound shows persistent hydronephrosis. Persistence of the radioactive label in the renal pelvis suggests UPJ obstruction.

What additional study is included to rule out vesicoureteral reflux?	Voiding cystourethrogram (VCUG)
What is the surgical treatment?	Pyeloplasty to enlarge the UPJ
When is antenatal intervention considered?	Only if ultrasound shows significant oligohydramnios, no cystic changes of kidneys, bilateral hydronephrosis, and impending pulmonary hypoplasia

VESICOURETERAL REFLUX

What is vesicoureteral reflux?	Retrograde passage of urine from the bladder into the ureter
What is the sex predilection?	Girls account for 85% of cases.
What are the complications?	1. UTI 2. Renal failure
What is the usual treatment?	Nonoperative management (including suppression antibiotics and close follow-up with urine cultures, cystourethrograms, and measurement of serum creatinine values) is successful in most patients.
What are the indications for surgery?	1. Recurrent UTI 2. Progressive renal injury 3. Noncompliance 4. Severe reflux
What is the surgical treatment?	Ureteral reimplantation with a long segment of the intravesicular ureter

URETHRAL VALVES

What are urethral valves?	Exaggerated forms of the normal small fold in the male urethra
What is the usual presentation?	UTI, bed wetting, poor urinary stream, urinary frequency, hematuria, and acute urinary retention
What is the diagnostic study of choice?	VCUG

What is the surgical treatment?	Endoscopic valve resection. If the infant is too small to permit use of the scope, temporary vesicostomy is performed until the infant is several months old.

EXSTROPHY OF THE BLADDER

What is exstrophy of the bladder?	Defect in the ventral abdominal wall coverage of at least part of the bladder, with pubic diastasis
Males have a 10-fold increased risk of what disorder?	Cryptorchidism
What hernia is common with bladder exstrophy?	Inguinal hernia
If untreated, all patients are at increased risk for what disorder?	Bladder carcinoma
What is the surgical treatment?	Multistage procedure: 1. Primary bladder closure (accompanied by herniorrhaphy and orchiopexy, if indicated), which causes incontinence 2. Epispadias repair during the next 3 years as bladder enlarges; bladder neck reconstruction to achieve continence at age 3–4

HYPOSPADIAS

What is hypospadias?	Anomaly in which the urethral meatus opens onto the ventral surface of the penis, proximal to the end of the glans
What is the incidence?	1:300 live male births
What is the etiology?	Defect in androgen stimulation of the developing penis, precluding complete formation of urethra and surrounding structures
What are the indications for surgical treatment?	All patients are offered surgical treatment for psychological reasons.

What is the timing of surgery?	Within the first year of life
What are the primary goals of surgery?	Straightening the penis and placing the meatus at the tip of the glans

PRUNE BELLY SYNDROME

What is the triad of physical findings?	1. Congenital absence or hypoplasia of abdominal wall musculature 2. Urinary tract abnormalities, with a large hypotonic bladder, dilated ureters, and dilated prostatic urethra 3. Bilateral cryptorchidism
What is another name for this syndrome?	Eagle-Barrett syndrome

TERATOMAS

What are teratomas?	Germ cell tumors containing elements of all 3 layers (endoderm, mesoderm, ectoderm). They contain tissue foreign to the anatomic location (formed from tissue that could not have resulted from metaplasia of cells normally found there).
What are the 5 common components?	1. Skin 2. Teeth 3. CNS tissue 4. Respiratory and alimentary mucosa 5. Cartilage and bone
Why do they cause symptoms?	Obstruction or compression of viscera
What are the 3 tumor markers?	1. hCG: Choriocarcinoma 2. α-Fetoprotein: Tumors containing yolk sac carcinoma and embryonal carcinoma; teratoma containing immature tissue 3. Lactate dehydrogenase isoenzyme 1: Yolk sac tumors (not specific)
Which type of teratoma:	
Is most common in neonates?	Sacrococcygeal

Is most common in adolescents?	Ovarian
Presents as a suprapubic mass?	Ovarian
Is extragonadal and is seen only in males?	Gastric
Is the most common extragonadal type?	Sacrococcygeal
What is the characteristic appearance of the sacrococcygeal type?	Protruding from the space between anus and coccyx, and usually covered with normal intact skin
What is included in the differential diagnosis of sacrococcygeal teratoma?	1. Myelomeningocele 2. Pilonidal cyst
What is the treatment of sacrococcygeal teratoma?	1. Surgical excision in continuity with excision of coccyx 2. If malignant, aggressive chemotherapy
What is the usual presentation of gastric teratoma?	Palpable epigastric mass and/or GI bleed
What is the treatment of gastric teratoma?	Surgical excision
What is the prognosis for gastric teratoma?	If excised completely, no additional therapy is required because these tumors are benign.
Which teratoma is often called a "dermoid" tumor?	Ovarian
What is the source of pain from this teratoma?	Volvulus of the ovarian pedicle
What must be included in the differential diagnosis?	Pregnancy
What is the treatment of ovarian teratoma?	Surgical excision, leaving functional ovarian tissue only if tumor is clearly benign

MISCELLANEOUS

What is a Breslow tape?	Tape used in trauma to estimate body weight of children based on height, IV fluid boluses, etc.
What is the #1 cause of death in children 1–15 years of age?	Trauma
What is the rule of 3's for barium reduction of intussusception?	3 feet high 3 tries

65

Plastic Surgery

What are the facial Langer's lines?

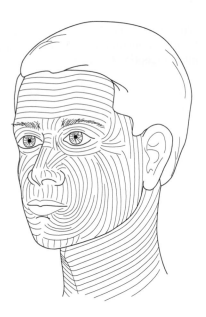

ABNORMALITIES OF WOUND HEALING

What is a hypertrophic scar?

A cicatrix that shows excessive deposition of collagen within the margins of the healing wound. The scar usually diminishes over time.

What is a keloid?

A scar with excessive deposition of collagen outside the margin of the healing wound; more common in African Americans than in Caucasians

What is the treatment of hypertrophic scars and keloids?

Excision can be attempted, but often results in recurrence. Corticosteroid injections and direct compression, sometimes combined with keloid excision, have had success in some patients.

What is crucial for successful excision?	Reapproximation of skin edges without tension
What is "proud flesh"?	Production of excessive granulation tissue in wound
What is the treatment of "proud flesh"?	Excision, chemical cautery (silver nitrate), and electrocautery are all effective.

FLAPS

What are the indications for the use of flaps?	1. Poor recipient bed vascularity 2. Full-thickness defects of eyelid, ear, nose, and lip 3. Exposed tendons 4. Tissue bulk needed for function or filling of dead space
What is a random pattern flap?	A flap that bases its blood supply on the dermal and subdermal plexuses. Its orientation is random because its blood supply does not rely on a particular anatomically defined vascular bundle.
What is an axial or arterial flap?	A flap based on direct cutaneous arteries perforating from an underlying artery
What is a fasciocutaneous flap, and where does it derive its blood supply?	A flap based on intermuscular septae. Its blood supply is derived from vessels that arborize within the septae to form plexuses.
What is a muscle flap?	A flap consisting of vascularized muscle. If it includes overlying subcutaneous tissue and skin, it is termed a musculocutaneous flap.
What are the advantages of a muscle flap?	The bulk supplied by the muscle and subcutaneous tissue aids in the reconstruction of large defects while offering durability in mechanically active areas.

TISSUE EXPANSION

How is tissue expansion accomplished?	Silastic prostheses are implanted beneath the tissue to be expanded; then saline is incrementally infused until tissue expansion is complete.

Can expansion damage tissue?	Gradual expansion preserves function and viability of all overlying structures. Damage is almost always the result of too rapid an expansion.
What are the signs of tissue damage?	Neurapraxia, loss of dermal appendages, necrosis of overlying skin, and ultimately exposure of the implant
What are common complications and their management?	1. Seroma—percutaneous aspiration. Use of suction drainage usually avoids seroma formation. 2. Hematoma—percutaneous drainage (rarely successful) followed by exploration for continued hemorrhage. Prevention through adequate hemostasis is crucial. 3. Infection—early infections mandating removal and replacement in 4–6 months. Late infections combined with or resulting from extrusion can be managed with low-volume frequent expansions until expansion is complete.
Why can an infected expander often be left in tissue?	Expanded tissue, including the implant capsule, has an extensive blood supply, giving it antimicrobial capabilities.

MAXILLOFACIAL TRAUMA

EMERGENCIES

What are the 3 commonly encountered emergencies of maxillofacial injuries?	1. Airway obstruction 2. Life-threatening hemorrhage 3. Aspiration
What are mechanisms of airway obstruction in maxillofacial trauma?	Soft tissue swelling, fractured teeth or denture fragments, blood, or gross anatomical disruption can all obstruct airflow.
What is the treatment?	Endotracheal intubation; in some cases, emergency cricothyroidotomy
Which maxillofacial injuries are commonly associated with serious hemorrhage?	Deep facial lacerations and closed maxillofacial injuries with associated fractures

What is the preferred treatment of hemorrhage in facial lacerations?	Direct pressure and circumferential pressure bandage
What is the danger in blind clamping of vessels through a facial laceration?	Damage to the facial nerve
What is the common source of bleeding in closed maxillofacial injuries?	Arteries and veins adjacent to the walls of fractured sinuses
What are the 4 common methods of controlling hemorrhage from these injuries?	1. Anterior-posterior (AP) nasal packing 2. External compression dressing 3. Selective arterial ligation 4. Maxillary fracture reduction
How is nasal packing frequently accomplished?	Two 30- to 50-mL Foley balloon catheters are inserted through the nares, inflated in the posterior pharynx, and pulled to occlude the posterior choanae. Antibiotic-soaked Vaseline gauze is then packed anteriorly through the nostrils.
Which arteries can be safely ligated to control life-threatening facial hemorrhage?	1. Internal maxillary artery 2. External carotid artery 3. Superficial temporal artery

SOFT TISSUE WOUNDS

What is the optimal time for facial wound closure?	Due to the excellent blood supply, closure can be performed up to 24 hours after the wound occurs.
What are the standard methods of wound cleansing?	Pressure irrigation, scrubbing or mechanical removal of debris, and sharp débridement
What are the long-term sequelae of retained debris?	Nidus for infection and "tattooing" of skin (foreign material can be incorporated into the forming scar). Later revision is usually unsatisfactory.
What are the common guidelines for extent of débridement?	Conservative resection (1–2 mm) is the rule. "Devitalized" tissue often survives in the facial region.

Are there any exceptions to débridement?	Resection should be avoided in the area of the vermilion, oral commissures, eyelid margin, nostrils, and distal nose.
What are the indications for prophylactic antibiotics?	1. Lacerations of oral cavity, including compound fractures 2. Fractures involving teeth 3. Sinus fractures 4. Animal bites
What is the postoperative wound care?	Suture lines are cleansed with 1:1 peroxide/saline on cotton-tip applicators, followed by bacitracin (facial) or bacitracin ophthalmic ointment tid (periorbital).
What is the postoperative care for intraoral wounds?	Irrigation every 4 hours with bactericidal mouthwash or 1:1 peroxide/saline
Is early scar revision commonly indicated?	No. Despite the appearance of initial scarring, revision is indicated only for functional problems (e.g., ectropion or obvious malalignment). Maturation with cosmetic improvement occurs for up to 1–2 years.

FACIAL NERVE

What are the 6 terminal branches of the facial nerve and what muscles do they innervate?	1. Frontal-temporal—muscles of forehead and superficial temporal region, including orbicularis oculi and frontalis and excluding temporalis (trigeminal) 2. Zygomatic—muscles of lower orbit, midface, including orbicularis oculi, but excluding masseter (trigeminal) 3. Buccal—muscles of cheek and mouth, including orbicularis oris 4. Mandibular—muscles of lower lip and chin, including orbicularis oris 5. Cervical—platysma, distal anastomosis to mandibular branch 6. Posterior auricular—occipitalis, auricularis posterior
Which facial nerve lacerations require repair?	Proximal to a line drawn from the lateral canthus to the nasolabial sulcus, all lacerations of facial nerve branches should be repaired, under magnification, with fine sutures. Distal to the line, the branches are too small. The cervical branch requires no repair.

What components of the facial nerve contribute to lacrimation, salivary secretion, and taste?

1. The chorda tympani passes through the petrotympanic fissure, supplies taste to the anterior two-thirds of the tongue, and innervates the submandibular and sublingual glands.
2. The greater petrosal nerve passes through the pterygopalatine fossa to innervate the lacrimal glands.

If facial paralysis is accompanied by loss of taste, lacrimation, or salivary secretion, how does this combination add to the diagnostic impression?

Because only the branchial motor branches and a sensory nerve to the posterior auricle exit the stylomastoid foramen, this would imply a more proximal lesion of the facial nerve.

TRIGEMINAL NERVE

Is the trigeminal ganglion intracranial or extracranial?

Intracranial

Where do the 3 branches of the trigeminal nerve exit the skull?

The superior orbital fissure (V1), the foramen rotundum (V2), and the foramen ovale (V3)

What muscles does the trigeminal nerve innervate?

Muscles of mastication (temporalis, masseter, and pterygoids), tensor tympani, tensor veli palatini, mylohyoid, and the anterior belly of the digastrics

What is the distribution of sensory innervation among the 3 branches?

Distribution corresponds to the 3 embryologic divisions of the face:
Frontonasal process is V1—forehead, nasal dorsum, innervation of frontal anterior dura
Maxillary process is V2—cheek, palate, and maxillary half of oral cavity
Mandibular process is V3—lower third of face, mandibular half of oral cavity, tongue

Are lacerations of the trigeminal nerve routinely repaired?

Yes. Because the motor function of the trigeminal is essential, repair of motor branches is usually undertaken.

Is sensory nerve repair necessary for protective sensation?

The majority of sensory innervation in the face has a high degree of overlap and does not mandate sensory nerve repair.

PAROTID GLAND

Which duct drains the parotid gland?	Stensen's duct
Where is the duct located?	Extends anteriorly from a point just anterior to the masseter and a finger's breadth below the zygomatic arch to the region of the second maxillary bicuspid
Is it imperative to repair lacerations of the parotid gland?	No. Salivary drainage from parotid trauma stops spontaneously unless Stensen's duct is involved.
How is the duct repaired?	Ductal lacerations are repaired with fine sutures under magnification over a stent.
What injury is commonly associated with ductal laceration?	Lacerations and blunt trauma to the buccal branch of the facial nerve, whose course parallels that of the duct

FACIAL FRACTURES

What are the common signs of facial fractures?	Contusions, bruises, or lacerations; pain or localized tenderness; anesthesia or paresthesia; paralysis; malocclusion; visual disturbances; facial deformity, often palpable, or asymmetry; crepitus
What radiographic evaluation should be performed?	CT scans with coronal reconstructions are the definitive diagnostic modality for facial trauma; however, plain film evaluation may be indicated or sufficient in certain cases.
What are the structures viewed on the following films?	
Waters'	Frontal, supraorbital, orbital, zygomaticomaxillary, and nasal areas
Towne's	Condylar and subcondylar region of mandible and floor of orbit
Lateral and AP skull	Sinuses, frontobasilar, and nasoethmoidal areas
AP and lateral oblique mandible	Body, symphysis, condylar, and coronoid mandible areas

Panorex	Entire mandible and lower maxilla
What additional study should be obtained before the reconstruction of fractures involving the occlusion?	Maxillary and mandibular dental impressions
What are the specific signs of a nasal fracture?	Lateral nasal deviation, retrusion, or flattening; dislocation of septum; difficulty breathing; nasal or periorbital hematomas; lacerations over the bridge; bleeding
What treatment is indicated for an isolated nasal fracture?	Closed reduction and manipulation
What are the 5 anatomic attachments of the zygoma?	1. Posterior—temporal bone 2. Anterior/superior—frontal bone 3. Medial—sphenoid bone 4. Anterior—maxillary bone 5. Anterior/inferior—maxillary alveolus
What are the 10 common signs of zygoma fractures?	Periorbital and subconjunctival hematoma; depression of lateral canthus; recession of malar prominence; step-off or tenderness of inferior orbital rim, anterior maxillary wall; unilateral epistaxis (through maxillary antrum); orbital entrapment inferiorly; infraorbital nerve numbness; globe dystopia or enophthalmos; intraoral hematoma of superior buccal sulcus; difficulty chewing due to impingement of the arch on the coronoid process
What is a nasoethmoidal orbital (NOE) fracture?	A fracture that includes the nose and medial orbital rim
What percentage of NOE fractures are bilateral?	66%
What are the common signs of an NOE fracture?	Depressed nasal dorsum; tenderness over medial canthal ligament; telecanthus (increased distance between eyes); eyelid "spectacle" hematomas; epistaxis; nasal laceration; mobility of medial orbital rim with direct pressure or intranasal traction

What is the Furnas traction test, and what does it test for?

The test is accomplished by palpating the medial canthal region while applying lateral traction on the eyelid. If the medial canthal ligament is intact, it should be palpable during this maneuver as a "bowstring."

What are the signs of a frontal sinus fracture?

Soft tissue trauma to forehead; epistaxis; depression of frontal bone

Which frontal sinus fractures require surgery?

Only displaced fractures require open reduction and fixation (wire and/or plates).

What is the treatment for comminuted frontal sinus fractures in which depressed fragments cannot easily be reduced and fixed?

Sinus obliteration or cranialization

What determines whether frontal sinus obliteration or cranialization is performed?

An intact posterior wall mandates sinus obliteration, whereas a severely disrupted wall dictates cranialization.

What is a common complication of frontal sinus fractures?

Mucocele (due to incomplete removal of sinus mucosa)

What are the common signs of supraorbital fractures?

Soft tissue trauma; depression or irregularity of superior orbital rim; numbness in supraorbital nerve distribution; eyelid ptosis; downward and outward protrusion of globe; superior orbital fissure or orbital apex syndrome

What are the common signs of an orbital floor fracture?

Periorbital and subconjunctival hematoma; anesthesia of infraorbital nerve; diplopia on upward or downward gaze (entrapment of inferior rectus and/or inferior oblique); enophthalmos; globe dystopia; orbital emphysema; ipsilateral epistaxis from maxillary sinus; positive forced duction

What is a forced duction exam, and what does it demonstrate?

Forced duction is performed by applying topical anesthetic to the globe, grasping the inferior conjunctiva, and testing whether upward movement of the globe is possible. If movement is restricted, it is likely due to entrapment of the inferior rectus within an orbital floor fracture.

CEREBROSPINAL FLUID RHINORRHEA

What fractures are commonly associated with CSF rhinorrhea?

50–75% of frontal basilar and NOE fractures; 25% of Le Fort II and III fractures

What is the bedside test for CSF rhinorrhea?

If bloody nasal drainage representing CSF is blotted onto a white paper towel, a clear ring extends out from a central spot of blood (double-ring sign).

What is the management of CSF rhinorrhea?

Fistulas associated with displaced fractures usually undergo direct repair. Those not associated with displaced fractures often resolve over a 2-week period.

Is antibiotic prophylaxis warranted?

Yes

What routine measures should be avoided in the setting of a CSF fistula?

Nasal packing and nasogastric tubes, which block nasal drainage and encourage bacterial growth

MANDIBLE FRACTURE

What are the labeled regions of the mandible?

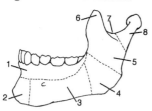

1. Alveolar process
2. Symphysis
3. Body
4. Angle
5. Ramus
6. Coronoid process
7. Mandibular notch
8. Condylar process

What is the anatomic distribution of fractures of the mandible?

A third in the condylar-subcondylar area, a third at the angle, a third in the body-symphysis.

What percentage of mandible fractures are bilateral?

> 50%

Do mandible fractures more commonly compound externally or intraorally?

Most compound intraorally; thus, a thorough exam of the oral cavity is essential.

| What are the common signs of a mandible fracture? | Intraoral or external soft tissue trauma; occlusal abnormality; numbness in distribution of mental nerve; bleeding from a tooth socket; fractured or missing teeth; trismus; open bite, abnormality of arch, or intercuspation of teeth; bleeding from the ear (laceration of anterior wall of ear canal from condylar fracture); intraoral odor |

RECONSTRUCTIVE PRINCIPLES

What are the indications for exploration of orbital floor or medial wall fractures?	Diplopia of primary or downward gaze persistent for 2 weeks; enophthalmos > 3 mm; other upper facial fractures requiring surgery
What is the primary goal of orbital wall reconstruction?	Restoration of globe support and reestablishment of normal proportions of bony volume to orbital content. This combination almost always requires an implant of the orbital floor, using alloplastic or autogenous materials.
Which complicating factors make nasoethmoidal fractures particularly challenging?	1. Fragility of the bones makes comminution and bone loss common. 2. Associated injuries to the lacrimal system, medial canthal tendon, and cranial cavity
What is the basic approach to reconstruction of the NOE fracture?	Interosseous plating or wiring with bone grafting as needed. Telecanthus is corrected by transnasal canthopexy.
Do nondisplaced fractures of the zygomatic arch or zygoma require treatment?	No, unless subsequent displacement is noted.
What is the basic approach to displaced zygoma fractures?	Depressed arch fractures require elevation alone. The remainder require reduction and fixation to the maxillary and frontal articulations.
What is intermaxillary fixation (IMF)?	Two arch bars are conformed to fit the maxillary and mandibular teeth and then fastened with circumdental wires. The arch bars are then wired to each other to restore the proper occlusal relationship.

If used alone, how long is IMF left in place?	6–8 weeks
What is the general goal of maxillary fracture treatment?	Restoration of the articulations with the 3 maxillary buttresses (zygomatic, nasofrontal, and pterygomaxillary), to reestablish the normal occlusal relation
How is this accomplished?	Using IMF, reestablish the occlusion. Plate and screw fixation of fracture fragments, with and without bone grafting, restores the maxillary buttresses.
What is the general goal for mandibular fracture treatment?	Restoration of normal occlusion
How is this accomplished?	With IMF. However, because the incidence of multiple mandible fractures is high and the muscles of mastication exert considerable force on fracture fragments, open reduction and fixation with heavy plates and screws may be needed to achieve stability of the arch.
Which mandibular fractures are rarely treated with open reduction-fixation, and how are they managed?	1. Ramus and coronoid fractures (rarely displaced due to muscle protection)—brief IMF or soft diet is the rule 2. Condylar fractures—if isolated, IMF for 3 weeks only, followed by physiotherapy to restore temporomandibular joint (TMJ) function 3. Alveolar fractures—often treated with a single arch bar, with IMF added if unstable

HAND SURGERY

ANATOMY

How does the skin of the hand differ on dorsal and ventral sides, and what are the functional implications?	Palmar skin is thick, tethered, irregularly surfaced, and moist; subcutaneous fat beneath provides padding, stability, and friction, for a strong grip. Dorsal skin is thin and mobile, with little fat; provides freedom for motion of the various joints.

What is the function of the tendon synovial sheaths?	The sheaths (consisting of tenosynovium) act as a mesentery, providing nutrient blood flow and lubrication for gliding of the tendons.

EXTRINSIC FLEXORS OF THE HAND

What are the extrinsic flexors of the hand?	Digital—flexor pollicis longus (FPL) Flexor digitorum profundus (FDP) Flexor digitorum superficialis (FDS) Wrist—palmaris longus (PL) Flexor carpi radialis (FCR) Flexor carpi ulnaris (FCU)

Where do the extrinsic flexors have their insertions?

FPL and FDP	Volar base of distal phalanx
FDS	Volar middle phalanx
FCU	Pisiform and hamate bones
FCR	Volar base of second and third metacarpal
PL	Superficial palmar fascia

How is each extrinsic flexor tested?

FPL	Flexion of thumb interphalangeal joint with metacarpophalangeal (MCP) joint extended
FDP	Flexion of distal interphalangeal joint with proximal interphalangeal (PIP) joint held in extension
FDS	Flexion of PIP with other fingers held in extension
FDP	Ulnar 3 FDP tendons share muscle belly and must be eliminated through extension of other digits during FDS testing
FCU, FCR, PL	Wrist flexed while tendons palpated

Where are the tendon sheaths of the flexors located?

The proximal sheaths start 1 finger breadth proximal to the flexor retinaculum and reach to the proximal transverse palmar crease. The separate sheaths unite during development to form a common sheath, except for the sheath of the thumb. Distal sheaths begin at the palmar (volar) plate of the MCPs and extend to the distal insertion of the flexor tendons. For the thumb and small fingers, the distal and proximal sheaths are continuous.

Does the sheath of the thumb communicate with the other flexor sheaths?

Yes, in 50% of individuals

What are the structure and function of the fibro-osseous tunnels of the flexor tendons?

In each digit, the tunnel is a fibrous sheath that runs from the metacarpal head to the insertion of the tendon on the distal phalanx. Thickenings, known as pulleys, guide the tendon during excursion. There are 5 annular (A–A5) and 3 cruciate (C–C3) pulleys.

Which pulleys are considered the most functionally important?

The A2 and A4 pulleys, over the proximal and middle phalanges, respectively

Extrinsic Extensors of the Hand

How many dorsal compartments and extensors are present in the hand?

6 dorsal compartments, which contain the 9 separate extensors

What are the extrinsic extensors of the hand (compartment: extensors [radial to ulnar])?

First

Abductor pollicis longus (APL), extensor pollicis brevis (EPB)

Second

Extensor carpi radialis longus (ECRL), extensor carpi radialis brevis (ECRB)

Third

Extensor pollicis longus (EPL)

Fourth	Extensor digitorum communis (EDC), extensor indicis proprius (EIP)
Fifth	Extensor digiti minimi (EDM)
Sixth	Extensor carpi ulnaris (ECU)

What are the insertions of the extensors?

APL	Base of thumb metacarpal
EPB	Base of proximal phalanx
ECRL	Base of index metacarpal
ECRB	Base of middle metacarpal
EPL	Base of distal phalanx thumb
EDC	Base of both middle and distal phalanges
EIP	Dorsal expansion of index finger, which inserts as above
EDM	Dorsal expansion of small finger, which inserts as above
ECU	Base of small finger metacarpal

How is each of these muscles tested?

APL or EPB	Abduct or extend, respectively, the thumb while palpating radial side of anatomic snuff-box.
ECRL and ECRB	Extend closed fist and palpate the 2 adjacent tendons.
EPL	Extend thumb while palpating ulnar side of snuff-box; lift thumb off table with hand flat on palm.
EDC	Straighten fingers, watch for MCP extension.
EIP	Extend index finger only, with hand closed in a fist.

EDM	Extend small finger only, with hand closed in a fist.
ECU	Extend and ulnar-deviate wrist with closed fist; palpate tendon just distal to ulnar head.
Where are the synovial sheaths of the extensors?	They extend proximally 1 finger breadth from underneath the extensor retinaculum and distally 1 finger breadth onto the dorsum of the hand. There are 6, 1 corresponding to each of the 6 compartments.
What is extrinsic extensor tightness?	If extensors limit the range of passive flexion of MCP and PIP joints combined, extrinsic tightness exists.
How is extrinsic extensor tightness tested?	By passively flexing the PIP joints with MCP joints, first in extension and then in flexion. If flexion of PIP joints is decreased by MCP flexion, tightness has been demonstrated.
What are the intrinsic muscles of the hand?	The muscles of the thenar and hypothenar eminences, the lumbricals, interossei, and adductor pollicis
What are the thenar muscles and their functions?	Abductor pollicis brevis—abducts the thumb with APL Flexor pollicis brevis—flexes thumb MCP Opponens pollicis—pulls thumb medially and forward across palm
How is thenar function evaluated?	Thumb and small fingertips are brought together with nails parallel (apposition); the thumb is raised 90° above the plain of the palm (abduction). The thenar eminence is observed for contraction and symmetry with the opposite side.
What is the function of the adductor pollicis, and how is it tested?	Thumb adduction. Test by holding a piece of paper between the thumb and radial index proximal phalanx—if weak, the interphalangeal (IP) of the thumb flexes, known as "Froment's sign."
What is the function of the lumbricals?	Flexion of MCPs and extension of IPs

How are the lumbricals tested?	By simultaneously accomplishing both MCP flexion and IP extension
What are the functions of the interossei (dorsal and palmar)?	Palmar interossei (PIO) **ad**duct digits; dorsal interossei (DIO) **ab**duct digits.
How are the interossei tested?	The most stringent test is to place the palm flat on the table, hyperextend the digits, and then abduct and adduct them. The first DIO can be palpated during the abduction of the index finger.
What are the muscles of the hypothenar eminence?	Abductor digiti minimi, flexor digiti minimi, and opponens digiti minimi (like the thenar eminence)
How are the hypothenar muscles tested?	To test abduction, abduct the small finger while observing for dimpling of the eminence. Opposition can be tested as described above for the thenar eminence.
What is intrinsic muscle tightness?	Limited PIP passive flexion during MCP flexion, which puts tension on the intrinsics. It is relieved by MCP extension, which relaxes the intrinsics.

NERVES OF THE UPPER EXTREMITY

What are the 3 primary nerves innervating the upper extremity?	Median, ulnar, and radial nerves
What is the anatomic course of the median nerve in the forearm?	The median nerve enters the forearm through the pronator teres and gives off the anterior interosseous branch in the proximal forearm. It then runs between the flexor digitorum profundus and sublimis, entering the radial side of the carpal tunnel at the wrist.
What is the anatomic course of the ulnar nerve in the forearm?	The ulnar nerve runs behind the medial epicondyle of the humerus, between the 2 heads of FCU, and lies between the FDP and FCU. It branches from the dorsal cutaneous branch in the distal forearm and then enters Guyon's canal at the wrist ulnar to the ulnar artery.

What is the anatomic course of the radial nerve in the forearm?

The radial nerve enters the cubital fossa between the brachialis medially and the brachioradialis and the ECRL laterally, and divides into superficial and deep branches at the lateral epicondyle of the humerus. The deep branch runs between superficial and deep layers of the supinator, entering the posterior compartment of the forearm. The superficial branch runs under the brachioradialis and above the supinator and pronator teres muscles, eventually coursing dorsally at the wrist.

What muscles are innervated by the median nerve in the forearm?

Pronator teres, FCR, PL, FDS, FDP (radial), FPL, and pronator quadratus

What muscles are innervated by the ulnar nerve in the forearm?

FCU, FDP (ulnar)

What muscles are innervated by the radial nerve in the forearm?

ECRB, supinator, EDC, EDM, ECU, APL, EPL, EPB, EIP, anconeus°, brachioradialis°, ECRL°, and triceps° (°innervated above the elbow)

How is sensory testing of the fingers best accomplished?

Tactile gnosia (tested by 2-point discrimination) is the best indicator of nerve function. Two prongs (e.g., a paper clip) are pressed against the skin while the patient identifies the sensation as a single or double point. This test is done with the probes both stationary and moving, and the minimal distance at which 2 points can be distinguished is determined. Abnormal is defined as > 6 mm static or > 3 mm moving required for detection of 2 points.

What is the best substitute in the uncooperative or unresponsive patient, or the child?

The immersion test (place the hand in water for 5–10 minutes, and then observe for wrinkling of the glabrous skin). Denervation of the skin prevents wrinkling.

What is the course of the median nerve in the hand, and what are the structures that it innervates?

The median nerve exits the carpal tunnel, branching into the thenar motor branch, common digital nerves (to the thumb, index finger, middle finger, and radial half of ring finger), the first and second lumbricals, and the sensory branches to the radial palm.

What is the course of the ulnar nerve in the hand, and what are the structures that it innervates?

The ulnar nerve exits Guyon's canal and divides into deep and superficial branches. The deep branch supplies the hypothenar muscles, the interossei, the third and fourth lumbricals, adductor pollicis, and deep flexor pollicis brevis. The superficial branch supplies the palmaris brevis, the common digital nerves (to small and ulnar half of ring finger), and sensation to the ulnar palm.

What is the course of the radial nerve in the hand, and what are the structures that it innervates?

After traveling beneath the brachioradialis tendon, the superficial branch of the radial nerve provides sensation to the radial half of the dorsum of the hand, to the entire dorsum of the thumb, and to the index and radial half of the middle finger dorsum proximal to the PIP joints.

HAND EMERGENCIES

TRAUMATIC AMPUTATIONS

What is the general cause of life-threatening hemorrhage in the forearm and hand?

Usually a partially transected artery. (Completely transected arteries can retract into the surrounding tissue and initiate vasospasm effectively, thus reducing the risk of life-threatening hemorrhage.)

What are the treatment options?

1. Direct pressure and elevation usually stop severe bleeding.
2. A tourniquet 100–150 mm Hg above systolic blood pressure can be applied as a temporizing measure for 30 minutes at a time, with 5-minute rests in between to assess for control of bleeding and for patient comfort.

What are the indications for replantation of an amputated digit?

1. Thumb amputations (especially if proximal to IP joint)
2. All amputations in children
3. Clean amputations (sharp division) at the hand, wrist, or distal forearm

Is replantation commonly limited by technical considerations?

No. Although restoration of blood supply is not always possible in a severely injured amputated part, more often reattachment and viability are possible. (Note: If the reattached part will offer no significant functional advantage over amputation, replantation should be avoided.)

What are the relative contraindications to replantation?

1. Severe crush or avulsion
2. Amputation between MCP and PIP joints of a single digit
3. Heavily contaminated wound

What are the absolute contraindications to replantation?

1. Severe medical problems or associated injuries increasing the risk of surgery
2. Multilevel injury to the amputated part
3. Inability to stop smoking for 3 months post replant
4. Psychiatric illness that precipitated self-amputation

What is the preoperative preparation in a patient with an amputated digit?

Débridement of stump with irrigation and dressing with nonadherent gauze, tetanus prophylaxis, IV antibiotics, and IV hydration

What is the preparation of the amputated part?

Débridement with irrigation, wrapping in gauze moistened with lactated Ringer's solution (LRS) or normal saline, and placement of wrapped part in sealed container immersed in an ice bath

How is an incompletely amputated part prepared?

The treatment is identical, with the additional step of detorquing intact vessels to restore blood supply. The attached part is cooled in insulated ice packs instead of in an ice bath.

What is the initial treatment of mangled parts that are unlikely to regain function, but maintain an adequate blood supply? Why?

Mangled parts (e.g., a severely injured finger) are often left intact because they are an excellent source for autologous grafting of skin, bone, articular surface, nerve, artery, and tendon.

COMPARTMENT SYNDROME

What is the mechanism of compartment syndrome?	Accumulation of fluid (either blood or exudate) in a fascial compartment builds pressure that obstructs venous outflow. As arterial inflow continues, the pressure increases until arterial inflow is decreased, causing ischemia and further progression of the fluid accumulation as tissue injury worsens.
What compartments can be affected in the forearm and hand?	Volar or dorsal compartments in the forearm; intrinsic muscle compartments in the hand
What are the cardinal signs of a compartment syndrome?	1. Gross appearance—Swollen, tense, tender hand or forearm 2. Muscles—Tender and increased pain on passive extension 3. Nerves—Pain (early), followed by paresthesias (later), followed by anesthesia (late) 4. Pulselessness (late!)
How can compartment syndrome be distinguished from simple swelling?	Compartment pressures can be measured; > 30 mm Hg is considered a true compartment syndrome. However, because pressures can evolve rapidly, a high clinical suspicion should lead to repeat measurements or prophylactic fasciotomies even with "normal" pressures.

HERPETIC WHITLOW

What is a herpetic whitlow?	A herpes simplex vesicle or ulcer on the finger (often seen in dental or medical personnel who do not use adequate precautions)
What tests may be used for diagnosis?	**Tzanck** smear of lesional fluid, scrapings for giant cells, fluorescent antibody testing of lesion fluid, or culture of the lesion for virus

What is the treatment?	Topical acyclovir ointment applied every 3 hours for 48 hours, with 5 days of oral acyclovir to start simultaneously. Incision and débridement should be avoided. Antibacterial antibiotics are indicated only in cases of suspected bacterial superinfection.

COMPLEX INFECTIONS OF THE HAND

SUPPURATIVE TENOSYNOVITIS

What is suppurative tenosynovitis?	A bacterial infection of the tendon sheath usually following penetrating trauma
Is it more common in extensor or flexor tendon sheaths?	Flexor
What are Kanavel's 4 signs of flexor tenosynovitis?	1. Flexed posture of affected digit 2. Tenderness along the sheath with erythema 3. Pain on passive extension of DIP joint 4. Fusiform swelling (sausage-like finger)
Which sign is the strongest indicator of tenosynovitis?	Pain on passive extension of the DIP joint
What is a horseshoe infection?	Suppurative tenosynovitis that has spread in a horseshoe pattern from either ring or small finger through palm to affect the other digit. May develop because the small finger and thumb tendon sheaths both extend from the palm and often communicate.
What is the immediate treatment of suppurative flexor tenosynovitis?	Incisions are made over the proximal sheath and at the level of the middle phalanx. A No. 5 French catheter is inserted between the A4 and A5 pulleys, and the sheath is irrigated with a bacitracin solution.
What additional treatment accompanies operative drainage?	IV antibiotics, splinting in the intrinsic plus position with elevation, and irrigation of the sheath every 4–6 hours with bacitracin solution through an indwelling catheter until the infection resolves

DEEP-SPACE INFECTIONS

What are the 2 areas for deep-space infections of the hand?	1. Midpalmar (between the flexor tendons and metacarpals of the ulnar 3 digits) 2. Thenar (between the flexor tendon of the index finger and the adductor pollicis)
What is the treatment?	1. Incision and débridement with drain placement. The midpalmar space is drained with a palmar incision between the third and fourth rays, the thenar space through a dorsal incision of the thumb web space 2. IV antibiotics
What are the common sources of septic arthritis?	1. Direct inoculation from penetrating trauma 2. Hematogenous spread
What are the common pathogens for penetrating trauma?	For trauma, especially of the MCP joint, the infection is often the product of human tooth penetration and inoculation. *Staphylococcus aureus* is the most common, but mixed gram-positive and gram-negative cultures are frequent.
Which organism is classically associated with human bites?	*Eikenella corrodens,* a gram-negative bacillus
What are the common pathogens for hematogenous spread?	Although any pathogen can cause septic arthritis in this manner, *Neisseria gonorrhoeae* must always be considered.
What is the treatment of septic arthritis?	Incision and débridement with drain placement. Antibiotic coverage includes a penicillin with activity against *S. aureus* and an aminoglycoside.
How is mycobacterial infection usually contracted?	From a puncture wound in the setting of soil or water

What is the usual presentation of mycobacterial arthritis?	Synovitis of a tendon sheath or joint develops approximately 6 weeks post-trauma.
How is mycobacterial arthritis diagnosed and treated?	Culture or the finding of multinucleated giant cells confirms the diagnosis. Long-term antibiotic therapy is required.

TENDON LACERATIONS

What flexor tendon injuries can be treated in the emergency department 4 (ED) setting?	None! Although careful inspection is acceptable in the emergency room, virtually **all** flexor tendon injuries require operative exploration, therapy, or both.
What extensor tendon injuries can be treated in the ED?	Any laceration in which both ends can be easily visualized for repair. Multiple tendon injuries or those with difficult exposure (i.e., more proximal) should be attempted only in the OR.
What are the zones used to describe flexor tendon lacerations?	Zone I—Midfinger pad to distal half of middle phalanx Zone II—Proximal half of middle phalanx to MCP joint, inclusive of the MCP Zone III—Distal palmar crease to midpalm Zone IV—Midpalm to wrist crease, carpus included Zone V—Wrist crease and proximal
Which zone is also called "no man's land"?	Zone II
What is the usual mechanism of a Zone I flexor injury?	Avulsion of the tendon insertion during grasping
Why is flexion often intact in a Zone I flexor injury?	The vinculum, a mesentery for the tendon, often stays connected to the distal phalanx.

Why are functional results of flexor tendon repair notoriously poor in Zone II?

Zone II requires smooth gliding of the FDS and FDP tendons in the narrow confines of the fibro-osseous tunnel of the tendon sheath. Repair without significant adhesion formation is difficult and often requires revision.

Injury to what structures often accompanies Zone III flexor injuries?

The superficial transverse vascular arch, the median nerve at its division into terminal branches, and the thenar motor branch of the median nerve

Why is operative exploration mandatory for Zone IV flexor injuries?

Exposure is technically demanding because it is located in the carpal tunnel.

Why are Zone V flexor lacerations, which are easily repaired, usually devastating injuries?

Tendon healing (which is generally good) often is overshadowed by a severe accompanying nerve injury (which generally recovers only partially).

What are the initial steps taken before operative repair of flexor tendons?

Débridement, loose closure, splinting in the intrinsic plus position except with the wrist in slight flexion

How long can surgical repair be delayed?

Although some controversy exists on the exact timing, repair within 6 days prevents significant contraction.

What is the usual method of tendon reapproximation?

A modified Kessler suture is widely used because of its good tensile strength, placement of the knot within the repair, and relatively small amount of ischemia induced.

What are the 3 major complications of partial tendon lacerations?

1. Delayed rupture
2. Trigger phenomenon
3. Decreased range of motion

Which partial tendon lacerations should be repaired?

Any laceration > 50% of the diameter or near the proximal pulley should be repaired. (Note: Controversy exists over indications for repair, because rates of rupture may be higher in repaired tendons and tensile strength may be decreased.)

How is the tendon repaired?

Approximation of the epitenon with fine sutures

What are the zones used to describe extensor tendon lacerations?	Zones I and II—Distal phalanx, DIP joint Zones III and IV—Central slip or lateral slips of the long extensor tendon, fibers of the intrinsic expansion, and the oblique and transverse fibers of the extensor aponeurosis Zone V—MCP region Zone VI—Digits proximal to MCP and area of extensor retinaculum
What is the usual mechanism for Zone I and II extensor injuries?	A blow to the extended digit, forcing flexion of the DIP joint and avulsion of the tendon with or without a fragment of bone
What is the resultant deformity?	Mallet finger (DIP joint flexion). Eventually the PIP joint becomes hyperextended through a proximal shift in the action of the extensors after distal rupture, and a swan-neck deformity results.
What is the most common resultant deformity of a Zone III or IV injury?	Boutonnière deformity (PIP joint flexion, DIP joint hyperextension)
What is the general treatment of extensor tendon injuries?	Open lacerations—direct repair of the tendon with subsequent splinting for 6–8 weeks (K wire for fixation of joint(s); closed rupture—splinting in neutral or hyperextension for 6–8 weeks ($\pm$ K-wire fixation)
How are lacerations to the extensor aponeurosis treated?	Splinting as previously described, with or without suture closure of the defect

NERVE INJURIES

What happens to peripheral nerves proximal to the site of injury?	Retrograde degeneration of axons (1–2 cm) with Schwann cell proliferation; degenerative changes of the neuronal cell body (may reverse in 40–120 days); axonal sprouting within 1 week that grows centrifugally from the site of transection

What happens to peripheral nerves DISTAL to the site of injury?

Wallerian degeneration (axonal disintegration progressive to the entire length of the distal segment); removal of debris by macrophages; Schwann cell proliferation within the neural tube and outside of the distal stump

Which types of nerve injuries mechanistically have the best prognosis?

From best to worst: laceration, crush, stretch (corresponds to size of the zone of injury)

What other factors worsen prognosis?

More proximal injuries (due to increased length of wallerian degeneration) and older age of patient

What is the initial treatment of nerve injuries?

Thorough débridement and closure (if possible) to best preserve integrity of divided nerve stumps

What is the best timing of repair for nerve lacerations?

Either primary repair or delayed primary repair, in 7–10 days

What is the indication for delayed repair, and how long can the patient wait without significant worsening of functional recovery?

Cases where nerve function may return (i.e., closed injury such as a crush or stretch injury). Delays of 5–6 months are possible.

What are the principles of nerve repair?

Tensionless reapproximation with minimal suturing; the least undermining possible; accurate fascicular alignment

What is the indication for nerve grafting?

When tensionless reapproximation is not possible

What nerves are usually used for grafting?

Sural and superficial radial nerves

FRACTURES OF THE HAND

EXTRA-ARTICULAR FRACTURES OF THE HAND

What is the standard treatment for nondisplaced extra-articular fractures of the metacarpals and phalanges?

Splinting in the intrinsic plus position with guarded motion to commence in 10–14 days. Stable phalangeal fractures may then be placed in a digital splint or "buddy taped" for 2–3 weeks. Metacarpal fractures remain splinted for 2–3 weeks.

When can displaced metacarpal and phalangeal fractures be treated with closed reduction?	Whenever closed reduction is able to correct for angulation or rotational deformity
What is boxer's fracture?	A fracture of the fifth metacarpal neck
How is this metacarpal fracture unique?	Usually volar angulation is not well tolerated in the metacarpals; however, because of the mobility of the fifth metacarpal, up to 40° of volar angulation can still give acceptable function.

INTRA-ARTICULAR FRACTURES OF THE HAND

What features of intra-articular fractures must be considered in deciding the most appropriate treatment?	1. Ligamentous injury and consequent joint instability 2. Integrity of the articular surface, which will greatly influence long-term functional recovery
What is the significance of small bone fragments seen on radiographs of intra-articular fractures?	Frequently these fragments point to an avulsion of a ligamentous attachment, which may have important consequences for joint stability.
What are the similarities and differences between a Bennett's fracture and a Rolando's fracture?	Both are intra-articular fractures of the base of the thumb metacarpal. A Bennett's fracture is by definition unstable because the APL displaces the shaft proximally and radially away from the other intra-articular fracture fragment. A Rolando's fracture is a Y- or T-shaped fracture of the base.
What is the treatment of these fractures?	Usually requires open reduction and internal fixation (ORIF)
What is the treatment of PIP intra-articular fractures?	Splint if < 25% of articular surface; ORIF if > 25% and unstable
What are the indications for ORIF in DIP intra-articular fractures?	1. > 30% of articular surface involved 2. Palmar subluxation of distal phalanx 3. Proximal displacement of fracture fragment (may result in extensor lag)

What is the nonoperative treatment of an intra-articular fracture of the DIP?	Splinting of the digit in the intrinsic plus position with progression to a digit splint or "buddy taping" for 2 or 3 weeks

DISLOCATIONS OF THE HAND

Which are the most typical dislocations of the DIP, PIP, and MCP joints?	DIP and PIP—Dorsal and lateral MCP (including thumb)—Usually dorsal
What is the treatment of these dislocations?	Closed reduction and splinting (degrees of flexion depend on joint)
What is the next step if instability of the joint persists?	Closed reduction and percutaneous fixation, followed by ORIF if this is unsuccessful
What is gamekeeper's thumb?	Disruption of the thumb's ulnar collateral ligament; usually incurred by lateral stress while grasping an object
How is degree of instability assessed?	Radiographic stress views under digital block for analgesia (Note: A fracture must first be ruled out with x-ray before stressing is allowed.)
What is the treatment of gamekeeper's thumb?	Thumb spica cast if < 40° of instability or a nondisplaced fracture; ORIF required for > 40° of instability or a displaced fracture.
What is the treatment of carpal–metacarpal (CM) dislocation?	Usually the ligamentous disruption is significant and requires at least percutaneous fixation after reduction.
Which CM dislocations are frequently associated with fracture?	Thumb dislocations (Bennett's fracture)

FRACTURES AND DISLOCATIONS OF THE WRIST

How is a scaphoid fracture diagnosed?	Snuff-box tenderness. Multiple radiographic views of the wrist, especially an oblique, are often needed for diagnosis.

What should be done if fracture is suspected, but x-ray examination is negative?

Potential scaphoid fractures should be treated expectantly and followed up with repeat imaging and exams.

How is a nondisplaced scaphoid fracture treated?

Cast with wrist in neutral and thumb in abduction for 4–6 weeks. Continue close radiographic follow-up.

What is a classic complication of proximal scaphoid fractures?

Avascular necrosis of the proximal fragment; can be prevented because union can often be obtained with conservative management

What is the usual mechanism for a hook, or hamate, fracture?

Striking a solid object while grasping a solid object

What is the treatment of hook, or hamate, fracture?

4–6 weeks of cast immobilization. Excision of the hook is indicated for nonunion.

What is Kienböck's disease?

Traumatic malacia of the lunate. Susceptible individuals undergo avascular necrosis in response to single or multiple traumas.

What is the treatment of Kienböck's disease?

Complex reconstructive techniques, including bone grafting and fusions

How is a lunate dislocation diagnosed?

Lateral wrist radiograph demonstrates volar displacement of the lunate. (Note: Dorsal lunate dislocations are rare.)

How is a perilunate dislocation diagnosed?

Lateral wrist radiograph demonstrates alignment of the lunate and dorsal displacement of the capitate and digits. (Note: Volar perilunate displacement is rare.)

How are lunate and perilunate dislocations treated?

Successful closed reduction followed by casting in thumb spica cast with 20° of wrist flexion. ORIF is often necessary.

What is scapholunate dissociation, and how is it diagnosed?

Disruption of the volar radioscapholunate ligament and the interosseous scapholunate ligament. Diagnosed by AP wrist radiograph showing a gap between scaphoid and lunate and an axially oriented scaphoid.

What is the treatment of scapholunate dissociation?	Closed reduction with K-wire fixation, or ORIF followed by immobilization in volar flexion

ULNAR NERVE COMPRESSION

What is the most common site of ulnar nerve compression?	At the elbow as the nerve passes through the cubital tunnel
What are the signs and symptoms?	Pain, paresthesias, numbness in the ulnar distribution; weakness of the interossei, adductor pollicis, FCU, and FDP to ring and small fingers
What is the nonoperative treatment of ulnar nerve compression?	Padding at the elbow
What is the operative treatment of ulnar nerve compression?	Release of the nerve from the cubital tunnel with rerouting anterior to the medial humeral epicondyle
As it is uncommon on its own, what other conditions often precipitate ulnar nerve compression at the wrist?	1. Ulnar artery aneurysm or compressing thrombosis 2. Repetitive trauma 3. Anterior dislocation of the ulnar head 4. Ganglion of the pisohamate joint (Note: The location of nerve compression, as with carpal tunnel, can be determined by nerve conduction studies and electromyography.)
Where is the radial nerve most susceptible to compression?	The mid-humerus posteriorly as it runs along the bone
What is the common mechanism of injury?	Prolonged pressure (e.g., "Saturday night palsy," trauma, heavy triceps use)
What are the symptoms?	Pain, paresthesias, numbness in radial distribution; weakness of wrist extension, digit extension at the MCPs, and thumb extension
What is the treatment?	Most ulnar nerve compressions respond to conservative therapy of a "cock-up" wrist splint.

FINGER-PAD DEFECTS

What is the treatment of tissue defects of the finger-pad with bone and soft tissue mostly intact?

The amputated pad can be used to fashion a full-thickness graft.

What are the options for larger defects?

Local V–Y advancement flaps or pedicle flaps derived from the thenar eminence or adjacent finger (cross finger flap)

When are the pedicle flaps divided postoperatively?

2 weeks

NAIL AND NAIL-BED INJURIES

What is the treatment of subungual hematoma WITHOUT severe disruption of the nail plate from the matrix?

Trephination—Holes are punched or burned through the nail plate to allow drainage.

Which injury commonly accompanies subungual hematomas?

Distal phalanx fractures

How does the risk of this concurrent injury alter management?

Radiographs should always be obtained, and sterile technique should be used for trephination (can convert a closed fracture into an open one).

What is the treatment of lacerations of the nail bed?

Repair with fine absorbable sutures. Exposed matrix may be covered with nonadherent gauze or the nail may be used as a splint.

What is the treatment of avulsions of the germinal matrix?

The germinal matrix should be replaced in the eponychial fold and either sutured in place or held with nonadherent gauze.

ARTHRITIS

RHEUMATOID ARTHRITIS

What are the common manifestations of rheumatoid arthritis in the hands?

1. Trigger fingers
2. Wrist tenosynovitis
3. Extensor tendon rupture
4. Carpal tunnel syndrome
5. Fibrosis and shortening of the intrinsics

What are the expected deformities as disease progresses?	1. Ulnar drift of the digits 2. Extensor lag at the MCPs 3. Swan-neck and boutonnière deformities 4. Degeneration of articular surfaces and bone mass
What is the treatment of arthritis?	In addition to systemic treatment with anti-inflammatory medications, attempts may be made to salvage function through reconstruction, replacement, and removal of diseased structures in selected patients.
In osteoarthritis, what are the most commonly involved joints of the hand?	IP joints of the digits; basal joint of the thumb
What are Heberden's and Bouchard's nodes?	Osteophytes of the DIP and PIP joints, respectively

MISCELLANEOUS HAND CONDITIONS

TRIGGER FINGER

What is the pathophysiologic mechanism of a trigger finger?	Triggering is caused by a discrepancy between the flexor tendons and the proximal sheath, specifically the A1 pulley.
What are the etiologies?	Idiopathic, tenosynovitis, post-traumatic, and rheumatoid arthritis
What is the treatment?	Steroid injections into the sheath with or without splinting of the IP joints in extension. If this fails, operative opening of the proximal sheath is performed.

DE QUERVAIN'S STENOSING TENOSYNOVITIS

What is de Quervain's stenosing tenosynovitis?	A tenosynovitis of the first dorsal compartment (APL and EPB), with or without triggering, secondary to the inflammation
What are the signs and symptoms?	Pain over the tendon sheaths with motion of the thumb; thickness and tenderness over the first compartment

What clinical tests are used to make the diagnosis?

1. Finkelstein's test—thumb is flexed and grasped by digits; then fist is ulnar deviated, which elicits pain over the radial styloid
2. Forceful abduction or extension of the thumb, which elicits pain

What other pathologic process can mimic the symptoms of de Quervain's? How can the two be distinguished?

Arthritis of the thumb carpometacarpal joint. This condition can be diagnosed by forcefully grinding the metacarpal on the trapezium, which elicits pain and crepitus in arthritis.

What is the treatment?

Steroid injections within the first dorsal compartment with or without splinting. If unsuccessful, operative release of the fibro-osseous sheaths of the first compartment is performed.

DUPUYTREN'S FASCIITIS AND CONTRACTURE

What is Dupuytren's fasciitis and contracture?

Painless thickening of the palmar fascia due to fibrous proliferation, which frequently begins as a nodule and may progress to a contracture of the MCP, PIP, or DIP joint with functional loss of the digit

Who does it typically affect?

Middle-aged patients, 7:1 ratio of men to women. Alcoholics, chronic invalids, epileptics, and patients with liver disease, diabetes mellitus, or pulmonary tuberculosis are at increased risk.

What are the most frequently affected regions of the hand?

1. Digits in order of decreasing frequency: ring, small, middle, thumb, index
2. Joints, in decreasing order: MCP, PIP, DIP

What is the treatment?

Lysis of constricting fascial bands provides temporary relief. To prevent recurrence, removal of the palmar fascia must be complete. Local corticosteroid injections are ineffective.

66

Otolaryngology Head and Neck Surgery

SALIVARY GLANDS

ANATOMY

What are the 3 major salivary glands?
1. Parotid
2. Submandibular
3. Sublingual

Where are the minor salivary glands?
The entire oral cavity and upper aerodigestive tract (600–1000 glands)

What is the general location for each major salivary gland duct?
1. Parotid—Stensen's (at 2nd maxillary molar)
2. Submandibular—Wharton's (in floor of mouth)
3. Sublingual—Multiple ducts (in floor of mouth)

What are the primary secretory cell types for each major salivary gland?
1. Parotid—Serous
2. Submandibular—Both serous and mucous
3. Sublingual—Mucous

Which intraoperative technique is most frequently used to find the facial nerve within the parotid gland?
Identification of the nerve at the stylomastoid foramen where it exits the skull and trace distally. Alternatively, a branch may be identified peripherally and traced proximally.

What are the 5 motor branches of the facial nerve?
1. Temporal
2. Zygomatic
3. Buccal
4. Mandibular
5. Cervical
(Cranial nerve [CN] VII supplies innervation to all muscles of facial expression.)

Which 3 nerves are in close proximity to the submandibular gland?	1. Marginal mandibular nerve (CN VII) → Superficial 2. Lingual nerve (CN V) → Deep and superior 3. Hypoglossal nerve (CN XII) → Deep to anterior belly of digastric muscle

SALIVARY GLAND TRAUMA

How is traumatic disruption of the extratemporal facial nerve managed?	Immediate primary repair
Which disruptive extratemporal facial nerve injuries do NOT require repair, and why?	Those lying medial to a vertical line through the lateral canthus or involving the cervical branch. The nerve will regenerate spontaneously.
How is a Stensen's duct injury managed?	Repair over polyethylene stent (6–0 to 7–0 monofilament); leave stent in place for 10 days
Which childhood salivary gland neoplasm is the most common?	Hemangioma (Capillary hemangiomas tend to occur in infancy, whereas cavernous hemangiomas are seen in older children.)
What are the 4 physical signs of parotid malignancy?	1. Facial nerve paralysis 2. Lymphadenopathy 3. Skin changes 4. Pain

SIALADENITIS

What is sialadenitis?	Inflammation of the salivary gland
What causes sialadenitis?	1. Infection 2. Obstruction of duct by calculi, stricture, or mucus plug

INFECTIOUS SIALADENITIS

How does infectious sialadenitis present?	Unilateral gland pain, fever, swelling, pus from duct orifice, and leukocytosis
What are the causes of infectious sialadenitis?	1. Viral—CMV, Coxsackie virus, mumps 2. Bacterial—Anaerobes, *Escherichia coli*, *Haemophilus influenzae*, *Staphylococcus aureus*, and *Streptococcus*

Which of these infectious etiologies are most common?	1. Mumps 2. *S. aureus*
What is the treatment of infectious sialadenitis?	1. Hydration, massage, sialogogues (agents that stimulate secretion of saliva, e.g., lemon juice), and warm compresses for symptomatic relief 2. Antibiotics for bacterial etiologies 3. Surgical excision if refractory
What are the relative indications for surgery?	1. Failure of antibiotics after 1 week of therapy 2. Recurrences 3. Multiple stones
What is the most common cause of acute suppurative parotiditis?	*S. aureus*
Which group of patients is at risk for acute suppurative parotiditis?	Debilitated patients who have a tendency toward dehydration and do not maintain good oral hygiene
What is the treatment of acute suppurative parotiditis?	Same as that of sialadenitis. Surgical drainage may be required if abscess develops.

SIALOLITHIASIS

Which salivary gland is most commonly affected by calculi?	Submandibular—80% (versus parotid only 20%)
What percentage of salivary gland calculi are radiopaque?	Depends on location (90% of calculi in submandibular gland versus only 10% in parotid). Overall, approximately 75% are radiopaque.
What are the symptoms?	Recurrent swelling and pain associated with eating
How is the condition diagnosed?	Plain films, sialography (injection of contrast dye through duct orifice), ultrasound, or CT scan
What is the initial treatment?	Conservative—Oral hydration (to stimulate salivary flow) and sialagogues

What is the treatment of chronic sialadenitis?

1. Stone removal (if distal) via duct papillotomy or excision of papilla
2. Gland excision (if proximal)

What are the numbered structures in this midsagittal view of the right larynx?

1. Epiglottis
2. Body of hyoid bone
3. Median thyrohyoid ligament
4. Vestibular ligament
5. Vocal ligament
6. Cricothyroid membrane
7. Tracheal ring
8. Cricoid cartilage
9. Arytenoid cartilage
10. Corniculate cartilage
11. Thyroid cartilage
12. Foramen for superior laryngeal nerve and artery
13. Superior horn of thyroid cartilage
14. Thyrohyoid membrane
15. Greater horn of hyoid bone

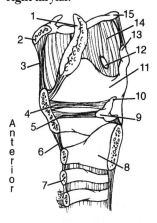

RECONSTRUCTIVE AND REHABILITATIVE LARYNGEAL SURGERY

What are the common non-neoplastic causes of hoarseness in adults?

Vocal cord (VC) nodules and polyps

What is the cause of VC nodules?

Voice abuse

What is the cause of VC polyps?

Smoking, gastroesophageal reflux, and voice abuse

What is the histologic appearance of VC nodules?

Epithelial hyperplasia and submucosal connective tissue fibrosis

What is the histologic appearance of VC polyps?

Subepithelial edema

What is the treatment of nodules and polyps?

Medical: Removal of offending agents, voice therapy
Surgical: Microsurgical excision

What is the result of unilateral VC immobility?

1. Voice disturbance
2. Airway protective deficits

What is the rehabilitative therapy for these entities?	1. VC injections (temporary medialization possible with Gelfoam) 2. Medialization thyroplasty

NOSE, PARANASAL SINUSES, AND FACE

ANATOMY

What are the paranasal sinuses?	1. Maxillary sinuses 2. Ethmoid (anterior and posterior) sinuses 3. Frontal sinuses 4. Sphenoid sinuses
What is the first sinus to develop?	Maxillary
At what age do the sinuses reach their final size?	Maxillary: Present at birth; biphasic growth age 3 and 7–18 Ethmoid: Present at birth; full size by age 12 Frontal: Rarely demonstrable radiographically before age 2; full size by 16–19 Sphenoid: Pneumatizes at age 4–5; full size by age 12–15
Which sinus is aplastic in > 5% of patients?	Frontal
Where is each paranasal sinus ostia located?	Maxillary: Middle meatus Anterior ethmoid: Middle meatus Posterior ethmoid: Superior meatus Frontal: Middle meatus Sphenoid: Sphenoethmoidal recess
Where is the lacrimal gland ostium located?	Inferior meatus
What are the components of the cartilaginous framework of the nose?	Upper lateral cartilages, lower lateral cartilages, cartilaginous septum, and sesamoid cartilages
What structures contribute to formation of the nasal septum?	Quadrangular cartilage, perpendicular plate of the ethmoid, vomer, maxillary crest, and palatine bone

What is the arterial supply of the nose and their sources?	1. Anterior and posterior ethmoid arteries (branches of the ophthalmic artery from the internal carotid artery) 2. Sphenopalatine and greater palatine arteries (branches of the internal maxillary artery from the external carotid artery) 3. Superior labial artery (branch of the facial artery from the exterior carotid artery)
Why are the veins of the face likely to propagate septic emboli to the brain?	Facial veins are valveless.

TRAUMATIC SEPTAL HEMATOMA

What is the treatment of traumatic septal hematoma?	Urgent incision and drainage
Why?	To prevent cartilage necrosis and resulting saddle-nose deformity

FACIAL CELLULITIS

What is the treatment of facial cellulitis?	Hospital admission, IV antibiotics, and close observation
Why is this treatment chosen?	To facilitate early detection of intracranial propagation of bacteria via valveless facial veins

APNEA

What is apnea?	Absence of respiration for 10 or more seconds
What are the 3 types of apnea?	1. Obstructive—Lack of airflow with continued effort 2. Central—Absence of effort 3. Mixed—Both
In patients with obstructive sleep apnea (OSA), what is the predominant site of obstruction?	Oropharynx. Obstruction can result from tongue, soft palate, tonsillar, adenoid, and pharyngeal wall.

How is OSA diagnosed?	1. History—Loud snoring, restless sleep, periods of apnea, and daytime somnolence 2. Physical exam—Associated with obesity, macroglossia, micrognathia, retrognathia, adenotonsillar hypertrophy, shallow palatal arch, large palate 3. Diagnostic study—Sleep study (polysomnogram)
What is the treatment of pediatric OSA?	Adenotonsillectomy
What is the treatment of OSA in adults?	1. Medical therapy—Continuous positive airway pressure (CPAP) masks, weight loss, avoidance of CNS depressants, and protriptyline 2. Surgery—May include tonsillectomy and adenoidectomy, uvulopalatopharyngoplasty and tracheotomy, midline glossectomy, mandibular advancements or osteotomy, and hyoid advancement
What malformations are found in Pierre Robin syndrome?	1. Glossoptosis 2. Micrognathia 3. Cleft palate These children often present with inadequate oral intake and aspiration that may require tracheostomy and gastrostomy tube.
What malformations are found in Apert's syndrome?	Midface hypoplasia with a small retrodisplaced maxilla, orbital hypertelorism, and a short widened skull
What is Ludwig's angina?	The spread of an infectious process into the sublingual, submandibular, and submental spaces
What is the most concerning complication?	Rapid progression of airway compromise (with floor of mouth edema displacing tongue posteriorly)
What are the signs and symptoms?	Limited movement of tongue, swelling of floor of mouth and submental region, fluctuance, and pain on movement of tongue

What is the most common source?	Dental infection (especially mandibular)
What are the most common pathogens?	Mixed oral flora
What is the treatment?	Same as for peritonsillar abscess

ACUTE RHINITIS

What are the symptoms of acute rhinitis?	Nasal stuffiness, rhinorrhea, sneezing, mild fever, headache, and general malaise; obstruction and thickened/purulent nasal discharge may follow
What are the findings on physical examination?	Swollen, erythematous nasal mucosa with a watery mucus discharge
What is the course/treatment?	Usually lasts 5–7 days; antihistamines and decongestants may help symptoms; interferon shortens the course of the virus.

OTHER OROPHARYNGEAL ABSCESSES

What is the location of a parapharyngeal abscess?	Fascial space between pharyngeal constrictor muscles and superficial layer of deep cervical fascia
What is the location of a retropharyngeal abscess?	Fascial space between posterior pharyngeal wall and prevertebral fascia
What are the complications?	1. Airway obstruction 2. Hemorrhage due to erosion into vessels of neck (e.g., carotid) 3. Intracranial infections 4. Aspiration 5. Spread to thoracic cavity (e.g., mediastinitis)
What is the treatment?	IV antibiotics, incision, and drainage
Should the procedure be performed under local or general anesthesia?	Local. General anesthesia can be dangerous with these abscesses because of sudden airway obstruction. Even with local anesthesia, the surgeon must be prepared to perform tracheostomy.

EARS

ANATOMY

What are the labeled landmarks of the external ear or auricle?	1. Helix
	2. Scaphoid fossa
	3. Triangular fossa
	4. Concha
	5. Antihelix
	6. Tragus
	7. Antitragus
	8. Intertragic incisure
	9. Lobule

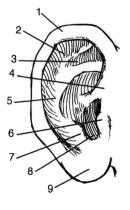

Which nerves travel within the internal auditory canal (IAC)?

Vestibulocochlear and facial nerves

Define conductive hearing loss.

Loss of conduction of sound from external ear canal to cochlea (e.g., cerumen, otitis media, ossicle destruction)

Define sensorineural hearing loss.

Damage to cochlea and hair cells/auditory neurons

What 2 tests use tuning forks to analyze hearing loss?

Weber's and Rinne's

Define the 2 hearing tests.

Weber's test

Tuning fork to forehead = normal = maximal sound center of head

Rinne's test

Tuning fork against mastoid until no sound → then tuning fork 2 cm from external canal = normal = sound 2× as long in air conduction

Describe the tuning fork analysis for hearing loss conditions.	*Test*	*Rinne's*	*Weber's*
	Normal bilateral	+/+	Middle
	Unilateral conductive loss	+/−	Lateralization to affected ear
	Bilateral conductive loss	+/−	Lateralization to worst ear
	Unilateral sensorineural loss	+/+	Lateralization to best ear
	Bilateral sensorineural loss	+/+	Lateralization to best ear

SENSORINEURAL HEARING LOSS

What are the signs?

Air conduction is better than bone conduction, but Weber's lateralizes to unaffected ear. Audiogram loss in high frequencies.

INFECTIONS OF THE EAR

SEROUS OTITIS MEDIA

What is serous otitis media?

Usually an acute response to temporary ventilatory dysfunction of the eustachian tube

What are the precipitating factors?

Nasopharyngeal inflammation; often allergic rhinitis or the common cold

What more serious lesion may have a similar presentation?

Nasopharyngeal carcinoma; be especially suspicious in the adult with prolonged unilateral serous otitis

What are the symptoms?

Sensation of otic fullness, tinnitus, hearing loss

What are the findings on examination?

Amber-colored tympanic membrane (TM) and often a visible fluid line or air bubbles behind the TM, which may be retracted with decreased mobility

What is the treatment?

Most cases resolve without treatment; antihistamines may help; myringotomy with aspiration of fluid has a high certainty of cure but is rarely necessary.

MUCOID OTITIS MEDIA

What age group is most affected?

Usually seen in children

With what other condition is it associated?	Chronic dysfunction of the eustachian tube, a common sequela of acute otitis media
What is the most common sequela?	Acquired hearing loss in children
What are the symptoms?	Often asymptomatic, though impaired hearing is common
What are the findings on examination?	Otoscopy may reveal a dull, retracted, immobile TM.
What is the treatment?	Search for underlying etiology; antihistamine-decongestant combinations are not efficacious; watch for 2–3 months for spontaneous resolution; myringotomy with tube insertion is necessary if there is no resolution; audiogram is indicated to document hearing loss.

VESTIBULAR NEURITIS

What is vestibular neuritis?	Severe attack(s) of prolonged vertigo; thought to have a viral origin
What is the typical history?	Healthy adult (30–60 years old) who has had an upper respiratory infection or sinusitis prior to an acute vestibular crisis characterized by severe vertigo, nausea, vomiting, and nystagmus
What is the course?	Symptoms usually last 3–7 days, with progressive improvement noted following a single episode; recurrences (usually less severe) may occur in the ensuing weeks.
What is the treatment?	IV phenothiazine given slowly will usually stop severe vertigo, nausea, and vomiting; diazepam or meclizine (vestibulosuppressives) may be helpful; mainstay of treatment is early, aggressive vestibular rehabilitation exercises once symptoms have been controlled.

TUMORS OF THE EAR

Glomus Tumors

What percentage of glomus tumors are bilateral?	10%

What are the symptoms?	By location: Pulsatile tinnitus, hearing loss, vertigo, CN palsy
What are the signs?	Conductive hearing loss, mass behind ear drum, CN deficit
What are the steps in evaluation?	Examination, audiogram, CT, MRI, angiogram

POSTERIOR FOSSA TUMORS

What are posterior fossa tumors?	Most commonly (90%) acoustic neuromas, which are benign schwannomas of CN VIII; less common primary tumors are meningioma, cholesteatoma, arachnoid cyst, cholesterol granuloma
Which site is most commonly affected?	Cerebellopontine angle
What are the early symptoms?	Tinnitus, hearing loss, vertigo
What symptoms occur later?	May involve CN IX, X, XI (caudal tumor growth), cerebellum by compression
How is the diagnosis made?	T1 MRI with contrast (gadolinium) is the gold standard. Audiometry, brainstem-evoked potentials, radiology (CT and MRI)
What is the treatment?	Surgical resection Gamma knife for poor operative candidates

CONGENITAL LESIONS OF THE EAR

What ear lesions are examples of major malformations?	1. Microtia (rudimentary pinna) 2. Atresia (lack of formation of external auditory canal with bony plate)
What is the treatment?	Repair of atresia follows repair of microtia. Microtia—Staged auricular reconstruction begins with contralateral costochondral cartilage. Atresia—Once conchal position is established with microtia repair, the atretic canal can be drilled out.

NECK

ANATOMY

Major Muscular Structures

What is the thin sheet-like muscle lying beneath the skin in the anterolateral neck?	Platysma muscle
What muscle divides the neck into anterior and posterior triangles?	Sternocleidomastoid (SCM) muscle
What muscle defines the posterior extent of the neck dissection?	Trapezius muscle
What group of muscles in the anterior neck acts to elevate and depress the larynx?	Strap muscles
What group of muscles defines the deep limit of the neck dissection?	Scalene muscles
What muscle serves to stabilize the scapula and allows abduction beyond 90°?	Trapezius muscle
In what plane are skin flaps raised for neck surgery?	Subplatysmal plane

MAJOR VASCULAR STRUCTURES

What landmark roughly approximates the site of the bifurcation of the common carotid artery?	Upper border of the thyroid cartilage
What are the branches of the internal carotid artery in the neck?	There are none.

| **What are the branches of the external carotid artery in the neck?** | 1. Superior thyroid artery
2. Ascending pharyngeal artery
3. Lingual artery
4. Facial artery
5. Occipital artery
6. Posterior auricular artery
7. Superficial temporal artery
8. Maxillary artery |

FASCIAL COMPARTMENTS

| **What are the layers of the deep cervical fascia?** | 1. Superficial layer—Surrounds entire neck; encloses trapezius, SCM, and omohyoid muscles
2. Middle (visceral) layer—Surrounds visceral structures of anterior neck
3. Deep (paravertebral) layer—Surrounds paraspinous muscles and vertebral column |
| **Which layers contribute to the formation of the carotid sheath?** | All of the above |

OTHER ANATOMIC TOPICS

| **What 3 structures are within the carotid sheath?** | Carotid artery, jugular vein, and vagus nerve |
| **What are the lymphatic zones in the neck?** | Zone 1—Submental and submandibular
Zones 2, 3, and 4—Equal thirds of the internal jugular chain, with Zone 2 being the most superior
Zone 5—Posterior cervical triangle |

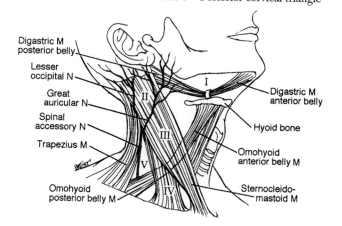

Describe the location of:

Jugular vein	Lies lateral to carotid artery, deep to SCM
Thoracic duct	Joins the venous system at the junction of the left internal jugular and subclavian veins
Vagus nerve (CN X)	Exits skull at jugular foramen; travels within the carotid sheath
Spinal accessory nerve (CN XI)	Exits skull at jugular foramen, passes deep to the posterior belly of digastric muscle, enters SCM about 4 cm below mastoid process, exits SCM 1 cm superior to Erb's point (greater auricular nerve meets SCM), and enters trapezius 2 finger breadths above clavicle
Hypoglossal nerve (CN XII)	Exits skull through hypoglossal canal, deep to digastric muscle in the submandibular triangle
Phrenic nerve	Runs lateral to medial on the surface of the anterior scalene muscle
Brachial plexus	Passing between the anterior and middle scalene muscles on the way to axilla

What spinal levels contribute to the:

Phrenic nerve?	C3, 4, and 5 (think "C3, 4, 5 keeps the diaphragm alive")
Brachial plexus?	C4–8 and T1

Identify the numbered structures in this cross-section of the neck.

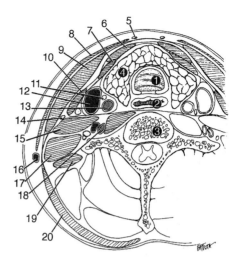

1. Trachea
2. Esophagus
3. Cervical (C7) vertebral body
4. Thyroid gland
5. Anterior jugular vein
6. Sternohyoid muscle
7. Sternothyroid muscle
8. Platysma muscle
9. SCM muscle
10. Omohyoid muscle
11. Vagus nerve
12. Internal jugular vein
13. Common carotid artery
14. Phrenic nerve
15. Scalenus anterior muscle
16. External jugular vein
17. Scalenus medius muscle
18. Vertebral artery
19. Scalenus posterior muscle
20. Trapezius muscle

HEAD AND NECK RECONSTRUCTION

What are the 3 pedicled myocutaneous flaps used in head and neck reconstruction?

1. Latissimus dorsi
2. Pectoralis major
3. Trapezius

Which flap is most commonly used?

Pectoralis major

What pedicled fasciocutaneous flap is used?	Deltopectoral flap
What is the vascular pedicle for each of the previously described flaps?	1. Pectoralis major → Thoracoacromial artery 2. Latissimus dorsi → Thoracodorsal artery 3. Trapezius → Descending branch of the transverse cervical artery and dorsal scapular artery 4. Deltopectoral flap → Anterior thoracic perforators of thoracoacromial artery
What are the FREE flaps commonly used for head and neck reconstruction?	Radial forearm, fibula, jejunum, scapula, iliac crest, and rectus abdominis
What tissue source may be used in cases of significant injury to the pharynx and esophagus?	Gastric pull-up
Where is the blood supply for this "pedicle"?	Right gastric and gastroepiploic vessels

MISCELLANEOUS TOPICS

Where is the most common neck mass?	Reactive lymph node
What is "quinsy"?	Paratonsillar abscess secondary to acute tonsillitis
What is the most common type of teratoma in the head and neck?	Epidermoid cyst
What is leukoplakia?	White patch in oropharynx
When is biopsy indicated in leukoplakia?	For smokers or alcoholics (high risk of head and neck carcinoma)
What is the most common type of branchial cleft anomaly?	Second cleft

What type of schwannoma arises from CN VIII?	Acoustic neuroma
What is the most common benign laryngeal lesion in both children and adults?	Laryngeal papilloma
What tumors of skeletal muscle have a predilection for the head and neck?	Rhabdomyomas
What is Bezold's abscess?	Cervical abscesses secondary to ear infection
What is the most common cause of facial paralysis?	Bell's palsy (etiology uncertain)
What is a maxillary torus?	Benign bony growth found midline in the palate
What is the most common bone tumor in the head and neck?	Osteogenic sarcoma (however, rarely seen in the head and neck)
Which parotid tumor accounts for 70% of all bilateral salivary tumors?	Warthin's tumor
What is an esthesioneuroblastoma?	Rare tumor that develops in the olfactory epithelium
Which facial fracture is characterized by complete craniofacial separation?	Le Fort III
What is odynophagia?	Painful swallowing
What is dysphagia?	Difficulty swallowing
What is Ménière's disease and the classic triad of presentation?	Disorder of membranous labyrinth. The triad is tinnitus, hearing loss, and vertigo.
What is a glomus jugulare?	Neoplasm arising from jugular bulb and often extending into the middle ear

What is median rhomboid glossitis?

A congenital defect caused by improper fusion of posterior third of tongue to anterior two-thirds; resembles neoplasm

What is the most common infection of the neck in children?

Acute cervical lymphadenitis

What is the most common infection of the neck in adults?

Acute cervical lymphadenitis

What is the most common head and neck tumor in children?

Hemangioma

What is vestibular neuritis?

Severe attacks of vertigo thought to be secondary to viral infection

What is ankyloglossia?

Limited movement of tongue because of shortened frenulum

What is a perilymphatic fistula?

Fistula (communication) between:
1. Middle ear and
2. Inner ear through round window or stapes footplate

Define presbycusis.

Sensorineural hearing loss due to gradual degenerative changes over a lifetime.

67

Thoracic Surgery

ACQUIRED LESIONS

CHEST WALL TUMORS

What are the most common benign chest wall tumors?

Chondroma, fibrous dysplasia, and lipoma

What are the most common malignant chest wall tumors?

Locally invasive malignancies (e.g., breast, lung) and metastases (e.g., kidney, colon), versus most common primary chest wall tumors, which are fibrosarcoma and chondrosarcoma

What percentage of benign versus malignant tumors present as painful, palpable mass?

Benign—66% (versus malignant—95%)

What is next on differential diagnosis of a painful chest mass?

Pulmonary infection with invasion into chest wall (i.e., *Actinomyces,* nocardiosis)

Which type demonstrates a classic "onion-peel" appearance on x-ray?

Ewing's sarcoma

Which type demonstrates a classic "sunburst" appearance on x-ray?

Osteogenic sarcoma (osteosarcoma)

What is the treatment of benign tumors?

Wide excision, because of difficulty determining malignant potential by histologic evaluation (Note: The "classic" 4-cm margin of excision is controversial and evolving.)

What is the treatment of malignant tumors?

Wide excision and occasionally resection of the entire involved bone (especially if high-grade tumor involves the sternum)

How is the resultant defect reconstructed?	Gore-Tex patch, methylmethacrylate plate and mesh "sandwich," or Prolene mesh. A muscle or musculocutaneous flap should also be rotated over the defect.
What is a pneumatocele?	Herniation of lung through defect in chest wall (due to trauma, surgery, or congenital defect)

TIETZE'S SYNDROME

What is Tietze's syndrome?	Nonsuppurative inflammation of the costochondral cartilages
What is the presentation and usual course?	Local pain and swelling; often resolves spontaneously

PLEURAL EFFUSION

What are the 2 types of effusions and their etiologies?	1. Transudative—Congestive heart failure, nephrotic syndrome, and cirrhosis 2. Exudative—Malignancy, trauma, infection, pancreatitis, and infarction
What are the most common causes of the following biochemical findings of an effusion?	
Glucose < 60 mg/100 mL	Malignancy, TB, pneumonia, or rheumatoid
Elevated amylase	Pancreatitis, esophageal rupture, or malignancy
pH < 7.2	Pneumonia, esophageal rupture (especially if < 6.5), malignancy, tuberculosis, systemic acidosis, rheumatoid, or hemothorax
Treatment of effusion varies depending on the etiology. If thoracentesis is performed, why should a massive effusion be evacuated in stages?	Although rare, flash pulmonary edema or circulatory collapse may occur if too large a volume is drained. A safe limit to remove at one time is about 1500 mL.

EMPYEMA

What is empyema?	Pleural effusion due to infection
What are the 3 empyema phases?	Exudative, fibropurulent, and chronic (or organized)
What is the time course of these phases?	Exudative: 0–24 hours Fibropurulent: 24–72 hours Organized: > 72 hours
What are the fluid characteristics of each of these phases?	Exudative—Thin, serous; pH > 7.3, normal glucose, protein < 2.5, WBC < 15,000 Fibropurulent and organized— Progressively more thick and purulent; pH < 7.3, low glucose, increased protein, and WBC > 15,000
Which characteristic gross feature develops as the untreated empyema matures?	Fibrous peel or rind around lung (resulting in the classic "trapped" lung, preventing lung reexpansion)
What is the most common etiology of empyema?	Pneumonia (develops in 1% of cases)
What are the most common associated organisms?	*Staphylococcus aureus* (most common), *Streptococcus*, and gram-negative organisms (e.g., *Pseudomonas, Klebsiella, Escherichia coli*)
Which infection classically develops into empyema early in the course of the pneumonia and rapidly progresses to the fibropurulent phase?	*Streptococcus pneumoniae*
Which infection is characterized by extreme clinical toxicity?	*Klebsiella*
What is the classic CXR finding of empyema?	Multiple air-fluid levels due to loculation of empyema by fibrous septae (these loculations frequently complicate drainage by tube thoracostomy)

What is the treatment of empyema in the exudative phase?	IV antibiotics and complete drainage via thoracentesis
What should be done if fluid reaccumulates after drainage of exudative-phase empyema?	Place tube thoracostomy for drainage.
What is the treatment of empyema in the fibropurulent phase?	Controversial. Many surgeons advocate attempting chest tube drainage before surgical intervention, whereas others favor surgery first.
What are the surgical options for drainage of fibropurulent empyema?	Thoracoscopic drainage; limited thoracotomy or Eloesser flap
What is the treatment of empyema in the organized phase?	Decortication—Removal of fibrous peel, empyema, and pleura in affected regions via thoracotomy (Note: Decortication may be necessary in the fibropurulent phase if trapped lung is discovered at surgery.)
What is a favorite option for surgical management of organized empyema in high-risk patients?	Eloesser flap (open pleurocutaneous fistula)—Remove rib, unroof empyemic cavity, and sew flap of skin to parietal pleura
What is the current management of empyema following pneumonectomy?	Drain pleural space, give IV antibiotics, and evaluate status of bronchial stump (leak versus intact) by bronchoscopy to determine if surgical repair is necessary.

CHYLOTHORAX

What is chylothorax?	Pleural effusion composed of lymphatic fluid or chyle due to disruption of thoracic duct
What is the course of the thoracic duct?	Cisterna chyli in the abdomen; aortic hiatus right side of vertebral column crosses to left side at T5 to T7; empties into left subclavian vein

What is the normal volume of flow per day through the duct?

Two liters! (Accounts for frequency of massive effusions in chylothorax)

What are the etiologies of chylothorax?

Iatrogenic injury during operative dissection along anterior vertebral surface (esophageal, aortic, or orthopedic surgery) or in left neck, blunt trauma, malignancy, and central venous catheter placement

How is the diagnosis made?

Biochemical and microscopic evaluation of pleural fluid (lipid/lymphocytes in chylothorax); lipid load test (high-lipid meal results in increased volume and milky appearance of pleural fluid); lymphangiogram (visualize leak)

What is the conservative treatment of chylothorax?

NPO with parenteral hyperalimentation or PO medium-chain triglycerides (absorbed directly into blood rather than lymphatics)

Reexpansion of lung and drainage of fluid with chest tube (or repeated thoracentesis)

What complications may arise during conservative therapy?

Dehydration, malnutrition (chyle contains lipid absorbed from bowel), and immunocompromise (due to loss of lymphocytes)

When should surgical intervention be considered?

After 3–4 weeks of unsuccessful conservative treatment

Chest tube output > 1000 mL/24 hours for > 1 week

What are the surgical options?

Pleurodesis (e.g., with talc)

Open or thoracoscopic ligation of thoracic duct (extensive collaterals permit chylous return from gut)

Pleuroperitoneal shunt (i.e., Denver)

Where should the ligation be performed?

Low in the mediastinum. Ligate the bundle of tissue between the aorta and azygous vein on the right side of the vertebral column near the diaphragm.

TRACHEA

ANATOMY

Which nerves are most likely to be injured during tracheal surgery?	Recurrent laryngeal nerves
What is the blood supply to the trachea?	Inferior thyroid artery (upper trachea) and bronchial arteries (lower trachea)
Why is the safest surgical approach in the AP plane?	Blood supply enters via lateral walls, and recurrent laryngeal nerves run along the lateral walls.
What percentage of the tracheal length may be safely resected in children versus adults?	Children, 33%; adults, 50–60%

TRACHEAL STENOSIS

What are the etiologies?	Intubation injury, tracheal tumors, and trauma
What is the criterion for a "critical stenosis" in an adult?	Intraluminal diameter < 4 mm
What is the usual presentation?	Cough, stridor, dyspnea, wheezing
Why are many patients with tracheal stenosis on steroids preoperatively?	Because the wheezing that frequently accompanies the stenosis is misdiagnosed as "asthma"
Should a flexible or rigid bronchoscope be used for preoperative evaluation in most cases, and why?	Rigid bronchoscope, because it can provide immediate airway (also allows better suctioning, larger biopsies, and dilating techniques)
What is the primary cause of technical problems with the tracheal anastomosis?	Excessive tension on the anastomosis
What maneuvers can be performed to reduce this problem?	Cervical flexion (secure chin to chest with **heavy suture**), suprahyoid laryngeal release, and mobilization of bilateral lung hila

What should be done to reduce the risk of tracheoesophageal fistula?	Interpose muscle flap between tracheal suture line and esophagus
What is the most common acute complication of tracheal surgery?	Laryngeal edema
What is the management?	Restrict fluids, administer racemic epinephrine and brief course of steroids
What is the most common late complication of tracheal surgery?	Granulations at suture line
What is the appropriate management?	Bronchoscopic removal of granulations ± exposed suture; ± short course of steroids
Where are postintubation tracheal stenoses most commonly found?	1. At the level of the endotracheal tube or tracheostomy cuff 2. At the level of the tracheostomy stoma
What tracheal lesion is often seen between these stenoses?	Segment of tracheomalacia
What is the consequence of this lesion?	With inspiration, the malacic segment collapses (exacerbates the airway obstruction).
What is the etiology of the cuff stenosis?	Circumferential mucosal ischemia with resultant fibrosis
What is the standard treatment of postintubation tracheal stenosis?	Resection with end-to-end anastomosis
What are the treatment options for high-risk patients?	Repeated dilations, laser ablation, or stent placement (i.e., trach tube or Silastic T-tube)

TRACHEAL TUMORS

What is the incidence of malignant tracheal tumors in children versus adults?	Children: < 10%; adults: > 80%!
What are the most common malignant types in adults?	1. Squamous cell carcinoma 2. Adenoid cystic carcinoma

What is the most common benign type in adults?	Squamous papillomas
What is the most common type in children?	Hemangioma
Which tumor classically presents with extensive proximal and distal submucosal spread?	Adenoid cystic carcinoma
What is the usual presentation of tracheal tumors?	Cough, dyspnea, stridor, hemoptysis, hoarseness, and wheezing
Why are distant metastases infrequent?	Patients often die early because of asphyxia from tracheal obstruction
How is the diagnosis usually confirmed?	Bronchoscopic biopsy
When is this diagnostic technique contraindicated?	1. Highly vascular tumors (e.g., hemangiomas, carcinoids) 2. Critical tracheal stenosis
How can the bronchoscope be used to temporarily stabilize the critically stenosed airway?	Core out intraluminal tumor with bronchoscope tip or endoscopic dilation
What is the treatment of malignant tumors?	Resection ± radiation therapy (pre- or post-op)
What is the best treatment for high-risk patients?	Placement of Silastic (Montgomery) T-tube stent
Compare incisions used for upper versus lower tumors.	Upper—Collar incision ± vertical sternal extension Lower—Posterolateral thoracotomy

ACQUIRED ESOPHAGORESPIRATORY FISTULAE

What is the usual presentation of small fistulae?	Chronic cough, weight loss, and recurrent lung infections
What is the usual presentation of large fistulae?	Paroxysmal coughing after eating or drinking (Ono's sign)

NONMALIGNANT FISTULAE

What are the most common etiologies of nonmalignant fistulae?

Erosion by the tracheal tube cuff and blunt chest trauma

What are the usual infectious etiologies?

Tuberculosis and histoplasmosis

What is the surgical treatment for nonmalignant fistulae?

Divide fistula, repair esophageal and tracheobronchial defects, and separate the repairs with muscle, pleural, or pericardial flap

MALIGNANT FISTULAE

What are the most common etiologies of malignant fistulae?

Esophageal (85%) and lung (10%) carcinoma

What are the surgical treatment options in the setting of esophageal carcinoma?

1. Esophageal exclusion (suture or staple proximal and distal ends) and bypass (usually with stomach or colon anastomosed to cervical esophagus)
2. Esophageal intubation with endoprosthesis (for high-risk patient) (Note: Resection of the fistula is contraindicated in the setting of carcinoma.)

What is the prognosis in the setting of malignancy?

80% mortality in 3 months (i.e., fistulae develop late in the disease course)

TRACHEOINNOMINATE ARTERY (TA) FISTULAE

What is the etiology?

Erosion into innominate artery by tracheostomy tube

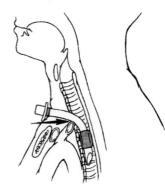

How can the potential for the future development of TA fistulae be dramatically reduced at the time of tracheostomy?	Place tracheostomy no lower than the third tracheal ring.
How can the risk in patients with chronic tracheostomy be reduced?	Avoid cuff overinflation
What sign occurs in 50% of patients before massive hemorrhage?	Transient sentinel bleed (especially significant if 1–2 weeks after tracheostomy)
What is the emergency (bedside) treatment?	Hyperinflate cuff and apply suprasternal pressure. If still massively bleeding, bluntly dissect innominate artery off trachea via the cutaneous stoma, and compress artery anteriorly against sternum.
What is the digital compression maneuver called?	Utley maneuver
What is the definitive surgical treatment?	Median sternotomy, resect innominate artery segment in contact with trachea, oversew the arterial stumps (bypass rarely indicated due to extensive collateral flow), and secure muscle flap over stumps. (Note: Tracheal defect is allowed to granulate closed.)

TRACHEOSTOMY

What are the indications?	1. Chronic respiratory failure 2. Copious tracheobronchial secretions 3. Upper airway obstruction or injury
When should a tracheostomy be performed in a ventilator-dependent patient?	Controversial; however, most experts now agree that if longer term ventilatory (> 14 days) support is necessary, tracheostomy shouldbe performed within 7 days.
Where should the incision be made in the trachea?	Second and third cartilages
What are the possible long-term complications?	Sepsis, hemorrhage, and tracheal stenosis

LUNG

ANATOMY

What is the blood supply to the lung?	Pulmonary arteries (primarily for gas exchange) and bronchial arteries from aorta and intercostal aorta (supply lung parenchyma)
What is the most common accessory lobe?	Azygous lobe (due to the developing lung forming a pleural mesentery-like structure around the azygous)
What is the location of this accessory lobe?	Right upper lobe region
Which is the "eparterial bronchus" and why is it so named?	Right upper bronchus. It is the only bronchus that lies superior to the pulmonary artery.
Which nerve runs anterior to the hilum?	Phrenic nerve
Which nerve runs posterior to the hilum?	Vagus nerve
Which vessel must be divided for adequate exposure of right bronchus or carina from right thoracotomy?	Azygous vein

CONGENITAL LUNG LESIONS

What is the most common etiology of lung hypoplasia?	Diaphragmatic hernia (herniated bowel preventing normal growth of lung)
What are the 2 classic lesions of congenital cystic lesions of the lung?	1. Bronchogenic cysts 2. Lung sequestration

BRONCHOGENIC CYSTS

What is a bronchogenic cyst?	Congenital cyst in lung (or mediastinum) likely secondary to failure of canalization of bronchial system with associated dilation of more proximal bronchi

What is the usual presentation in an infant or child?	Respiratory insufficiency, compression atelectasis, and pneumothorax
What is the usual presentation in an adult?	Recurrent pneumonia and sepsis
What is the classic CXR finding?	Smooth density extending from mediastinal border at the level of carina (fluid- and/or air-filled)

BRONCHIECTASIS

What is bronchiectasis?	Chronic dilation of distal bronchial tree (usually the second–fourth-order segmental bronchi)
What is the most common etiology?	Destructive pneumonia (bacterial or viral)
What rare congenital syndrome includes bronchiectasis in its triad of lesions?	Kartagener's syndrome (triad also includes situs inversus and sinusitis)
What is the usual presentation?	Chronic cough productive for characteristic copious, purulent, fetid sputum (especially in morning)
What is the gold standard for diagnosis?	Bronchogram (Note: Although thin-cut CT is gaining in popularity, a bronchogram still defines the anatomy best and should be done in any potential candidate for surgery.)
What are the indications for surgery for bronchiectasis?	1. Recurrent pulmonary infections 2. Significant hemoptysis 3. Brain abscess due to bacterial emboli
What is the procedure of choice for bronchiectasis?	Resection of affected regions (Note: The diffuse nature of the disease prevents most patients from undergoing surgery.)

TUBERCULOSIS (TB)

What is the responsible organism and route of transmission?	*Mycobacterium tuberculosis* by aerosolized droplets

What percentage of infected individuals have clinically significant TB?	Only 5–15%
What is the most common region of lung to be affected?	Apices of lung
What is the evolution of the parenchymal lesion?	Pulmonary infiltrate—caseous necrosis—fibrosis and calcification (granulomas)
What is a Ghon complex?	Parenchymal lesion plus enlarged hilar lymph nodes
What is a Rasmussen aneurysm?	Dilated branch of pulmonary artery within or near a TB cavity
What is the usual presentation of these aneurysms?	Hemoptysis
What are the indications for surgical resection for TB?	Failure of anti-TB medical therapy (e.g., isoniazid, rifampin, pyrazinamide) as manifested by persistently positive sputum, massive or recurrent hemoptysis, bronchopleural fistula, or mass lesion in a region of TB (to exclude malignancy)

MYCOTIC INFECTIONS

What are the most common mycotic infections in the United States?	Histoplasmosis (most common), coccidioidomycosis, *Aspergillus,* and blastomycosis
What organism has traditionally been grouped with fungal infections but is bacterial in origin?	Actinomycosis
Which of these infections is associated with:	
Dental abscesses?	Actinomycosis
Thin-walled cavity with air–fluid level?	Coccidioidomycosis
Chronic papulopustular skin ulcers?	Blastomycosis

Abscesses containing "sulfur granules"?	Actinomycosis
What is a mycetoma?	Classic "fungus ball" composed of *Aspergillus*
What is the usual predisposing lesion of a mycetoma?	Cavity secondary to *M. tuberculosis*
What is the classic finding on upright CXR?	Radiolucent crescent (small ball in larger round cavity)
What is the medical treatment of pulmonary fungal infection?	Amphotericin B for all infections except actinomycosis, which requires penicillin
What are the indications for surgical intervention for mycotic pulmonary infections?	Most agree that excision is indicated for cavitary lesions refractory to medical treatment and recurrent hemoptysis.

MASSIVE HEMOPTYSIS

What are the etiologies?	Lung abscess, bronchiectasis, trauma, and, much less frequently, tumor
What is the most common etiology?	Mycetoma (see Mycotic Infections section)
What is the usual cause of death?	Asphyxia (not hemorrhagic shock)
What is the acute management of massive hemoptysis?	Protect the nonbleeding lung! Place patient on side (with bleeding side down if known pathology on one side); use rigid bronchoscopy to determine side of bleeding (right vs. left); insert Fogarty venous occlusion catheter into bleeding bronchus and endotracheal tube into trachea or nonbleeding bronchus (the latter may require flexible bronchoscope).
What is the definitive treatment of massive hemoptysis?	Lobectomy or pneumonectomy

What is an option for high-risk patients?	Selective bronchial artery embolization (Note: Rebleeding rate is significant, and many surgeons believe that elective resection is prudent if patient's condition improves.)

BENIGN LUNG TUMORS

Benign lung tumors account for what percentage of primary lung tumors?	< 1%
What are the 4 different types?	1. Hamartoma 2. Carcinoid 3. Adenoid cystic 4. Mucoepidermoid
Which are actually low-grade malignant tumors?	Carcinoid, adenoid cystic, and mucoepidermoid (Note: These types were traditionally called "bronchial adenomas.")
Which type is most common?	Carcinoid (accounts for 85% of low-grade malignant tumors)
Carcinoids arise from what origin cell?	Kulchitsky's cell (neuroendocrine argentaffin cells)
What are the features of the carcinoid syndrome?	Cutaneous flushing, diarrhea, bronchoconstriction, and right-sided valvular disease (tricuspid, pulmonary)
What percentage of patients develop this syndrome?	Only 3%
What is the appearance of carcinoid on bronchoscopy?	Red (very vascular tumors)
What is the usual presentation of benign lung tumors?	Central tumors—Cough, pneumonia, dyspnea, or hemoptysis Peripheral tumors—Characteristically asymptomatic (found incidentally on CXR as a well-defined, slightly lobulated mass)

What is the treatment?
Central tumors—Sleeve resection
Peripheral tumors—Wedge resection or enucleation

What is a sleeve resection?
Removal of segment of bronchus (and accompanying lobe) followed by end-to-end anastomosis of remaining proximal and distal bronchial ends

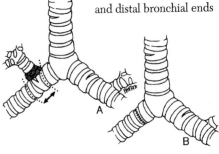

What is the benefit of a sleeve resection?
Preservation of uninvolved distal lung

METASTATIC LUNG TUMORS

What percentage of patients with carcinoma develop metastases to the lung?
30%

What are the most common sources?
Colon (30%), breast (15%), and kidney (7%)

What are the primary criteria in consideration for potential resection?
1. Metastatic disease isolated to the lung
2. Primary carcinoma controlled
3. Metastases potentially resectable (technically and in terms of patient's predicted reserve after resection of lung parenchyma)

Which groups of carcinomas preferentially metastasize to the lung?
1. Soft tissue sarcomas
2. Osteogenic sarcomas
3. Renal carcinomas

Some metastases may be so small that they are undetectable at surgery. What is the reported increased risk associated with a later, second resection?
No increased risk; postoperative survival same

SEGMENTAL ANATOMY OF THE LUNG (JACKSON AND HUBER NOMENCLATURE)

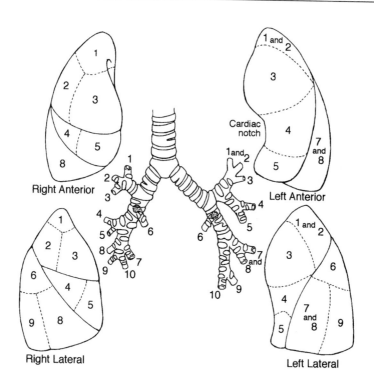

Right

Upper lobe:
1. Apical segment
2. Posterior
3. Anterior

Middle lobe:
4. Lateral
5. Medial

Lower lobe:
6. Superior
7. Medial basal
8. Anterior basal
9. Lateral basal
10. Posterior basal

Left

Upper lobe:
1. & 2. Apical segments
3. Anterior
4. & 5. Superior and inferior (lingular)

Lower lobe:
6. Superior
7. & 8. Anteromedial basal
9. Lateral basal
10. Posterior basal

During a bronchoscopy how do you tell right from left?

The posterior trachea is identified by the membranous tissue versus the anterior cartilage

MEDIASTINUM

ANATOMY

What are the anatomic compartments of the mediastinum?

Anterior (and superior), middle, and posterior

What are the major landmarks between these compartments as noted on lateral CXR?

A = plane between sternal angle and disc between T4 and T5; B = plane just anterior to pericardium; C = plane posterior to heart and between trachea and esophagus

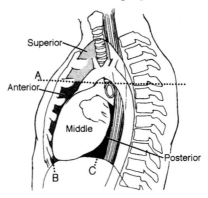

MEDIASTINAL MASSES

Which tumor is associated with the following findings?

Vertebral anomalies

Enteric cyst

Radiologic evidence of tooth within mass

Teratoma

Hypoglycemia and why

Neurosarcoma; secretes an insulin-like substance; called the Doege-Potter syndrome

Gynecomastia

Nonseminomatous germ-cell tumors

Characteristic fever pattern	Hodgkin's lymphoma (Pel-Ebstein fever)
Hypertension	Pheochromocytoma and chemodectoma
Red-cell aplasia	Thymoma
Cushing's syndrome	Thymoma, primary carcinoma, and carcinoid (mediastinal)
Ulceration into bronchus, esophagus, or lung	Enteric cyst (gastric mucosa subtype)
Large size, and why	Mesenchymal tumors. These tumors characteristically do not fix to or invade adjacent structures, so they remain asymptomatic until late.
Identified chromosomal abnormalities (Klinefelter's syndrome, 5q deletion, trisomy 8)	Nonseminomatous germ-cell tumors
Ptosis and diplopia	Thymoma with associated myasthenia gravis
Increased levels of VMA (vanillylmandelic acid) and HVA (homovanillic acid) in urine	Pheochromocytoma
Increased uptake with 131I-MIBG (metaiodobenzylguanidine) scan	Pheochromocytoma
Cerebellar and truncal ataxia with darting eye movements	Neuroblastoma; called opsomyoclonus
Night sweats and pruritus	Lymphoma
Cells from all 3 germ layers: endo-, meso-, and ectoderm	Teratoma
Eaton-Lambert syndrome	Thymoma (Note: Thymomas are associated with more systemic syndromes than are any other mediastinal mass.)

ESOPHAGUS

ANATOMY

What are the anatomic narrowings of the esophagus?	Upper esophageal sphincter (UES), midthorax (due to external compression by left bronchus and aortic arch), and lower esophageal sphincter (LES)
Which is the most narrow?	UES
Which type of muscle makes up the muscularis layer?	Skeletal muscle (upper third), smooth muscle (lower third), mixed smooth and skeletal (middle third)
Which named muscle forms the UES?	Cricopharyngeal muscle
At what tracheal and vertebral level is it located?	Cricoid cartilage and T1 vertebra
Unlike most of the gastrointestinal tract, the esophagus lacks what gross feature?	Serosa
What is the arterial supply of the esophagus?	1. Inferior thyroid artery 2. Bronchial arteries 3. "Esophageal arteries" from aorta 4. Inferior phrenic artery 5. Left gastric artery
Which named nerves travel with the esophagus?	Right and left vagus nerves
Which of these nerves is located on the anterior surface?	Left
Which nerves form the intramural autonomic nervous system of the esophagus?	Auerbach's plexus (between the longitudinal and circular muscle layers) and Meissner's plexus (within submucosa)

ESOPHAGEAL MOTILITY DISORDERS

What are the types of primary motility disorders?	1. Oropharyngeal dysphagia 2. Achalasia 3. Diffuse esophageal spasm

What is the classic type of secondary motility disorder?	Scleroderma
What is the most common symptom?	Dysphagia (difficulty swallowing), notably of both solids and liquids
Which type is associated with increased risk of carcinoma?	Achalasia
What diagnostic tests should be administered?	1. Barium esophagogram 2. Manometry
Which feature of these disorders often makes diagnosis difficult?	Intermittent nature of symptoms. During asymptomatic intervals, esophagogram and manometry findings are usually normal!

OROPHARYNGEAL DYSPHAGIA

What is the physiologic lesion in oropharyngeal dysphagia?	UES does not relax during swallowing.
What are the general groups of etiologies?	Neurogenic disorders (e.g., stroke, brain tumor, multiple sclerosis); myogenic disorders (e.g., muscular dystrophy, myasthenia gravis); structural causes (Zenker's diverticulum); mechanical causes (e.g., webs, tumors); postoperative scarring; and gastroesophageal reflux
What are the symptoms?	Cervical dysphagia, intermittent hoarseness, weight loss, and excessive saliva expectoration
What is the finding on barium esophagogram?	Prominent posterior cricopharyngeal bar
What is the treatment?	Varies widely depending on the etiology
What must be confirmed before surgery, and why?	Competence of LES (by manometry and acid reflux test). Myotomy makes the UES incompetent, and in the presence of LES incompetence, tracheobronchial aspiration occurs.

If surgery is undertaken, which procedure is performed?	Cervical esophagomyotomy (longitudinal incision of muscular layers of the esophagus) to reduce resistance to swallowing
What incision is used?	Oblique left cervical incision, parallel to the anterior border of sternocleidomastoid muscle
Why is it important to avoid disruption of mucosa during the procedures for treatment of esophageal motility disorders?	1. Perforated mucosa increases incidence of postoperative strictures and infection. 2. Risk of life-threatening mediastinitis
What is the management of intraoperative injury to esophageal mucosa?	Primary repair of mucosa. Esophagogram on postop day 1. If leak present or if esophageal emptying unsatisfactory, drains (neck drain or chest tube and nasogastric tubes) should remain in place and parenteral hyperalimentation initiated; then, on postop day 10, perform follow-up esophagogram to confirm closure of leak before removal of drains. If esophagogram is normal, follow routine postoperative management.

SCLERODERMA

What percentage of patients with scleroderma have symptoms referable to esophageal involvement?	> 50%
What characteristic pathologic changes occur in the esophagus?	Atrophy of muscularis and fibrotic replacement of the smooth muscle (distal two-thirds of esophagus)
What is the resultant physiologic lesion?	Weak, nonpropulsive contractions of distal esophagus and loss of LES tone
What are the symptoms?	Heartburn (due to reflux), epigastric fullness, and sensation of slow emptying of esophagus
What is the treatment?	Antireflux procedure (fundoplication); in advanced cases, esophagectomy may be required.

ESOPHAGEAL DIVERTICULA

What are the general mechanisms of esophageal diverticula formation?

Pulsion—Pushing out of segment of esophageal wall by intraluminal force
Traction—Pulling out of segment by external traction

What are the most common primary etiologies of diverticula due to each mechanism?

Pulsion—Abnormal esophageal motility
Traction—Inflamed mediastinal lymph nodes

What are specific examples of each type of diverticula?

Pulsion—Pharyngoesophageal (Zenker's) and epiphrenic diverticulae
Traction—Midesophageal (parabronchial) diverticulae

Which are "true" versus "false" diverticula?

Pulsion types are false diverticula (mucosa and submucosa protrude through a defect in muscular portion of wall).
Traction types are true diverticula (mucosa, submucosa, and muscular portion of wall).

What are the symptoms?

Dysphagia, retrosternal chest pain, regurgitation of undigested food, cough, severe halitosis, and gurgling sounds in throat

Which diagnostic study is indicated?

Barium esophagogram (Note: Avoid esophagoscopy because of the increased risk of perforation.)

What other study should also be done as part of workup?

Manometry (to assess the esophageal motility disorder in pulsion types)

What are the indications for treatment?

All symptomatic patients should undergo surgical repair.

Which type rarely requires treatment?

Midesophageal (because rarely symptomatic)

PHARYNGOESOPHAGEAL (ZENKER'S) DIVERTICULUM

What is the specific location in the esophagus?

Posterior midline within inferior pharyngeal constrictor between thyropharyngeus and cricopharyngeal muscles (Killian's triangle)

Which anatomic landmark is used to locate the sac intraoperatively?	Cricoid cartilage
What motility disorder is associated with pharyngoesophageal diverticulum?	Oropharyngeal dysphagia
What is the current standard surgical treatment?	Diverticulotomy and cricopharyngeal myotomy
What alternative surgical procedure is gaining popularity, and why?	Diverticulopexy (mobilize, invert, and tack pouch to the anterior spinal fascia); significantly reduced risk of postoperative leak/fistula
What occurs if myotomy is not performed?	Diverticulum recurs.

EPIPHRENIC DIVERTICULUM

What is the location in the esophagus?	Distal esophagus (usually within 10 cm of cardia)
What motility disorder is associated with epiphrenic diverticulum?	Diffuse esophageal spasm and achalasia
What is the treatment?	Diverticulectomy; long esophagomyotomy or modified Heller myotomy; ± antireflux procedure (controversial)
Which incision should be used?	Left posterolateral thoracotomy (best access to distal esophagus)

ESOPHAGEAL PERFORATION

What is the most common etiology?	Iatrogenic (esophageal endoscopy or dilatation procedures, paraesophageal surgical procedures)
What are the other etiologies?	Boerhaave's syndrome (most common non-iatrogenic etiology), trauma, swallowed foreign body, and caustic injuries

Why does the esophagus tend to rupture at lower pressures than the remainder of the gastrointestinal tract?

Lacks serosa (Collagen fibers of serosa provide considerable strength to alimentary tract wall.)

What is the usual presentation?

Chest pain, dysphagia, nausea, fever, tachycardia, and (not infrequently) hypotension

What is the classic sign of cervical rupture?

Subcutaneous (SQ) emphysema in neck and anterior thorax (crepitus)

What is the classic sign of intrathoracic rupture?

Hamman's crunch (crackles auscultated as heart beats against emphysematous mediastinum)

Why may the patient with esophageal rupture become acutely unstable?

1. Tension pneumothorax (due to concurrent tear in mediastinal pleura)
2. Hypovolemic shock (Rates of fluid accumulation in the mediastinum as high as 1 L/h have been reported.)

What is the first study performed if perforation is suspected?

CXR

What are the classic findings on this study?

Subcutaneous or mediastinal emphysema, or both; widened mediastinum; ± pleural effusion or pneumothorax (if pleura torn)

What is the diagnostic study of choice?

Contrast esophagogram (first, use water-soluble Gastrografin)

What biochemical test from thoracentesis sample of effusion would suggest perforation?

Elevated amylase (especially if isoenzyme from salivary glands)

What life-threatening condition develops with esophageal perforation?

Mediastinitis (primarily due to the virulent oral flora bacteria free in the mediastinum)

What is the key prognostic factor?

Duration between event and corrective surgery

Why?

Infection usually does not establish until 18–24 hours after the event (but once it develops, treating resultant empyema and suppurative mediastinitis is very difficult).

What is the treatment of cervical esophageal perforations?

Surgical exploration, drainage of retropharyngeal space and upper mediastinum with Jackson-Pratt drains, repair of perforation (if located), and IV antibiotics

What is the postoperative management regimen of cervical perforations?

Closely follow for evidence of mediastinitis; on day 5–7, perform contrast esophagogram with Gastrografin, then barium. If no leak, drains may be removed and PO intake initiated.

In the treatment of thoracic (and abdominal) esophageal perforations, what is the most important factor in determining the course of treatment?

Interval between perforation and diagnosis

Why?

With late diagnosis, mediastinitis is well established, and any esophageal repair will likely break down because of inflammation, tissue friability, and infection.

What are the generally accepted intervals for "early" versus "late" diagnosis?

Early: < 8 hours
Late: > 24 hours
(The interval between 8 and 24 hours is controversial and best left to the surgeon's judgment.)

What is usually recommended for early diagnoses?

Direct repair of esophageal leak plus drainage (mediastinal and pleural tubes); ± definitive treatment for any underlying esophageal pathology (e.g., myotomy for achalasia)

What procedure can reduce the risk of fistula when primary repair is performed?

Reinforce esophageal suture line with flap of pleura, intercostal muscle, or diaphragm.

What procedure is usually recommended for late diagnoses (controversial)?	**Drainage** plus diversion-exclusion of esophagus (end cervical esophagostomy [spit-fistula]), distal cervical esophagus stapled (cardioesophageal junction ligation, gastrostomy/jejunostomy tubes)
What are Cameron's criteria for use of nonoperative treatment for patients with thoracic perforation?	1. Contained leak (isolated within mediastinum) 2. Self-draining back into esophagus 3. Minimal symptoms 4. No (or minimal) signs of clinical sepsis
What are the components of nonoperative management?	NPO, parenteral hyperalimentation, and IV antibiotics

IATROGENIC PERFORATION

What are the most common sites of iatrogenic perforation?	Just proximal to upper esophageal sphincter, gastric cardia, or an esophageal pathology (e.g., stricture)
Are iatrogenic perforations usually diagnosed earlier or later than those in Boerhaave's syndrome?	Earlier, because the procedure forces the surgeon to consider perforation early in the symptomatic patient (perforation is often initially missed in Boerhaave's syndrome because of the relative infrequency of the disease)

BENIGN ESOPHAGEAL TUMORS

Benign esophageal tumors account for what percentage of esophageal tumors?	Only 1%
What are the 2 most common types?	1. Leiomyoma (66%) 2. Congenital esophageal cyst (also called enteric cyst or esophageal duplication cyst) (See Mediastinal Masses section.)
How is the diagnosis made?	1. Barium esophagogram 2. Esophagoscopy (to rule out carcinoma)

Leiomyoma

What are the symptoms?	Dysphagia, chest pain (if < 5 cm in size, often asymptomatic)
What is the classic finding on barium esophagogram?	Smooth narrowing of lumen with intact mucosa (intramural mass)
How is esophagoscopic protocol different with leiomyoma versus carcinoma, and why?	Mass is **not** biopsied.
What are the indications for treatment?	1. Symptomatic patient (chest pain, dysphagia) 2. Mass > 5 cm in size
What is the procedure?	Surgically enucleate from esophageal wall via extramucosal approach.
What incision should be used?	Posterolateral thoracotomy (right if in upper two-thirds, left if in lower one-third)
Why should endoscopic removal be avoided?	Increased risk of esophageal rupture and late stricture (due to disruption of mucosa)

CORROSIVE ESOPHAGEAL INJURIES

How are these burns classified?	First degree—Only mucosal erythema and edema Second degree—Erythema, edema, and ulceration (partial esophageal circumference) Third degree—Circumferential esophageal ulceration and mucosal sloughing
Which diagnostic studies should be performed on initial evaluation?	Esophagoscopy followed by barium esophagogram
What contraindicates the first study?	Evidence of laryngeal or pharyngeal burn (stridor, hoarseness, dyspnea). Admit and monitor for airway obstruction (maximal edema sometimes delayed 6–24 hours!) before diagnostic evaluation of esophagus.

What is the treatment of each type/degree of burn?

First degree—Brief observation; continue PO intake, and discharge home

Second degree—Antibiotics for 3 weeks; continue PO intake, follow up with endoscopy after 3 weeks

Third degree—Same as second, plus large gastrostomy (Note: Some also advocate steroid therapy to reduce incidence of stricture formation.)

What are the late sequelae of corrosive injury?

Stricture formation (most common), malignant degeneration, and hiatal hernia (fibrotic esophagus retracting stomach into chest)

What is the treatment of the most common sequela?

Repeated bougie dilatation of stricture (safest approach being retrograde through gastrostomy); alternatively, balloon dilatation

How long is this treatment continued?

Until a permanently patent lumen develops or 6 months of unsuccessful conservative treatment (Then consider esophagectomy.)

OTHER ESOPHAGEAL LESIONS

Esophageal Webs

What is the most common symptom?

Dysphagia

What are the types and general location of each in the esophagus?

Plummer-Vinson syndrome (PVS) web— Upper esophagus

Schatzki's ring—Distal esophagus (at squamocolumnar junction)

What is the etiology of each type?

Uncertain; presumed etiology for PVS is iron deficiency, and for Schatzki's gastroesophageal reflux.

What is the target population of PVS?

Middle-aged women

What are the characteristic findings on physical exam of this population?

Edentulous, spoon-shaped fingers with brittle nails, and atrophic oral mucosa

What is the treatment?   Dilation of web plus iron supplements in
                               PVS; antireflux procedure in Schatzki's

BARIUM ESOPHAGOGRAM

**What is the most likely
diagnosis for each of the
following line drawings of
various barium studies?
(Several possibilities are
present; try to pick the best.)**

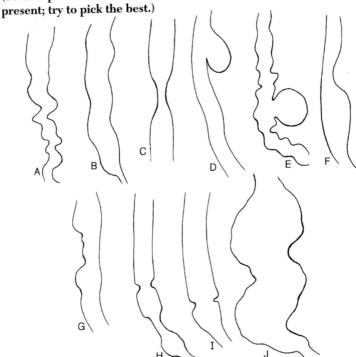

A. Diffuse spasm
B. Achalasia (moderate)
C. Carcinoma: Annular type
D. Zenker's diverticulum
E. Diffuse spasm with epiphrenic
   diverticulum
F. Leiomyoma
G. Carcinoma: Fungating type
H. Sliding hiatal hernia (type I) with
   Barrett's esophagus and esophageal
   stricture due to reflux
I. Schatzki's ring
J. Achalasia (severe)

THORACIC TRAUMA

TRACHEOBRONCHIAL TRAUMA

What is the most common mechanism of injury?	Motor vehicle accidents (hyperextended neck striking dashboard or steering wheel)
What are the classic findings on physical exam?	Subcutaneous emphysema (especially with cervical tracheal injury), auscultation of mediastinal emphysema (Hamman's crunch)
What are the associated CXR findings?	Pneumomediastinum, pneumothorax (PTX), and subcutaneous emphysema
What would significantly increase suspicion of tracheobronchial disruption after placement of tube thoracostomy?	1. Persistent air leak 2. Incomplete reexpansion of lung 3. Worsening respiratory status/symptoms when tube placed to suction because of resultant increase in flow through tracheobronchial lesion (almost pathognomonic)
How is definitive diagnosis made?	Bronchoscopy
What is the acute management of tracheobronchial trauma?	Establish a secure airway via intubation (use flexible bronchoscope to guide endotracheal tube if tracheal injury present).
What are the indications for surgical repair?	1. Persistent air leak 2. Large air leak with respiratory compromise due to incomplete expansion of lung
What procedure is used?	Primary repair and pleural or muscular flap wrap around the suture line
What procedure can be performed if primary repair of trachea is not feasible at time of injury?	Bronchoscopic placement of a silicone tracheal T-tube (Montgomery)
What is the major chronic sequela of unrecognized tracheobronchial disruption?	Stricture formation with increased risk of necrotizing infection (seen more frequently in partial obstruction than complete)

PULMONARY TRAUMA

PULMONARY CONTUSION

What is the mechanism?

Blunt chest trauma—increased pulmonary capillary pressure—extravasation of blood cells, plasma, and serum proteins into interstitium and alveoli

What is the physiologic result of this injury?

Intrapulmonary shunting (and hypoxia), reduced pulmonary compliance (and hypercarbia due to hypoventilation)

What is the classic finding on CXR?

Hazy infiltrate in region of blunt trauma

How long after injury before CXR findings become evident?

Variable: within several minutes in 70% of cases; up to 6 hours in 30%. Regardless, over next 24 hours, size and density often **dramatically** increase.

What may mimic pulmonary contusion on CXR in the trauma patient?

1. Atelectasis distal to aspiration of foreign body (e.g., tooth, dentures, food)
2. Hemothorax in supine patient (generalized haziness over entire lung field)

What is the treatment of pulmonary contusion?

Most cases require only supplemental oxygen; +/− mask continuous positive airway pressure (CPAP), intubate and ventilate as needed; judicious use of IV fluids

TRAUMATIC ASPHYXIA

What is the mechanism of injury?

Crush injury to the thorax

What is the classic triad of physical findings?

1. Facial and upper torso edema with cyanotic appearance
2. Subconjunctival hemorrhage
3. Petechiae (due to retrograde flow through valveless veins of upper body associated with sudden increase in intrathoracic pressure)

What is the treatment?	Supportive, head elevation, and supplemental oxygen

TRAUMATIC AIR EMBOLISM

What is the most common cause?	Penetrating wound to chest resulting in injury to abutting pulmonary vessel and tracheobronchial lumen
What dramatically increases the risk of air embolus?	Positive pressure ventilation
What is the presentation?	1. Cerebral ischemia (e.g., seizures) and cardiac ischemia (infarction, arrhythmias) due to the resultant air emboli and platelet—fibrin aggregates 2. Coagulopathy and bronchospasm due to activation of inflammatory cascades
What is the treatment?	Left lateral decubitus position, feet elevated 30°–60° (unfortunately often difficult in the trauma patient); aspirate air from CVP line(consider cardiopulmonary bypass or hyperbaric oxygen)

MISCELLANEOUS

What is the differential diagnosis for thoracic outlet syndrome?	Cervical spine Ruptured intervertebral disk Osteoarthritis Spinal cord tumors Peripheral neuropathy (e.g., carpal tunnel syndrome) Brachial plexus palsy Arterial Aneurysm Embolism Occlusive disease Thromboangiitis obliterans Raynaud's disease Venous Thrombophlebitis Vasculitis, collagen disease

What are the types of bronchial adenomas?	Carcinoid, mucoepidermoid carcinoma, mucous gland adenoma, adenoid cystic carcinoma
What is the most common bronchial adenoma?	Carcinoid (85%)
Are bronchial adenomas benign?	No, it is a misconception. Most can be malignant.
Name 3 causes of vena cava syndrome other than malignant tumors.	1. Chronic mediastinitis 2. Benign tumors 3. Thrombosis (often resulting from a long-term central line)
What may aggravate the symptoms of superior vena cava (SVC) syndrome?	Lying flat or bending over
What is the clinical course of SVC syndrome?	Depends on rapidity of onset. Rapid onset of severe obstruction with no time to develop collateral circulation leads to severe symptoms and possibly fatal cerebral edema; chronic onset, as in fibrosing mediastinitis, may be very insidious and mild as collateral drainage develops.
How is the diagnosis of SVC syndrome made?	1. Measure upper extremity venous pressure. 2. Venography localizes the obstruction. 3. CT scan evaluates for tumor. 4. Obtain MRI/MRA.
Name 4 tumors of the anterior mediastinum.	"Four **T**s": 1. **T**hymomas 2. **T**eratomas 3. **T**hyroid tumor 4. **T**errible lymphomas
What are the classic locations of aspiration pneumonia?	RUL—Posterior segment RLL—Superior segment
What bronchus is inadvertently intubated most often?	The right main stem (less of an angle from the trachea than the left)

68

Cardiovascular Surgery

CONGENITAL HEART DISEASE

What 3 general physiologic disturbances are associated with congenital heart disease?	Left to right (L to R) shunts, R to L shunts, and ventricular outflow obstruction
What are the 3 most common defects and their relative frequencies among all congenital heart defects?	Ventricular septal defect (VSD; 30–40%) Atrial septal defect (ASD; 10–15%) Patent ductus arteriosus (PDA; 10–20%)
What are the most common general INITIAL presentations of congenital heart lesions?	CHF, cyanosis, and poor peripheral perfusion
Which presentation is classic for each of the classes of lesions?	CHF (acyanotic): L to R shunt, ventricular outflow obstruction Cyanosis: R to L shunt CHF and cyanosis: Complex defects. Rarely, shunts may also eventually develop into CHF, but cyanosis is the presenting sign.
How are these presentations diagnosed in the child?	CHF: Failure to thrive, tachycardia, tachypnea, hepatic enlargement (unlike adults, rales develop late) Cyanosis: Discoloration of mucous membranes and skin
Which class of defects is characteristically associated with increased versus decreased pulmonary blood flow (PBF)?	Increased PBF: L to R shunts Decreased PBF: R to L shunts

Which shunt classically reverses if untreated, and what is the syndrome called?	L to R shunts; Eisenmenger's syndrome (discussed later)

CYANOTIC CONGENITAL HEART DISEASE

What is the most common cyanotic congenital defect?	Tetralogy of Fallot (TOF; 50% of cyanotic lesions)

SEQUELAE OF CYANOTIC HEART DISEASE

What are the classic sequelae of cyanotic heart disease?	Hypertrophic osteoarthropathy (clubbing), polycythemia, hypercyanotic spells, cerebrovascular accidents, brain abscesses, coagulation disorders, and endocarditis
What are hypercyanotic (or hypoxic) spells?	Abrupt increase in cyanosis associated with cerebral anoxia that may result in unconsciousness, seizure, or death
What is the usual mechanism of these spells?	Infundibular muscle spasm in the right ventricular outflow tract, resulting in a sudden reduction in blood flow to the lungs
Why are brain abscesses common in patients with cyanotic heart disease?	R to L shunt permits venous blood to bypass the lungs, which are an important filter for bacteria.
What are the most common organisms in these abscesses?	Gram-positive cocci (staphylococcus and streptococcus)
Brain abscesses are most often seen with which anomaly?	TOF
What is the hallmark physical finding of CHF in a child?	Hepatic enlargement

VENTRICULAR SEPTAL DEFECTS

What is the anatomic lesion?	Abnormal communication between the left and right ventricles
What are the locations ("types") of VSD?	Infundibular or canal septum (beneath the semilunar valves), membranous septum, inlet septum, and muscular septum

Which type is most common?	Membranous septum (80–85%)
What is a "large" VSD?	Diameter $\geq$ aortic orifice
What percentage of patients with VSD have additional congenital cardiac lesions?	> 50%
What is the main physiologic problem in VSD?	L to R shunt, resulting in increased pulmonary blood flow
What classic syndrome may develop if VSD is untreated?	Eisenmenger's syndrome
Describe the murmur associated with VSD.	Harsh pansystolic murmur at the left sternal border
When do infants with large VSDs become symptomatic, and why?	6 weeks to 3 months. Pulmonary vascular resistance (PVR) must decrease from its high fetal baseline value before L to R shunt is possible. (PVR does not reach the normal adult level until after 3 months of age.)
What are the complications of VSD?	Large VSD: CHF and pulmonary hypertension Small VSD: Increased risk of endocarditis
Why is nonoperative management initially warranted in many cases?	Many patients (25–50%) have spontaneous closure. The chance of closure decreases with increasing age at presentation (80% of defects noted at 1 month versus only 25% noted at 12 months).

ATRIAL SEPTAL DEFECTS

What is the anatomic lesion?	Abnormal communication between the right and left atria
What are the types and the general location of each type in the septum?	Sinus venosus: High in the atrial septum Ostium secundum: Middle (fossa ovalis region) Ostium primum: Low
Which type is the most common?	Ostium secundum (80%)

What is the main physiologic problem in ASD?

L to R shunt

Why is this problem minimal during the first few years of life?

Right ventricular hypertrophy of infancy takes time to subside. In infancy, compliance of the right ventricle (RV) is similar to that of the left ventricle (LV), thus minimizing the shunt.

What are the primary factors that determine the degree of shunting in ASD?

Compliance of the ventricles, PVR, and size of the ASD. Size is less important than in VSD.

What percentage of the general population has a patent foramen ovale (PFO)?

10–25%

Why is PFO not considered an ASD?

It usually permits only unidirectional (R to L) shunt because of the relation between the remnants of the septum primum and the septum secundum.

At what age do UNTREATED patients with isolated ASD become symptomatic?

30–40 years old (usually asymptomatic until then)

At what age do UNTREATED patients with ASD show a clear increase in mortality rate?

20 years old. The survival rate (untreated) is 85% at 20 years, 40% at 40 years, and 25% at 50 years.

How does ASD present?

CHF (e.g., dyspnea)

Describe the murmur associated with ASDs.

Systolic ejection murmur at the left sternal border

What is the primary contraindication to surgery?

Irreversible pulmonary hypertension (> 10 Wood units)

What corrective procedure is performed?

Closure of ASD by primary closure or patch (prosthetic or pericardial)

What is the main operative complication?

Injury to the conduction system

PATENT DUCTUS ARTERIOSUS

PDA is the embryologic remnant of what structure?	Sixth left aortic arch
What is the normal function of the ductus arteriosus?	Acts as R to L shunt in the fetus to bypass the uninflated lungs (blood oxygenated at the placenta)
When does it usually close?	In the first few days of life (96% closed by 48 hours). Complete closure, through fibrosis and intimal proliferation, to form the ligamentum arteriosus takes several months.
What stimulates this initial closure?	It is theorized that increased arterial oxygen tension may constrict the muscle in the ductus.
What physiologic conditions may prevent closure of the ductus?	Hypoxia and increased levels of prostaglandins
PDA is common in what group of infants?	Premature infants, especially girls
Describe the murmur associated with PDAs.	Continuous "machinery" murmur with a late systolic peak, widely transmitted to the precordium and neck. The diastolic component of the murmur is absent in infancy because of elevated PVR (normal physiology); thus, it often is not continuous until 1 year of age.
What is the other classic finding on cardiovascular physical exam?	Wide pulse pressure with bounding pulse (large PDAs only)
What are the most common causes of death in adults with UNTREATED PDA?	CHF and bacterial endocarditis, especially *Streptococcus viridans*
What is the medical treatment of PDA?	Indomethacin (prostaglandin E_1 inhibitor). If unresolved in 1 week, surgery is indicated.

In which patients is medical treatment ineffective?	Full-term infants; children
What is the surgical treatment?	Ligation, clipping, or division of the PDA
Care is taken to avoid injury to what nerve that courses close to the PDA?	Left recurrent laryngeal nerve
When is surgery performed?	If the PDA is large and CHF develops, surgery is performed immediately, regardless of patient age. Otherwise, surgery is performed at 1–2 years of age or thereafter whenever the diagnosis is made.
What is the primary contraindication to surgery, and why?	Cyanosis caused by an untreated cyanotic cardiac anomaly or severe pulmonary hypertension, both of which depend on the patency of the ductus for patient survival (one as a source of blood to the lung, the other as a means to shunt blood away from the high-pressure pulmonary bed)

TRUNCUS ARTERIOSUS

What is the anatomic lesion?	Single large vessel that straddles the ventricular septum (instead of a separate aorta and pulmonary artery), with a 3- to 6-leaflet truncal valve

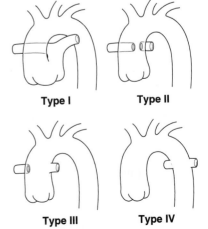

Type I   Type II

Type III   Type IV

What additional congenital cardiac lesion is always seen in these patients?

VSD, usually immediately under the truncal valve

What is the palliative surgical procedure?

Pulmonary artery banding to permit growth for infants with severe concurrent noncardiac disease (rarely used)

What is the corrective procedure?

Excision of the origin of the pulmonary artery from the main truncus and closure of the aortic defect, placement of a conduit (homograft or porcine composite graft) to establish continuity between the RV and pulmonary artery, and closure of the VSD

TETRALOGY OF FALLOT

What are the 4 classic anatomic features?

1. Overriding aorta (dextroposition of the aorta)
2. Obstruction to right ventricular outflow (infundibular or valvular pulmonic stenosis)
3. VSD
4. Right ventricular hypertrophy

① Overriding aorta
② Valvular and infundibular pulmonary stenosis
③ Large ventricular septal defect
④ Hypertrophic right ventricle

What is the pentalogy of Fallot?

TOF plus ASD

What is the surgical procedure for TOF?

Palliative systemic to pulmonary shunt (i.e., Blalock-Taussig subclavian artery to pulmonary artery shunt). Traditionally, a corrective procedure is performed 6 months to 2 years later to correct pulmonary outflow obstruction and close the VSD. Some surgeons now prefer early total correction without an intervening palliative shunt.

EBSTEIN'S ANOMALY

What is the basic anatomic lesion?

Tricuspid valve is positioned abnormally low within the RV (with a large "sail" anterior leaflet and septal and posterior leaflets originating from the wall of the RV). The RV is divided into a thin "atrialized" supravalvular portion and a normal trabeculated apical and infundibular portion. ASD is also usually present.

What is the surgical treatment?

Tricuspid valvuloplasty, followed by reconstruction with plication of the atrialized portion of the RV, followed by ASD closure. Occasionally, tricuspid valve replacement (the procedure of choice in the past) is necessary.

TRANSPOSITION OF THE GREAT VESSELS

What is the anatomic lesion?

Ventriculoarterial discordance (e.g., aorta originates from the RV; the pulmonary artery from the LV) with AV concordance (ventricles are connected to the appropriate atria). This condition results in parallel, rather than serial, systemic and pulmonary circulations.

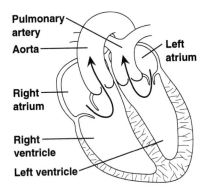

What is the claim to fame of this condition?

Most common congenital defect that causes cyanosis and CHF in the newborn period (> 90% by day 1)

What is the palliative surgical procedure?

Balloon atrial septostomy. Palliative septectomy (Blalock-Hanlon procedure) is now virtually obsolete.

What are the options for corrective procedure?

Atrial switch procedure: Intra-atrial baffle to redirect venous blood toward the appropriate great vessel (i.e., Mustard procedure)

Arterial switch procedure: Switching of the aorta and pulmonary artery and reimplantation of the coronary arteries into the aorta (Jatene procedure)

TOTAL ANOMALOUS PULMONARY VENOUS CONNECTION (TAPVC)

What is the general anatomic lesion?

No pulmonary veins directly drain into the left atrium (LA) ± pulmonary vein stenosis.

What are the 3 types and their relative frequencies?

Supracardiac: Pulmonary venous drainage into the SVC (50%)

Intracardiac: Pulmonary venous drainage into the coronary sinus or right atrium (RA)

Infracardiac: Pulmonary venous drainage into the IVC

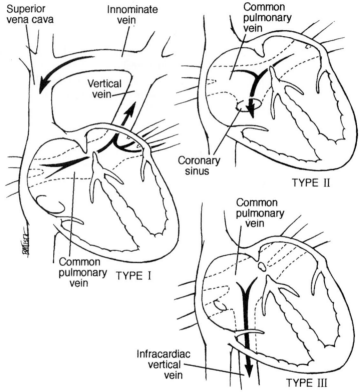

What is a partial APVC (PAPVC)?

Some, but not all, pulmonary veins empty into the LA.

What is scimitar syndrome?

PAPVC in which the pulmonary veins from the right lung join to form a single vertical vein that curves downward to join with the IVC

HYPOPLASTIC LEFT HEART SYNDROME

What is the anatomic lesion?

Aortic valve atresia or severe hypoplasia (primary lesion), LV hypoplasia, mitral valve atresia or hypoplasia, and ASD. The interventricular septum is usually intact.

VASCULAR RINGS

What is the embryonic origin of a vascular ring?	Anomalous development of the aorta and pulmonary artery from the embryonic aortic arches
What is the most common type?	Double aortic arch
What is the most prominent symptom?	Stridor as a result of compression of the trachea by vascular rings
Although a variety of anomalies and multiple operative techniques exist, what is the basic surgical procedure?	The compressive arteries are divided, and bypass performed if necessary

ANEURYSM OF THE SINUS OF VALSALVA

What are the sinuses of Valsalva?	Outpouchings of the aortic root corresponding to leaflets (indentations where commissures meet the aortic wall)
What are the etiologies of aneurysms of these sinuses?	Congenital: Aortic wall media does not meet the aortic annulus Acquired: Endocarditis, myxomatous degeneration, syphilis, and chronic aortic dissection

EISENMENGER'S SYNDROME

What is Eisenmenger's syndrome?	Reversal of a long-standing untreated L to R shunt (i.e., becomes an R to L shunt)
Why does it occur?	L to R shunt increases pressure in the right side of the heart. Reactive changes (e.g., medial hypertrophy, sclerosis) occur in the pulmonary arterioles, followed by pulmonary hypertension. Eventually, the shunt reverses.
What is the most common cardiac lesion associated with this syndrome, if left untreated?	VSD
What is the usual presentation?	New onset of cyanosis in a patient with L to R shunt

What is the most common cause of death?	Massive hemoptysis. Patients often die by 30–40 years of age.
What is the treatment?	Heart-lung transplant; thus, the condition is considered inoperable by many.

ACQUIRED CORONARY ARTERY DISEASE

CORONARY ANATOMY

Identify the labeled arteries.

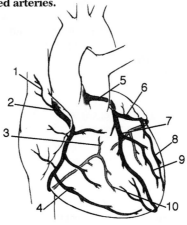

1. Sinoatrial nodal artery
2. Right coronary artery
3. AV nodal artery
4. Right marginal artery
5. Left main coronary artery
6. Circumflex artery
7. Left anterior descending (LAD) artery
8. Obtuse marginal arteries
9. Diagonal arteries
10. Posterior descending artery

What percentage of patients with CAD have "triple-vessel disease"?	> 50%. These patients have significant atherosclerosis in all 3 primary coronary arteries (right, LAD or left main, and circumflex).
Are most individuals right or left "dominant," and what does this designation mean?	90% are right dominant (posterior descending artery originates from the right coronary circulation). In left-dominant individuals, the posterior descending artery originates from the circumflex artery.

What are the multiple secondary branches off the LAD and the circumflex artery?	LAD: Septal and diagonal arteries Circumflex: Marginal arteries
Coronary arteries arise from what aortic region?	Sinuses of Valsalva
Which coronary artery supplies the sinus node versus the AV node?	Both are usually supplied by the right coronary artery.
Most atherosclerotic lesions are located in what general region of the coronary arteries?	Proximal one-third to one-half. This feature permits coronary artery bypass, except in the occasional patient with severe distal disease.

CORONARY ARTERY BYPASS GRAFTING (CABG)

What is the main risk associated with using both internal mammary arteries for CABG?	Sternal wound infection and dehiscence
Which patients are at increased risk for this complication?	Obese patients and patients with diabetes
After CABG, what percentage of patients are free of ischemia:	
In the early postoperative period?	90%
At 5 years?	75%
At 10 years?	50%
What is the most common cause of recurrence of angina < 5 years versus > 7 years after CABG?	< 5 years: Progression of atherosclerotic disease in native coronary arteries > 7 years: Atherosclerotic disease in saphenous vein graft
What decreases the risk of future graft thrombosis?	Aspirin

What is the mortality rate for:

Elective CABG?	1–2%
Emergent CABG?	3–8% (often even higher in the setting of postinfarction angina)
Emergent CABG in the setting of cardiogenic shock?	> 50%
Elective redo CABG?	7–8%
Emergent redo CABG?	25%
Acute MI?	10–25% (e.g., surgery is worth the risk to prevent or delay MI)

MECHANICAL COMPLICATIONS OF ISCHEMIC HEART DISEASE

What type of patient typically has these complications?	Patients with single-vessel disease, no history of angina, and uncomplicated MI with acute decompensation in the early post-MI period

LEFT VENTRICULAR ANEURYSM

What is the most common etiology of left ventricular aneurysm?	Large transmural MI (infarcted tissue replaced by a fibrous scar that permits localized dilation of the ventricle)
What is the incidence of this complication?	5–15% of patients with MI
What region is most commonly involved?	Anterior-apical surface of the LV (LAD territory)
What is the most common presentation?	Left ventricular failure (LVF)
How is the diagnosis made?	Dyskinesia (paradoxic outward bulge of the region during systole) seen on ventriculogram or echocardiogram. (Because of transient functional changes associated with stunned myocardium, the diagnosis of left ventricular aneurysm cannot be made at the time of acute MI.)

What is the classic ECG finding?	Persistent ST elevation in the involved territory after MI (versus in pericarditis, ST elevations occur in almost all leads)
What are the usual complications?	LVF, arrhythmias, angina, and, infrequently, emboli from mural thrombus. These aneurysms rarely rupture.
What are the indications for surgery for left ventricular aneurysm?	Symptomatic patient Arrhythmias refractory to medical therapy Aneurysm > 5–6 cm
What is the surgical procedure?	Aneurysmectomy and CABG to the ischemic territory
What is the waiting period after MI for elective repair, and why?	At least 2 months, to permit the aneurysm to become well demarcated and the rim to become fibrotic (versus necrotic and difficult to suture)
What are the 5-year survival rates for treated versus untreated patients?	Treated: 75–80% Untreated: 20–30%

ACUTE VENTRICULAR SEPTAL DEFECT

When does acute VSD classically present?	5–7 days after MI
What is the classic presentation?	Acute CHF with a new, harsh pansystolic murmur and thrill at the left sternal border
What is the usual Swan-Ganz catheter finding?	"Step-up" of oxygen saturation (> 10%) between the LA (proximal port) and pulmonary artery (distal port)
What is the medical treatment?	Same treatment as acute ischemic mitral regurgitation (MR)
What is the surgical procedure for acute VSD?	Left ventriculotomy through the infarction with patch repair of VSD and patch closure of ventriculotomy. (Although repair was often delayed for several weeks in the past, it is now performed acutely.)

Compare the timing of surgery if cardiac output (CO) is normal versus decreased.	CO is artifactually increased in patients with VSD because the thermodilution curve is altered by the L to R shunt. CO does not affect timing.

ACUTE ISCHEMIC MITRAL REGURGITATION

What are the mechanisms of acute ischemic MR?	Papillary muscle dysfunction or stunning (most common), annular dilation, and papillary muscle rupture (rare)
What territory is usually involved in MI associated with MR?	Posterolateral territory with injury to the posterior papillary muscle (usually circumflex coronary artery territory)
What is the classic presentation?	CHF with a new holosystolic murmur radiating to the axilla
What are the Swan-Ganz catheter findings?	Large V wave on the pulmonary capillary wedge pressure (PCWP) tracing; no "step-up" of oxygen saturation
Acute ischemic MR accounts for what percentage of early MI deaths?	1%
What is the mortality rate in UNTREATED patients with MI complicated by ischemic MR?	70% in the first 24 hours; 90% in the first 2 weeks
What key question must be answered to guide patient management?	Will the etiology of MR likely resolve with supportive medical therapy (stunning), or is acute surgical correction required (ruptured papillary muscle)?
What is the hemodynamic goal of medical treatment?	Afterload reduction to minimize regurgitant flow by maximizing flow from the LV. This therapy is also used to temporarily stabilize the surgical patient before repair.
What is the treatment of the hypotensive patient?	Dobutamine and intra-aortic balloon pump (IABP)
What is the surgical procedure for acute ischemic MR?	Mitral valve replacement (MVR) and CABG to the infarcted territory (and other territories at risk)

ACQUIRED VALVULAR HEART DISEASE

AORTIC VALVE

What is the normal patent surface area of the aortic valve?	2.5–3.5 cm²
What gross changes occur in the heart as a result of aortic stenosis (AS) versus aortic regurgitation (AR)?	AS: Left ventricular hypertrophy (LVH) (concentric) because of pressure overload AR: Left ventricular dilation (and LVH) because of volume overload

Compare AS with AR:

Which is generally less well tolerated?	AS. Strain on the LV caused by increased intraventricular pressure is greater than that of volume overload.
Which has a male:female ratio of 8:1?	AS
Which may be associated with ascending aortic dilatation?	Both. In AS, it may develop as a result of poststenotic turbulence. An ascending aortic aneurysm with associated dilation of the aortic annulus may cause AR.
What studies are used to diagnose and quantify the severity of AS and AR?	Echocardiogram (with Doppler) and cardiac catheterization (ventriculogram)
What variables are measured with these studies?	AS: Transvalvular pressure gradient and valvular surface area AR: Severity of regurgitation Valvular surface areas are calculated with the Grolin formula, using estimates of flow and gradients. Thus, the criteria for severity of valvular lesions are rough guidelines; the patient's symptoms are far more important!
Which patients should also have a coronary angiogram?	Any patient > 35 years old or with symptoms of MI (angina), regardless of age
What cardiac structures are at risk for injury during aortic valve replacement (AVR)?	Coronary artery ostia and the bundle of His in the membranous ventricular septum, specifically at the commissure between the right and noncoronary cusps

Which patients are at greatest risk for postoperative ventricular failure after AVR?	Patients with a low preoperative ejection fraction ($< 40\%$)
What is the treatment of postoperative ventricular failure?	Vasodilators (for afterload reduction) and inotropic support, $+$ IABP until the ventricle recovers or adapts
What is the target systolic blood pressure (SBP) after AVR, and why?	Goal SBP is < 120 mm Hg to reduce the risk of bleeding from the aortic suture line. (The ascending aorta is incised to gain access to the valve.)
What conduction disturbance may occur after AVR?	Heart block, usually caused by edema around the bundle of His and therefore transient. Occasionally, permanent heart block occurs because of intraoperative mechanical trauma (i.e., suture through the bundle).
What is the treatment of postoperative conduction disturbances?	Temporary pacing with pacing wires (placed intraoperatively) until the edema resolves; a permanent pacer if heart block persists
What is the 10-year mortality rate for untreated symptomatic AS versus AR?	AS: $\cong 100\%$; AR $< 40\%$

VALVULAR AORTIC STENOSIS

What is the claim to fame of valvular AS?	Most common isolated valvular lesion
What are the etiologies?	Calcification of congenitally bicuspid aortic valve (50%), rheumatic fever (33%), and senile (idiopathic) calcification of a normal (trileaflet) aortic valve
What are the 3 nonvalvular etiologies of left ventricular outflow obstruction?	Hypertrophic cardiomyopathy (septal hypertrophy), subvalvular stenosis (focal LV outflow tract stenosis or web), and supravalvular stenosis (aortic narrowing or web)

When is valvular stenosis considered critical?

Transvalvular systolic pressure gradient > 50 mm Hg
Valvular surface area < 1.0 cm2

How is cardiac output maintained as stenosis progresses?

Gradual LVH to overcome increasing afterload

What is the usual age at initial presentation?

40–60 years if AS is caused by calcification of the bicuspid valve; otherwise, 60–80 years

What are the symptoms?

Angina, syncope, and exertional dyspnea as a result of CHF

What is the average life expectancy (if untreated) after the onset of each of these symptoms?

Angina: 3–5 years; Syncope: 2–3 years; Dyspnea: 1–2 years. Symptoms are characteristically late, and once they develop, there is rapid clinical deterioration if left untreated.

What is the usual mechanism of angina in AS?

Increased myocardial oxygen demand because of increased afterload plus decreased oxygen delivery because of LVH. (Angina may also be caused by concurrent CAD.)

AS is rarely symptomatic before the valve surface area is reduced to what size?

1.0 cm^2 (about one-third of the normal area)

Why may loss of sinus rhythm cause acute decompensation in AS?

LVH results in reduced ventricular compliance, and the synchronized atrial contraction of diastole becomes an important component of ventricular filling.

Describe the murmur associated with AS.

Crescendo-decrescendo systolic murmur in the second right intercostal space with radiation to the carotids. Intensity does not correlate with severity; in fact, the most severe cases often have barely audible murmurs.

What are the other classic findings of AS?	Pulsus parvus et tardus (delayed, slow carotid upstroke, with decreased amplitude); narrowed pulse pressure; paradoxic split of S_2 because of delayed closure of the aortic valve (A_2 follows P_2); decreased intensity of S_2; ejection click after S_1; LV lift or heave
What valvular lesion often masks the clinical findings of AS?	Mitral stenosis (MS)
What are the usual ECG findings?	Evidence of LVH: S (V1 or V2) + R (V5 or V6) > 35 mm, R (V5 or V6) > 27 mm, or R (AVL) > 11 mm Evidence of LV strain: Repolarization changes (ST depression with upward convexity and T wave inversion)
What are the usual CXR findings?	Normal cardiac silhouette, except for some rounding of the apex because of LVH, + calcifications at the level of the aortic valve, + widening of the cephalad mediastinum because of poststenotic dilatation of the aorta
When is echocardiography often inaccurate in its assessment of AS?	In the presence of concurrent MS (or AR) or low cardiac output
What is the most feared common complication of AS?	Sudden death because of ventricular fibrillation
What is the etiology of this complication?	Hypertrophy increases the risk of subendocardial ischemia and, thus, ventricular ectopy.
What are the indications for surgical treatment?	Symptomatic patient (angina, syncope, CHF) Critical AS The surface area criteria for surgery vary from 0.5–1.0 cm^2, depending on the surgeon as well as the patient's overall condition. Asymptomatic patients are rarely considered for surgery.

What is the surgical procedure?	AVR ± annuloplasty (incision of the annulus to accommodate placement of a larger prosthetic valve in a patient with a small aortic root)
What are the treatment options for the poor surgical candidate?	Percutaneous balloon valvuloplasty; unfortunately, 50–75% restenose in 6 months Palliative medical therapy for CHF + angina (i.e., digitalis, diuretics, nitrates)
What is the 5-year survival rate for patients who have had AVR for AS?	80–90%. If ventricular function is impaired at the time of surgery, the 5-year survival rate is reduced by 15–25%.

AORTIC REGURGITATION

What are the etiologies of AR?	Myxomatous degeneration (i.e., Marfan's disease), rheumatic fever, bacterial endocarditis, ascending aortic aneurysm or dissection with dilation of the aortic annulus, calcification of a congenitally bicuspid valve
What are the symptoms?	Uncomfortable palpitations as a result of arrhythmias, ectopic ventricular beats, or powerful contractions of the dilated LV against the chest wall; symptoms of left heart failure (e.g., dyspnea, orthopnea); and angina
What is the classic presentation of ACUTE AR?	Fulminant CHF (versus adaptive changes in the LV that permit gradual tolerance of chronic AR over time)
What is the classic blood pressure finding and the mechanism?	Wide pulse pressure (often 80–100 mm Hg) because of increased SBP associated with increased CO and decreased diastolic blood pressure associated with regurgitation
What is the classic character of the pulse?	Bounding because of collapse during diastole (Corrigan's pulse); double-peaked ("bisferious" pulse); "pistol shot" femoral pulse (excessively high femoral compared with brachial SBP; Hill's sign)

What are the usual ECG findings?	Evidence of LVH and strain, as in AS
What are the usual CXR findings?	Enlarged cardiac silhouette with downward displacement of the LV apex because of LV dilation, widening of the cephalad mediastinum if AR is caused by ascending aortic aneurysm
Why is the timing of surgical intervention more controversial than with AS?	AR causes more indolent deterioration of LV function.
What are the indications for surgical treatment of AR?	Acute significant AR Symptomatic patient with moderate exercise or at rest (New York Heart Association [NYHA] class III or IV) Asymptomatic patient with evidence of deteriorating LV function
What are the surgical options?	AVR ± tube graft for an ascending aortic aneurysm (often as a composite graft); occasionally, aortic valve repair (valve resuspension, replacement of leaflets, or simple suture closure of the cusp perforation)
What is the 5-year survival rate after AVR for AR?	75–80%. If ventricular function is impaired at the time of surgery, the 5-year survival rate is reduced by 15–25%.

MITRAL VALVE

What is the normal patent surface area of the mitral valve?	4–6 cm^2
Is MR or MS associated with LA enlargement?	Both are.
What are the classic signs of LA enlargement on anteroposterior CXR?	Double contour sign (round, double density noted within the cardiac silhouette), straightened left heart border, + elevated left bronchus

What is the classic ECG finding with LA enlargement?	P-mitrale: Broad, notched P wave in lead II
What systemic complication is associated with LA enlargement?	Systemic embolization (thrombus formation caused by stasis in the dilated low-pressure chamber)
What is the incidence of thromboembolism in MS and MR?	MS: 15–30%; MR: < 5%. (MS has the highest risk of thromboembolism of any valve lesion.)
What step is taken preoperatively to reduce the risk of thromboembolism?	Anticoagulation with warfarin (Coumadin)
What step is often undertaken intraoperatively to reduce the future risk of thromboembolism?	Ligation of the left atrial appendage, which frequently harbors a thrombus
What common arrhythmia is associated with LA enlargement?	Atrial fibrillation

MITRAL STENOSIS

What is the etiology of MS?	Rheumatic fever, which is noted in the patient's history only about 50% of the time because of the 20- to 30-year interval between infection and the symptoms of valvular disease
What is the criterion for critical MS?	Valve surface area < 1.0 cm²
What is the primary physiologic effect of MS?	Pulmonary hypertension
What are the symptoms of MS?	Dyspnea (most common), fatigue, orthopnea, and palpitations
Why may hemoptysis develop?	Chronic pulmonary hypertension causes dilation of the collaterals between the pulmonary and bronchial veins, forming submucosal varices in the bronchus.

What are the indications for surgery?	Multiple indications, including NYHA class III or IV, critical MS, CHF, pulmonary hypertension, atrial fibrillation, systemic emboli, endocarditis, and transvalvular gradient > 10 mm Hg
What is the first-line surgical procedure?	Open commissurotomy (sharp separation of fused leaflets)
When is this technique contraindicated?	Extensive calcification of the valve
What is the restenosis rate at 5 years?	Only 10%. Unlike in the aortic valve, mitral commissurotomy is effective in selected patients.
What procedure is usually performed if MS recurs?	MVR

MITRAL REGURGITATION

What are the etiologies of MR?	Rheumatic fever (40–45%), myxomatous degeneration, severe mitral valve prolapse, senile (idiopathic) calcification of mitral valve, infectious endocarditis, trauma, hypertrophic cardiomyopathy, and MI or ischemia (see Postoperative Myocardial Ischemia section)
What are the symptoms?	Fatigue, dyspnea, and palpitations. Symptoms are similar to those of MS, but are characteristically insidious and late, unless caused by MI.
Describe the murmur associated with MR.	Holosystolic at the apex, with radiation to the axilla
What is the characteristic finding on pulmonary artery catheter tracing?	Prominent V wave because of regurgitant systolic flow
What is the medical treatment of MR?	Salt restriction, diuretics, and digitalis; can be palliative for many years
What are the indications for surgical treatment?	Acute MR (i.e., ischemic MR) NYHA class III or IV status Progressive increase in regurgitant fraction

What are the surgical options?

MVR or mitral valve repair, including leaflet repair, annuloplasty (reducing size of dilated annulus with sutures or a prosthetic ring), chordae tendineae reconstruction, or reimplantation of ruptured papillary muscle

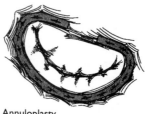

Annuloplasty

Why may LVF develop in the early postoperative period?

LV no longer has a low-pressure vent (LA) into which it can unload blood during systole. With correction of MR, LV ejects all of its volume into the high-pressure aorta.

What is the treatment of postoperative LVF?

Vasodilator therapy for afterload reduction; inotrope therapy + IABP (See the Mechanical Complications of Ischemic Heart Disease section for a discussion of MR caused by myocardial ischemia.)

MITRAL VALVE PROLAPSE

What is mitral valve prolapse?

Bulging of the mitral leaflets into the LA during systole because of redundant MV tissue ± chordae tendineae

What is the incidence in the general population?

3–4%

What is the target population?

Girls and women 15–30 years old. It is often seen in patients with myxomatous degenerative disorders, and thus appears to be genetic.

What are the symptoms?

Most patients are asymptomatic. The most common symptoms are fatigue, nonspecific chest pain, palpitation, and dyspnea.

What is the classic auscultatory sign?	Mid- to late systolic click
What percentage of these patients develop significant MR?	5–7%

TRICUSPID VALVE

Does tricuspid valve disease (TVD) present more frequently as tricuspid regurgitation (TR) or tricuspid stenosis (TS)?	TR (75%)
What is the most common etiology of isolated acquired TVD?	Infectious endocarditis caused by IV drug abuse. Venous return from injected veins slowly bathes the tricuspid valve before reaching the lungs, which filter many of the bacteria.
What is the most common etiology of primary acquired TVD?	Rheumatic heart disease (almost always accompanied by mitral stenosis)

PULMONARY VALVE

What is the most common acquired pulmonary valve lesion?	Functional pulmonary regurgitation caused by dilation of pulmonary annulus. It usually occurs secondary to pulmonary hypertension associated with MS.

RHEUMATIC HEART DISEASE

What is the etiology of rheumatic heart disease?	Systemic immune disease associated with antecedent hemolytic group A streptococcal pharyngitis (rheumatic fever). Patients have high antistreptolysin (ASO) titers.
What are the gross effects on the affected valve?	Leaflet fibrosis, shortening of the chordae tendineae, and commissural fusion
What are the most commonly involved valves?	Mitral valve: 85% of cases Aortic valve: 30% of cases Tricuspid and pulmonary valves: < 5% of cases

PROSTHETIC VALVES

Mechanical Valves

What are the most commonly used mechanical valves?	St. Jude (low-profile, bi-leaflet hinged valve), Starr-Edwards (caged ball valve)
What is the primary disadvantage of these valves?	Lifelong anticoagulation (Coumadin) because of the high risk of thromboembolism. Most institutions also anticoagulate tissue valves for 3–8 weeks postoperatively until Dacron and suture lines endothelialize.
What are the contraindications to the use of mechanical valves (i.e., indications for tissue valves)?	Absolute: History of major bleeding Relative: Unreliable noncompliant patient; patient > 65 years old (because of increased risk of stroke associated with anticoagulation); pregnancy (current or planned)

TISSUE VALVES

What is the most common type of tissue valve?	Xenograft (glutaraldehyde-fixed porcine valve) [porcine = pig]
What is the primary disadvantage of these valves?	Deterioration over time
When do 50% of the valves require replacement?	13 years
What are the contraindications to tissue valves (i.e., indications for mechanical valves)?	Rapid calcification of valve occurs in young patients (especially children, but anyone < 30 years old) and patients who are receiving renal dialysis
What 3 additional types of tissue valves are occasionally used?	1. Bovine pericardial valves 2. Homograft (human donor valve) 3. Autograft (autotransplant of valve)
What are the major disadvantages of homograft valves?	Limited supply; more difficult procedure, longer cross-clamp time
What is the valve autograft procedure?	Diseased aortic valve is excised. The pulmonary valve is excised and sutured into the aortic position. A bioprosthetic valve is sutured into the pulmonary position (i.e., Ross procedure).

Complications of Valve Replacement

What are the early postoperative complications of valve replacement?

Conduction abnormalities (the AV-His bundle travels close to the valvular annuli, and multiple sutures must be placed near this region), endocarditis, systemic thromboemboli, and ventricular failure

What are the late complications of valve replacement?

Systemic thromboemboli, endocarditis, and bleeding as a result of anticoagulation

What is the most common late complication of mechanical valves?

Cerebral thromboemboli

What is the incidence of this complication?

1–5% each year, even with anticoagulation. Incidence varies with the type of valve (e.g., for St. Jude valve, only 1–2% per year).

Cerebral thromboemboli occur most frequently with replacement of which valve?

Mitral valve

Three-Dimensional Relation Among Cardiac Valves

On CXR, the valve that was replaced can be identified by its position. In the illustrations of anteroposterior and lateral views of the heart on CXR, which valves would be placed in positions 1 through 8?

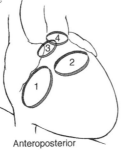
Anteroposterior

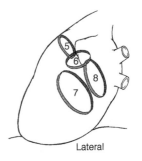
Lateral

1. Tricuspid
2. Mitral
3. Aortic
4. Pulmonary
5. Pulmonary
6. Aortic
7. Tricuspid
8. Mitral

INFECTIOUS ENDOCARDITIS (IE)

Which native valve is at greatest risk for endocarditis?	Mitral valve (accounts for 80% of cases)
What distinguishes acute from subacute native valve endocarditis (NVE)?	Acute: Rapid onset; usually caused by virulent organisms Subacute: Indolent onset; usually caused by less virulent organisms
Are normal or diseased valves the target in acute versus subacute NVE?	Acute: Normal, although some minor lesion must be present to cause the turbulence that permits the bacteria to invade the valve Subacute: Diseased (e.g., rheumatic heart disease, congenital bicuspid aortic valve)
A prosthetic valve in which position is at greatest risk for IE?	Aortic valve (accounts for 60% of cases)
Define early versus late prosthetic valve endocarditis (PVE).	Early: < 2 months after surgery Late: > 2 months after surgery
What is the incidence of PVE in tissue versus mechanical valves?	5–10% (same for both)
Why is aggressive therapy necessary for early PVE?	Mortality rate of 60–70%
What are the most common organisms responsible for IE in the following settings?	
Acute NVE	*Staphylococcus aureus* and group A streptococcus
Subacute NVE	*Streptococcus viridans*, enterococci
Early PVE	*Staphylococcus epidermidis, S. aureus,* and diphtheroids

Late PVE	*Enterococcus, S. aureus*, and gram-negative bacteria
Fungal endocarditis	*Candida* and *Aspergillus*
Right-sided endocarditis in IV drug abusers	*S. aureus, Candida*, and gram-negative bacteria (*Pseudomonas*)
What are the most common signs of IE?	Fever and new murmur
What are the classic findings on physical exam (in decreasing order of frequency)?	Skin and conjunctival petechiae (most common), nail bed splinter hemorrhages, Osler nodes (painful nodules on pads of digits), Janeway lesions (painless macular lesions on palms and soles), Roth's spots (pale oval lesions on retina with surrounding hemorrhage)
How is the diagnosis made?	Positive blood culture (3) Echocardiography: Detects vegetations, regurgitation, and paravalvular leakage caused by ring abscess
What is the medical treatment?	4–6 weeks of IV antibiotic therapy
What is the most common indication for surgery?	CHF
What are the other indications for surgery?	Early PVE, unstable (i.e., rocking) prosthetic valve caused by PVE, positive blood culture findings after 2 weeks of IV antibiotics, fungal infections, recurrent emboli, septic shock while receiving antibiotics, and conduction defects in heart because of ring abscess
What is the surgical procedure?	Excision of the valve and aggressive débridement of any surrounding infected necrotic myocardium, followed by valve replacement. The tricuspid valve may not require replacement if pulmonary hypertension is absent.
What is the reinfection rate of the new valve?	Only 5–10%

DISEASES OF THE GREAT VESSELS

THORACIC AND THORACOABDOMINAL AORTIC ANEURYSMS

What are the etiologies of thoracic and thoracoabdominal aortic aneurysms?

Atherosclerosis, myxomatous degeneration (i.e., Marfan's disease), aortic dissection, and infection (i.e., syphilis)

What is the incidence of aneurysms in the various thoracic aortic regions?

Ascending aorta: > 40%
Descending aorta: 35%
Aortic arch: 10% (thoracoabdominal aorta: 10%)

What is the most common etiology of ascending aortic aneurysms?

Myxomatous degeneration

What is the cardiac lesion most frequently associated with ascending aortic aneurysms?

Aortic insufficiency because of dilation of the aortic valve annulus (annuloaortic ectasia). It is rarely seen in patients with an atherosclerotic etiology.

What is the gross difference in appearance between atherosclerotic and myxomatous ascending aortic aneurysms?

Atherosclerotic: Fusiform shape
Myxomatous: Pear shape

Why are aortic arch aneurysms difficult to manage?

Because they involve the aortic arch vessels, the risk of intraoperative cerebral ischemia is significant.

What is the most common etiology of descending or thoracoabdominal aortic aneurysms?

Atherosclerosis

Which etiology is classically associated with saccular aneurysms?

Syphilis

What is the most common presentation of thoracic aneurysm?

Incidental finding on CXR in an asymptomatic patient

What is the most common symptom of thoracic aneurysm?

Chronic dull or "boring" pain in the back or precordium

What is the classic, although less common, presentation of:

Ascending aortic aneurysm?

CHF (e.g., dyspnea) because of aortic insufficiency

Descending aortic aneurysm?

Cough and dyspnea because of compression of left main bronchus

What is the primary complication of aortic aneurysms if untreated?

Rupture and death

How does the rate of expansion compare with that of abdominal aortic aneurysms?

More rapid expansion as well as greater risk of rupture

What is the 5-year survival rate if untreated?

20%

What diagnostic studies are performed?

CT scan with contrast, MRI, or aortogram. Some patients undergo surgery on the basis of MRI findings alone.

What are the indications for surgery for thoracic aortic aneurysms?

Symptomatic aneurysm
Asymptomatic aneurysm > 6–7 cm (in Marfan's disease, aneurysm > 5–6 cm)
Rapid increase in aneurysm size. Because of the rapid rate of enlargement and the tendency to rupture, many advocate earlier surgical intervention as morbidity and mortality rates of repair decline.

What is the usual surgical procedure?

Tube graft replacement (Dacron, homograft, or polytetrafluoroethylene [PTFE]) of diseased segment of aorta. Cardiopulmonary bypass (CPB) is usually required.

What procedure is often used for ascending aortic aneurysms caused by Marfan's disease?

Bentall procedure: Replacement of ascending aorta and aortic valve with a composite graft because of the frequency of dilation of the valve annulus

What is the Crawford, or inclusion, technique? Where is it used most frequently?

Incorporation or implantation of a group of arteries (as an island or cuff) into the prosthetic tube graft rather than multiple individual implantation sites; used primarily for arch vessels, visceral arteries, and intercostal-lumbar arteries

What technique is necessary to minimize cerebral ischemia during the repair of aortic arch aneurysms?

Deep hypothermic circulatory arrest

What are 2 alternatives to CPB in the repair of some descending and thoracoabdominal aortic aneurysms?

Simple cross-clamping of the aorta plus nitroprusside IV to control the resultant hypertension

Heparin-bonded Gott or tridodecyl-methylammonium chloride (TDMAC) shunt (aortoaortic or aortofemoral)

How are most saccular aneurysms managed?

Simple excision with repair of resultant aortic defect at base of aneurysm

What is the overall operative mortality rate?

< 10%

What is the most common cause of death?

MI

What are the postoperative complications?

Respiratory insufficiency (most common), MI, acute tubular necrosis, paraplegia, and stroke

What classic syndrome is associated with spinal ischemia?

Anterior spinal artery syndrome

Repair of which types of aortic aneurysm increases the risk of spinal ischemia?

Thoracoabdominal and descending aortic aneurysms

Why are these types at higher risk for spinal ischemia?

The primary blood supply to the anterior spinal cord is supplied by the artery of Adamkiewicz, a large intercostal or lumbar artery usually located between T8 and L4. To prevent back-bleeding into the surgical field, the intercostals and lumbars are often oversewn or ligated.

What are the signs and symptoms associated with the anterior spinal artery syndrome?	Paraplegia, incontinence (bowel or bladder), and sensory loss for pain and temperature
What long-term medical therapy is often prescribed after aortic aneurysm surgery?	Antihypertensive agents (often β-blockers)
What is the primary reason for close long-term follow-up?	Increased risk of development of dissection or aneurysm in any residual aorta
What is the 5-year survival rate after surgery?	50%

HEART TRANSPLANTATION

What are the indications for heart transplantation?	Ischemic cardiomyopathy ("end-stage" CAD), idiopathic (primary) cardiomyopathy (i.e., dilated, restrictive), secondary cardiomyopathy (i.e., viral, alcoholic, infiltrative, toxic, metabolic), some types of congenital heart disease, and retransplantation for severe acute or chronic rejection
What are the absolute contraindications to transplantation?	Pulmonary hypertension (> 6 Wood units and uncontrollable with oral pharmacologic therapy), active infection, active malignancy, irreversible hepatic disease, irreversible renal disease (if renal transplant is not possible), and age > 65 years (age criteria are institution dependent)
What is the major limiting factor in the number of heart transplants currently performed?	Scarcity of donor cardiac allografts
What are the potential future alternatives to allograft transplantation?	Long-term left ventricular assist devices (LVADs), xenotransplants (use of animal hearts), and artificial hearts

PREOPERATIVE PERIOD AND PROCEDURE

What interventions are used to support the patient who is awaiting transplantation?

Pharmacologic treatment to reduce volume overload and maintain CO (i.e., diuretics, digoxin, dopamine, dobutamine, amrinone), IABP, and mechanical circulatory assist devices (LVADs or biventricular assist devices, the "bridges to transplantation")

What criteria are used to match donors and recipients for heart transplantation?

ABO compatibility (because of shortage of donors and limits of myocardial preservation, human leukocyte antigen [HLA] matching is not feasible) and CMV status. In adults, size matching plays a minor role.

What is the accepted limit of ex vivo ischemic time for the donor heart?

Only 4–6 hours!

What are the 2 types of heart transplantation?

Orthotopic: Removal of recipient ventricles (accounts for > 95% of transplants performed)
Heterotopic: Piggybacking of donor heart onto recipient heart

How is the recipient heart excised?

The patient is placed on cardiopulmonary bypass and the aorta is cross-clamped. The aorta and pulmonary artery are transected, and a circumferential incision is made proximal to the AV groove, leaving most of the left and right atria in the recipient.

EFFECTS OF DONOR HEART DENERVATION

What does "denervation" of donor heart refer to?

Harvesting of a donor heart necessitates transection of its innervating fibers.

What are the important physiologic results of denervation?

Baseline tachycardia (90–110 beats/min) because of the loss of parasympathetic tone that normally inhibits the sinoatrial node
Delayed myocardial response to stress because of the exclusive dependence on circulating catecholamines from distant noncardiac sites for positive chronotropic and inotropic effects

What standard cardiac therapeutic interventions are ineffective with loss of autonomic innervation?	Atropine, digoxin, carotid sinus massage, and the Valsalva maneuver
How does denervation complicate the presentation of MI?	Heart transplant recipients do not have angina because of the lack of afferent sensory fibers. Several years after transplantation, a few patients apparently have reinnervation of the donor heart and experience angina, but these are rare and unpredictable exceptions.

EARLY POSTOPERATIVE HEMODYNAMIC COMPLICATIONS

What is the usual etiology of early postoperative low CO?	The newly transplanted heart is noncompliant and stiff because of the injury associated with harvesting, cooling, and ischemia. Fortunately, this dysfunction usually resolves during the first 3 days.
What is the treatment of early low CO?	Volume (to optimize preload in noncompliant ventricles), isoproterenol (to maintain heart rate [HR] at 100–125 beats/min), $\pm$ additional inotropic support with dobutamine
What are 2 additional complications and their first-line treatment?	Right ventricular failure (RVF): Isoproterenol Sinus bradycardia and junctional rhythms: Isoproterenol, not atropine
A patient moves to a chair on postoperative day 2 and promptly loses consciousness. What is the most likely etiology?	Orthostatic hypotension because of the loss of normal reflex tachycardia as well as a great dependence on preload
What is the most common cause of death in the first year?	Infection
What is the most common cause of death after the first year?	Rejection

INFECTIOUS COMPLICATIONS

What is the most common site of infections in heart transplant recipients?	Lungs
These patients are at risk for opportunistic infections in addition to the usual bacterial pathogens encountered in surgery. When is each type of infection most prevalent?	Bacterial: Acute infections ($<$ 1 month postoperatively) Opportunistic: Subacute infections ($>$ 1 month, especially 1–4 months)
What are the most common organisms in acute infections?	Gram-negative bacilli (*Pseudomonas, Escherichia coli,* and *Klebsiella*)
What are the most common organisms in subacute infections?	CMV, although some groups report *Pneumocystis* as the most prevalent
What are the 4 types of opportunistic infection?	Intracellular: *Listeria, Mycobacterium, Salmonella* Fungal: *Candida, Aspergillus* Viral: Herpes simplex, CMV Protozoal: *Pneumocystis, Toxoplasma*
What transplant is associated with the highest incidence of aspergillosis?	Heart transplant
What drug is given if a CMV-positive heart is transplanted into a CMV-negative recipient (CMV mismatch)?	Ganciclovir (also used to treat serious CMV infection)
What is the standard immunosuppressive maintenance regimen for heart transplantation?	Triple therapy: Cyclosporine, prednisone, and azathioprine (Imuran)
What is the most common type of rejection?	Acute rejection (days to months postoperatively). The highest incidence of rejection occurs in the first 3 months.

What percentage of patients have a rejection episode during the first few months?	80%!
What is the classic manifestation of chronic rejection (controversial)?	Accelerated coronary artery disease (ACAD). Some theorize that there are nonrejection etiologies for ACAD (e.g., CMV).
What is the most common presentation of rejection?	Usually asymptomatic, unless severe
What are the classic signs?	Fever; if severe, signs of RV and/or LV dysfunction (e.g., S3, S4, jugular venous distension [JVD], hepatomegaly, and arrhythmias)
What is the most reliable way to diagnose rejection?	Endomyocardial biopsy of the RV septum with a percutaneous bioptome
What is the most common treatment of rejection?	Corticosteroids: Short course of IV methylprednisolone (Solu-Medrol) on an outpatient basis, requiring a daily visit to the hospital, or increased dose of oral prednisone, if rejection is mild
What is the main complication of this treatment?	Increased risk of opportunistic infection. Over the last several years, the threshold for treatment of rejection has become steadily higher to avoid the more dangerous infectious complications of additional immunosuppression.
What additional immunosuppressive agents may be used if steroids fail?	The monoclonal antibody OKT3 or ATG (antithymocyte globulin)
What is the most common reason for retransplantation?	Chronic rejection, which accounts for 66% of cases
What are the most common neoplasms seen in heart transplant recipients?	Carcinoma of the skin and lip (i.e., squamous cell carcinoma); non-Hodgkin's lymphoma
What are the survival rates at 1 and 5 years?	1 year: 80–90% 5 years: 50–60%

CARDIOPULMONARY BYPASS

What are the functions of CPB?	Perfusion of the body with blood, gas exchange (oxygen added and carbon dioxide removed from blood), alterations of core temperature (decrease in temperature during surgery to reduce metabolic rate)
Compare total CPB with partial CPB.	Total CPB: All venous blood is bypassed to the pump Partial CPB: Some venous blood passes through the lungs
What are the components of the basic CPB circuit?	Venous cannula(e) from RA (or superior and inferior vena cava); heart-lung machine with pump apparatus, heat exchanger, and oxygenator; arterial filter; arterial cannula into the ascending aorta. (The femoral artery and vein occasionally are used for cannulation sites.)
How is the heart arrested so that surgery can be performed safely?	Infusion of cold, high-potassium solution (i.e., cardioplegia) into aortic root or directly into coronary arteries after cross-clamping of ascending aorta. Topical cold saline ($4°C$) helps to maintain myocardial temperature at $\cong 15°C$.
To what temperature is the patient usually cooled for a standard cardiac procedure?	28–$32°C$ (mild hypothermia)
What is deep, or profound, hypothermia?	$< 18°C$
How low may pump rate be reduced during profound hypothermia?	Pump may be turned off (i.e., hypothermic circulatory arrest)
For what procedures is profound hypothermia indicated?	Aortic arch surgery and complex congenital cardiac surgery
What step is necessary to prevent thrombosis in the pump?	Patient must be anticoagulated with heparin (activated clotting time is monitored intraoperatively)

A patient is not weaning from CPB (i.e., as the pump rate is decreased, the patient cannot maintain blood pressure). What steps are taken to permit successful discontinuation of CPB?	1. Intravascular volume (crystalloid or blood) is increased. 2. Vasopressor and inotropic support (infusions of dopamine, dobutamine, or epinephrine) is provided. 3. ± IABP is placed. 4. ± Left and/or right ventricular assist device (VAD) is placed. 5. Very rarely, heart transplant is performed.
Shortly after discontinuing CPB, severe pulmonary hypertension suddenly develops. What is the most likely etiology?	Protamine reaction. Protamine sulfate is used to reverse the activity of heparin after completing CPB.
What features of the patient history suggest the potential for protamine reaction?	Diabetes (protamine in insulin) Allergies to iodine or seafood Patient or family history of protamine reaction
What is "postperfusion syndrome" (PPS)?	End-organ effects of the "whole-body inflammatory reaction" associated with CPB, manifested as postoperative pulmonary insufficiency, renal failure, bleeding disorder, and/or myocardial dysfunction
What is the etiology of PPS?	Uncertain. Current evidence suggests that contact with the synthetic surfaces of the extracorporeal circuit activates the humoral (i.e., complement) and cellular (i.e., neutrophil) cascades of the acute inflammatory response, resulting in endothelial injury.
Which factor is activated at the onset of CPB and appears to initiate the various humoral cascades?	Factor XII (Hageman factor)
Which complement anaphylatoxins appear intimately involved in PPS?	C3a and C5a
What is the treatment of PPS?	Supportive therapy (e.g., ventilator, dialysis) until the patient recovers

POSTOPERATIVE INTENSIVE CARE MANAGEMENT

CARDIAC OUTPUT

What are the physiologic determinants of CO?	Preload (end-diastolic volume of the ventricle) Compliance (tendency of the ventricle to permit distension with blood) Afterload (the force opposing ventricular ejection) Contractility (intrinsic contractile performance, independent of other determinants of CO): $CO = SV \times HR$ (SV = stroke volume)
What is the cardiac index (CI)?	CO per body surface area expressed in meters squared
What are the normal values for CO and CI?	$CO = 4\text{--}8$ L/min $CI = 2.5\text{--}4$ L/min/m^2
What is the Frank-Starling relation?	Relation between resting muscle length (determined by preload) and tension achieved by the contracting muscle. Up to a point defined by the Frank-Starling curve of the ventricle, increases in preload augment stroke volume and thus CO.
What is the key determinant of CO in a heart with normal versus reduced compliance?	Normal compliance: Preload Reduced compliance: Afterload
Why is blood pressure an INSENSITIVE index of myocardial performance?	Blood pressure is the product of systemic vascular resistance and CO. If CO decreases, blood pressure is maintained initially by compensatory arterial vasoconstriction because of reflex sympathetic discharge; thus, a decrease in blood pressure is often a late sign of reduced myocardial performance.

LOW CARDIAC OUTPUT SYNDROME (LCOS)

What is the presentation of LCOS?	Cool, clammy skin; slow capillary refill; oliguria (< 0.5 mL/kg/h); restlessness; depressed mental status; tachypnea, metabolic acidosis

What are the etiologies of LCOS in the postoperative period?

Hypovolemia (third spacing, diuresis, bleeding, or relative hypovolemia because of reflex vasodilation associated with postoperative warming); elevated SVR (hypothermia, circulating catecholamines); myocardial dysfunction (ischemia, hypothermia, volume overload); pericardial tamponade; dysrhythmia; and increased intrathoracic pressure (positive end-expiratory pressure [PEEP], tension pneumothorax)

In what order are these determinants of CO addressed to improve CO?

1. HR (and arrhythmias)
2. Preload
3. Afterload
4. Contractility

For each determinant, what disturbance usually causes LCOS, and what are the therapeutic options and management?

Bradycardia: Atropine, isoproterenol, temporary pacer
Tachycardia: Fluids, oxygen, anxiolytics, morphine, esmolol (rarely)
Inadequate preload: Fluids, control of mediastinal bleeding (and rule out tamponade)
Elevated afterload: Warming lights or blanket, fluids, vasodilator therapy
Reduced contractility: Inotropic therapy, mechanical assist device (and rule out myocardial ischemia; see Postoperative Myocardial Ischemia section)

What are the first-line inotropic agents?

Dobutamine and dopamine

What are the second-line agents (e.g., used if first-line agents are ineffective)?

Epinephrine and amrinone (rarely used)

If LCOS persists despite second-line inotropic therapy, and all other determinants of CO are optimized, what mechanical assist is initiated?

IABP and/or VAD

What is the primary benefit of each mechanical assist device?	IABP: Can be placed percutaneously (VAD requires open-chest surgery) VAD: Completely replaces the pumping function of the heart (IABP only augments existing cardiac function)

POSTOPERATIVE MYOCARDIAL ISCHEMIA

What is the incidence of postoperative MI following cardiac surgery?	3–15%
When in the postoperative period is the patient at greatest risk of myocardial ischemia?	First 6 hours
What are the sequelae of myocardial ischemia?	MI, LCOS, arrhythmias, RVF, acute MR, acute VSD, and acute ventricular free wall rupture ($\pm$ pericardial tamponade)
What are the treatment goals, and how are they achieved?	Alleviation of myocardial ischemia: Oxygen, nitrates, $\pm$ surgery Treatment of ventricular dysfunction: According to LCOS treatment regimen Prevention or treatment of arrhythmias: Correct electrolyte disturbances, administer lidocaine or procainamide
When is surgery indicated for myocardial ischemia after cardiac surgery?	Patients who are hemodynamically or electrically unstable because of significant myocardial ischemia Mechanical complications of ischemia (i.e., acute MR or VSD) (See the Acquired Coronary Artery Disease section for a discussion of mechanical complications.)
What is the treatment of RVF?	Volume expansion (the foundation of treatment of RVF) Dobutamine, the overall pharmacologic agent of choice because it reduces pulmonary afterload and provides inotropic support

POSTOPERATIVE HYPERTENSION

What are the etiologies of postoperative hypertension?

Pain or anxiety, hypothermia, hypoxia, hypercarbia, LCOS (with reflex vasoconstriction), and hyperdynamic myocardium syndrome, fluid overload

What are the sequelae?

Myocardial ischemia, LCOS, cerebrovascular accident, increased postoperative bleeding, and aortic dissection

What is the goal of treatment?

Reduction of blood pressure while maintaining adequate visceral perfusion, especially coronary and cerebral. The target mean arterial pressure is 60–85 mm Hg (variable depending on patient's baseline blood pressure).

What is the first-line parenteral agent for vasodilation?

Sodium nitroprusside

POSTOPERATIVE HYPOTENSION

What are the most common etiologies in the postoperative cardiac surgery patient?

Hypovolemia, myocardial ischemia or infarction, cardiac tamponade, arrhythmias, and tension pneumothorax

What is shock?

Inadequate perfusion pressures to preserve visceral function (not hypotension per se)

What are the etiologies of cardiogenic shock?

Large MI (> 30–40% of LV), acute MR, acute VSD, RVF

What is the mortality rate associated with cardiogenic shock?

75%

HYPERDYNAMIC MYOCARDIUM SYNDROME

What is hyperdynamic myocardium syndrome?

Elevated CO caused by increased myocardial contractility ± tachycardia. The mechanism is uncertain, but may involve circulating catecholamines.

Which patients are at greatest risk for hyperdynamic myocardium syndrome?	Patients with compensatory hypertrophy of the LV because of preoperative systemic hypertension, AS, or idiopathic subaortic stenosis
What is the indication for treatment?	Significant tachycardia with untoward effects on diastolic ventricular filling or myocardial oxygen demand
What is the pharmacologic intervention of choice?	Esmolol (parenteral (β-blocker with a short half-life)

POSTOPERATIVE HEMORRHAGE

What is the medical management?	Increased PEEP on the ventilator, vasodilators for hypertension, protamine sulfate, fresh-frozen plasma (if prothrombin time or partial thromboplastin time is elevated), and platelets (if platelet count < 100,000), desmopressin acetate (DDAVP).
When is cryoprecipitate indicated?	Fibrinogen < 100 mg/dL
What are the indications for re-exploration?	Bleeding rate from chest tubes of 200 mL/h for 4–6 hours (> 1500 mL over 12 hours), evidence of pericardial tamponade, or sudden significant increase in chest tube output (300–500 mL)

PERICARDIAL TAMPONADE

How does pericardial tamponade reduce CO?	Preload reduction: Low pressure of venous return has difficulty overcoming the intrapericardial pressure gradient formed by the tamponade
What is the usual presentation of tamponade?	Tachycardia, hypotension, distended neck veins, and pulsus paradoxus, often in a patient with bleeding from the chest tube that is initially heavy and suddenly stops. However, freely draining chest tubes and tamponade are not mutually exclusive.
What is the classic finding on Swan-Ganz catheter readings?	Equalization of diastolic pressures in the heart (central venous pressure [CVP], RV end-diastolic pressure, pulmonary diastolic pressure, and PCWP), usually 18–22 mm Hg

What is the treatment?	Volume loading, inotropes, and elevation of the feet until an OR is available for re-exploration of the mediastinum. If the patient becomes unstable before surgery despite conservative measures, emergent bedside re-exploration is performed.

CARDIAC ICU

In patient management, trends, rather than absolute numbers, are key, but these values are guidelines. What are the normal values for the following parameters?

CO and CI	CO = 4–8 L/min CI = 2.5–4 L/min/m^2
CVP	CVP = 0–4 mm Hg
PCWP	PCWP = 12–15 mm Hg
SVR	SVR = 900–1400 dynes/sec/cm^2
PVR	PVR = 150–250 dynes/sec/cm^2

What is the general management regimen for each of the following classic clinical scenarios?

Decreased CO, decreased PCWP, increased or decreased SVR	Volume (i.e., crystalloid, blood)
Normal or increased CO, but decreased blood pressure, normal PCWP, decreased SVR	Vasopressor (i.e., phenylephrine)
Decreased CO, increased PCWP, normal or decreased SVR	Inotrope (i.e., dopamine, dobutamine)
Decreased CO, increased PCWP, increased SVR	Vasodilator (i.e., sodium nitroprusside) + IABP if blood pressure is too low for vasodilator therapy alone

What measurement is performed to evaluate oxygen delivery and the adequacy of tissue perfusion?	Mixed venous oxygen saturation. A sample is drawn slowly through the distal port of the Swan-Ganz catheter (the site of the most deoxygenated blood in the body, the pulmonary artery).
What is a normal value of this measurement?	65–75% saturation
What does an increase in oxygen saturation between the proximal port of the Swan-Ganz catheter (in the RA) and the distal port (in the pulmonary artery) suggest?	Intracardiac shunt (i.e., VSD)
How do patients with cyanide toxicity present initially?	Decreased contractility and CO
What are the classic LATE findings of toxicity?	Dilated pupils, headache, absent reflexes, nausea, mental status changes ± coma, death

INTRA-AORTIC BALLOON PUMP

What are the indications for IABP?	Refractory LVF after CPB (e.g., inability to wean from bypass pump) Unstable angina refractory to medical treatment CHF in a patient awaiting surgery (i.e., acute MR or VSD, transplant candidate) Cardiogenic shock caused by MI (now rare, unless the patient is a candidate for CABG or percutaneous transluminal coronary angioplasty [PTCA])
What are the contraindications to IABP?	Aortic aneurysm or synthetic thoracic aortic graft (may rupture with balloon inflation) Moderate or severe aortic regurgitation (IABP may worsen regurgitation)
What is the usual route of insertion?	Femoral artery, but the pump can be placed directly into the aorta at the time of median sternotomy if severe peripheral atherosclerosis precludes a femoral approach

Where does the balloon reside in the aorta?	Between the left subclavian artery and the diaphragm
What complication occurs if the balloon migrates?	Intermittent ischemia in territories supplied by vessels that are intermittently occluded by the inflated balloon (e.g., carotid, subclavian, renal, celiac)
How does the IABP work?	Balloon inflates during diastole, increasing pressure inside the aorta, which increases coronary and visceral perfusion; balloon deflates during systole, reducing afterload, which decreases cardiac work
What is the key benefit of IABP over medical treatment of hypotension or decreased CO?	No increase in oxygen consumption or demand, unlike (α- or β-agonists, which cause increased cardiac work because of increased afterload or HR and contractility, respectively
What are the complications of IABP?	Lower extremity ischemia because of occlusion of femoral artery. Monitoring distal pulses is imperative. Emboli caused by thrombosis around the balloon Bowel infarction, renal failure, and paraplegia caused by migration of the balloon Mechanical damage to formed components of the blood

LEFT VENTRICULAR ASSIST DEVICE

What are the indications for LVAD?	Intraoperative MI to reduce left ventricular work temporarily and allow the heart to recover more quickly "Bridge" for heart transplant candidates until a donor is available
Why is LVAD not true cardiopulmonary bypass?	Only a perfusion device, with no oxygenator in the circuit
How is the LVAD fundamentally different from the IABP?	LVAD provides "flow" and can fully replace pumping function of heart. IABP provides "pressure assistance" and only augments existing cardiac function.

| How is the LVAD different from extracorporeal membrane oxygenation (ECMO)? | ECMO includes a membrane lung apparatus and can also provide support for respiratory insufficiency; the inflow source is the RA. |

AUTOMATIC IMPLANTABLE CARDIOVERTER DEFIBRILLATOR (AICD)

What are the 3 components of the AICD?	Sensory leads to detect arrhythmia Anode-cathode titanium patches around the heart Pulse generator to terminate arrhythmia Newer devices also have pacing capability for bradycardia and asystole.
What is the indication for AICD?	Malignant ventricular arrhythmia refractory to medical therapy
What are the 1-year survival rates in treated patients and untreated historical control subjects?	AICD: 95–98%. Untreated: 30–40%. These patients are at high risk for sudden death syndrome.
Why is pharmacologic therapy necessary after AICD placement?	Episodes of nonsustained ventricular tachycardia and atrial fibrillation can cause discharge of the AICD.

CARDIAC TUMORS

What is the most common type of cardiac tumor?	Metastatic neoplasm (lung, breast, melanoma, and lymphoma) accounts for 65-70% of all malignant cardiac tumors.
What is the most common complication associated with this type of tumor?	Pericardial tamponade from bloody pericardial effusion
What are the 2 most common primary malignant cardiac tumors?	Sarcoma (i.e., rhabdomyosarcoma, angiosarcoma): 15–20% of all malignant cardiac tumors Melanoma: 5–10%
How do these tumors differ grossly from myxoma?	Intramural rather than intraluminal; thus, almost always unresectable
What is the most common cardiac tumor in children?	Rhabdomyoma (benign)

What is the most common primary tumor of the pericardium?	Mesothelioma
What aspect of the surgical intervention reduces the incidence of recurrence?	Resection of the origin of the stalk (part of the septal wall)

BENIGN CARDIAC TUMORS

What is the most common benign cardiac tumor?	Myxoma, which is also the most common primary cardiac tumor, accounting for 60–80% of all primary cardiac tumors
This tumor occurs most in which chamber?	LA: 75% (> 95% in atria)
What is the classic gross feature?	Pedunculated (stalk attached to atrial septal wall)
What complications are associated with this tumor?	LA outflow obstruction ("ball valve") and emboli (from the friable surface of the myxoma). Acute vascular obstruction in patients with no heart disease, especially if young, suggests this source.

69

Transplant Surgery

MAJOR HISTOCOMPATIBILITY COMPLEX (MHC)

What is the MHC?	Cluster of genes on the short arm of chromosome 6
What is this cluster called in humans?	Human leukocyte antigen (HLA)
What are the important characteristics of MHC (HLA) antigens?	1. Extreme polymorphism 2. Produced by closely linked subloci that form inheritable HLA haplotypes 3. Codominant expression of HLA (HLA antigens on the cell surface)
Where are the polymorphisms clustered?	Polymorphic amino acids are clustered in the peptide-binding site in the antigen-binding groove.
What are the 3 basic products of the MHC and the corresponding regions involved?	1. Class I antigen: HLA-A, -B, and -C 2. Class II antigen: HLA-D region, with DR, DQ, and DP 3. Class III antigens: Complement cascade
On what cell types are these MHC products expressed?	1. Class I antigens: All nucleated cells and platelets 2. Class II antigens: B-lymphocytes, activated T-cells, macrophages, and monocytes
What lymphocytes do not express class II antigens?	Resting T-lymphocytes
What causes allograft rejection?	Foreign histocompatibility antigens on the graft and tissue

What antigens are histocompatibility antigens?	Any antigen that causes tissue incompatibility between donor and recipient
What are the strongest transplantation antigens?	Antigens that express the MHC (HLA in humans)
What 2 tests detect HLA antigens?	1. Serologic testing with antigen-specific antisera 2. Mixed lymphocyte culture (MLC)
What does MLC detect?	Proliferative capacity of the host lymphocytes to antigens on the graft (MHC class II antigens, or D antigens)
Which classes of MHC genes significantly affect transplantation?	Classes I and II
What are the structures of class I and class II molecules?	Two polypeptide chains with variable and constant regions, similar to the immunoglobulin structure
What do class I genes encode for?	Transplantation antigens that are primary targets for cytotoxic T-lymphocytes (CTLs) in rejection; cell surface molecules that present certain antigens to CD8 T-cells (i.e., viral antigens)
What do class II genes represent?	Immune response genes
Class I gene products are the primary target of which cells?	CTLs
Class II gene products are the primary target of which cells?	T_h cells
What are the minor transplantation antigens?	Antigens that express genes on other chromosomes that are capable of weaker, slower rejection. They are presented by class I and class II MHC determinants.
Which antigens cause rejection of grafts between HLA-identical siblings?	Minor transplantation antigens

IMMUNOSUPPRESSIVE AGENTS

What is MMF?	Mycophenolate **mo**fetil
How does it work?	Inhibits T-cells and B-cells by inhibiting purine synthesis

FK-506 (TACROLIMUS)

What is the basic structure of FK-506?	Macrolide antibiotic
What is the source of FK-506?	Soil fungus (*Streptomyces tsukubaensis*)
What is the potency of FK-506 compared with that of cyclosporine A (CSA)?	FK-506 is 500 times more potent than CSA.
What is the typical dosing regimen for FK-506?	0.05 mg/kg PO every 12 hours
What is the therapeutic drug level?	10–15 ng/mL
What is the mechanism of immunosuppressive action?	Inhibits T-cell activation and maturation
What are the intracellular receptors for FK-506?	FK-binding proteins
What adverse side effects are associated with FK-506 administration?	1. Nephrotoxicity 2. Anorexia and weight loss 3. Neurotoxicity
What drugs increase FK-506 levels?	1. Verapamil 2. Ketoconazole 3. Erythromycin 4. Diltiazem 5. Fluconazole 6. Cimetidine
What drugs decrease FK-506 levels?	1. Phenytoin 2. Phenobarbital 3. Carbamazepine 4. Rifampin

RAPAMYCIN (RAPA)

What is the structure of RAPA?

Macrolide antibiotic

What is the mechanism of immunosuppressive action?

1. Inhibits B-cell and T-cell activation and proliferation
2. Inhibits activated T-cells
3. Blocks the ability of the interleukin (IL)-2 receptor to induce signal transduction

What intracellular receptor does RAPA bind?

FK-binding proteins

What action is inhibited by RAPA, but not by CSA and FK-506?

Activated cell proliferation induced by IL-2 and IL-4

LIVER TRANSPLANTATION

What factor significantly decreases morbidity and mortality rates of the anhepatic phase of the orthotopic liver transplant (OLTx) procedure (i.e., after hepatectomy and before the completion of implantation)?

Heparin-free veno-venous bypass. The cannula drains the IVC, and the centrifugal pump returns blood to the axillary vein.

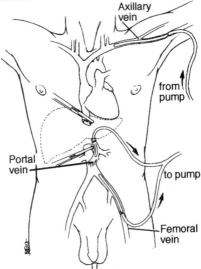

What standard anastomoses are used for OLTx?

1. Suprahepatic IVC and infrahepatic IVC anastomoses
2. Portal vein anastomosis
3. Hepatic (splenic) artery anastomosis
4. Anastomosis for biliary drainage

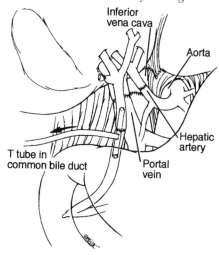

What is the veno-venous bypass during liver transplant surgery?

During the "anhepatic" phase of the transplant the blood from the portal vein and iliac vein are pumped back to the heart through the pump.

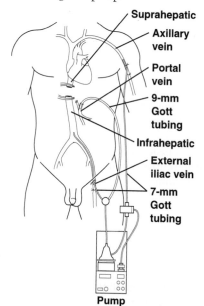

What is the most common anatomic liver arterial anomaly?

Double (or multiple) hepatic artery

What 2 other commonly encountered variations in hepatic artery anatomy are important during procurement and implantation of the allograft?

1. Left hepatic artery originating from left gastric artery (palpable in gastrohepatic omentum): 15% of individuals
2. Right hepatic artery originating from superior mesenteric artery (palpable posterior and to the right of portal vein in porta hepatis): (12–17%) of individuals

What is included in the differential diagnosis of abnormal coagulation parameters in a patient with OLTx?

1. Rejection
2. Ischemia
3. Infection
4. Obstruction
5. Cholangitis

Thrombosis is most common in what vessel?

Hepatic artery

What biliary complications are associated with acute versus chronic hepatic artery thrombosis?

Acute: Bile duct leak
Chronic: Bile duct strictures

What are the clinical signs of caval stenosis?

1. Lower extremity edema
2. Ascites
3. Renal insufficiency

Hepatic abscesses are a common presentation of what complication?

Hepatic artery thrombosis

What procedure differentiates among rejection, ischemia, viral infection, and cholangitis?

Liver biopsy

What histologic findings suggest rejection?

Mixed inflammatory cell infiltrate of the portal triads, bile duct injury, and endothelialitis

What histologic finding suggests cholangitis?

Polymorphonuclear neutrophil (PMN) infiltration of the portal triads

What is the most common cause of renal failure after OLTx?	**Preoperative** hepatorenal syndrome. Other causes include hypotension, sepsis, and CSA toxicity.
What paralytic agent is avoided during renal transplantation in patients undergoing dialysis, and why?	Succinylcholine. Hemodialysis breaks down serum cholinesterases (i.e., prolonged action of the agent).

GASTROINTESTINAL TRACT TRANSPLANTATION

What are cluster transplants?	Transplants of multiple abdominal viscera
Provide examples of cluster transplants.	1. Liver-intestine en bloc 2. Liver, duodenum, and pancreas
What are the indications for small bowel transplantation?	Patients with short gut unable to continue on TPN
What are the complications of chronic hyperalimentation?	1. Cirrhosis 2. Liver failure 3. Vascular access complications
What factor complicates rejection in small bowel transplantation?	In addition to classic allograft rejection, recipients may also experience graft-versus-host disease (GVHD) from donor lymphocytes.
How is the bowel pretreated to reduce the risk of GVHD?	Radiation
What is the complication of this therapy?	Radiation enteritis

IMMUNOSUPPRESSION

COMPLICATIONS

What is the most common complication of immunosuppression?	Infection
What is the most common cause of death in transplant recipients?	Infection

What are the other complications of immunosuppression?	1. Hypertension (HTN) 2. Cushing's disease (steroid-induced diabetes, cataracts, myopathy, hyperlipemia, osteoporosis, and hypercholesterolemia) 3. Thrombophlebitis 4. Malignancy 5. Pancreatitis 6. Avascular necrosis (femoral head)

INFECTION

What are the most common types of fungal infection in immunosuppressed patients?	1. *Candida albicans* 2. *Aspergillus*
What is the most common protozoan infection in immunosuppressed patients?	*Pneumocystis carinii*
What drug is given prophylactically for this protozoal infection?	Trimethoprim and sulfamethoxazole (Bactrim)
What is the typical chest x-ray finding in a patient with:	
Aspergillus **infection?**	Upper-lobe cavities
Pneumocystis **infection?**	Alveolar infiltrates
What are the most common viral infections in transplant recipients?	Herpes group of DNA viruses in descending order: CMV > herpes simplex > herpes zoster
What is the most common viral agent thought to elicit rejection?	CMV
What is the usual clinical presentation of CMV?	Fever, neutropenia, malaise, pneumonitis myocarditis, pancreatitis, and acute cecal ulceration
Which immunosuppressant increases the risk of CMV infection?	Antilymphocyte antibody

Which immunosuppressant decreases the risk of CMV infection, and why?	Cyclosporine, because of the sparing of sensitized T cells

MALIGNANCY

Which malignancies often occur in immunosuppressed patients?	1. Immunoproliferative malignancies (i.e., B-cell lymphomas) 2. Epithelial cancers 3. Malignancies with viral etiologies (i.e., cervical cancer)
What is the relative increased risk of these cancers in transplant patients?	1. Lymphoma: 350 × 2. Skin cancer: 40 × 3. Cervical cancer: 4 ×
What is the viral etiology of polyclonal B-cell lymphoproliferative disorder?	Epstein-Barr virus
What are 3 explanations for the increased risk of cancer associated with immunosuppression?	1. Decreased tumor immunosurveillance 2. Use of mutagenic immunosuppressive agents (i.e., azathioprine [AZA; Imuran]) 3. Increased susceptibility to herpes and increased exposure to viral promoters

REVIEW OF MECHANISMS OF REJECTION

What causes accelerated acute rejection?	T-cell mediated or antibody rejection
Describe the following mechanisms of rejection.	
Hyperacute	Secondary to recipient **pre**formed antibodies to donor ABO or HLA antigen
Accelerated acute	Humoral or cell-mediated
Acute	Cellular immunity
Chronic	Humoral or cellular immunity (or both)

70   Orthopaedic Surgery

ORTHOPAEDIC TERMS

Define the following terms.

Supination	Palm up
Pronation	Palm down
Plantarflexion	Foot down at ankle joint
Dorsiflexion	Foot up at ankle joint
Adduction	Movement toward the midline of the body
Abduction	Movement away from the midline of the body
Inversion	Foot sole faces midline
Eversion	Foot sole faces laterally
Autograft bone	Bone from patient
Allograft bone	Bone from human donor other than patient
Reduction	Maneuver to restore proper alignment to fracture or joint
Closed reduction	Reduction done without surgery
Open reduction	Surgical reduction
Varus	Extremity deformity with apex pointed away from midline

Valgus	Extremity deformity with apex pointed toward midline
Dislocation	Total loss of congruity between articular surfaces of a joint
Subluxation	Partial loss of congruity between articular surfaces of a joint
Arthroplasty	Total joint replacement
Arthrodesis	Joint fusion
Osteotomy	Cutting bone to help realign joint surfaces

COMMON EPONYMS

Name the following fractures or injuries.

Distal radial fracture with dorsal displacement	Colles', which usually occurs secondary to a fall on an outstretched hand
Lunate fracture	Kienböck's
Radial fracture at junction of middle and distal thirds, with distal radial-ulnar dislocation	Galeazzi's
Avulsion of the anterior glenoid labrum	Bankart's
Tarsal-metatarsal fracture or dislocation	Lisfranc's
Fifth metatarsal shaft fracture	Jones'
Radial head subluxation in a child	Nursemaid's elbow
Tibial tuberosity osteochondrosis	Osgood-Schlatter disease
Osteochondrosis of the navicular bone	Köhler's

Fracture of the distal fibula	Pott's
Fracture of the spinous process of C7	Clay shoveler's
Fracture of the pedicles of C2	Hangman's
Fracture of the metacarpal neck	Boxer's; classically, the fifth digit

COMMONLY MISSED ORTHOPAEDIC INJURIES

List some commonly missed orthopaedic injuries.

1. Carpal bone injuries, especially scaphoid
2. Radial head fractures
3. Posterior dislocation of the shoulder
4. Patellar tendon tears
5. Compartment syndrome
6. Rotational deformities of metacarpal and phalangeal fractures
7. Tendon injuries of the hand
8. Femoral neck fractures in the elderly

BASIC SCIENCE

What type of bone formation results in:

Long bones?	Endochondral ossification
Flat bones?	Intramembranous ossification

What type of bone growth determines long bone:

Length?	Interstitial
Width?	Appositional

What cell type:

Produces osteoid?	Osteoblasts
Resorbs bone?	Osteoclasts

What type of collagen predominates in:

    Bone?

Type I

    Articular cartilage?

Type II

What is the composition of articular cartilage?

1. Water (65%)
2. Collagen, type II (20%)
3. Proteoglycan (10%)
4. Chondrocytes (5%)

What are the systemic effects of:

    Parathyroid hormone?

1. Bone: Mobilizes calcium (Ca^{2+}) and phosphorus (Po_4^{2-})
2. Kidney: Resorbs Ca^{2+}, excretes Po_4^{2-}, and increases vitamin D level
3. Gut: Increases absorption of Ca^{2+} and Po_4^{2-} (through vitamin D)
4. Overall effect: Increases plasma Ca^{2+} level

    Vitamin D?

1. Bone: Mobilizes Ca^{2+}
2. Kidney: Resorbs Po_4^{2-}
3. Gut: Promotes Ca^{2+} and Po_4^{2-} absorption
4. Overall effect: Increases plasma Ca^{2+} and Po_4^{2-} levels

    Calcitonin?

1. Bone: Decreases mobilization of Ca^{2+} and Po_4^{2-}
2. Kidney: Decreases resorption of Ca^{2+} and Po_4^{2-}
3. Gut: Increases electrolyte secretion
4. Overall effect: Decreases plasma Ca^{2+} level

What are the 2 primary components of a sarcomere?

1. Thick filament: Myosin
2. Thin filament: Actin

BIOMECHANICS

What is stress?

Force per unit area

What is strain?	Change in length divided by the original length
What is the Wolfe law?	Bone is formed along the lines of stress and resorbed from areas without stress.
What is stress shielding?	A rigid implant removes the stress from an area of bone, and the bone weakens as a response to the Wolfe law.
Which of the following common orthopaedic materials most closely matches the rigidity of bone: stainless steel, titanium, polymethyl methacrylate (PMMA; cement), or polyethylene?	PMMA
What type of force does bone most strongly resist?	Compression
What type of force does ligament or tendon most strongly resist?	Tension

GAIT ANALYSIS

Where is the center of gravity for the human body?	Just anterior to sacral vertebra 2
How far does the center of gravity move during gait?	Horizontal and vertical oscillation of 5 cm
What is a concentric contraction?	Muscle fires while shortening (e.g., a person is about to jump)
What is an eccentric contraction?	Muscle fires while lengthening (e.g., a person is landing from a jump)
Are most muscles of the lower extremity most active during concentric or eccentric contraction?	Eccentric
What percentage of gait is spent in stance?	60%

What is the increased energy expenditure during gait with:	
Unilateral below-the-knee amputation?	25%
Bilateral below-the-knee amputation?	40%
Unilateral above-the-knee amputation?	> 60%

FRACTURES

GENERAL PRINCIPLES

Describe the physical exam in a fractured extremity.	1. Observe entire extremity (open, angulation) 2. Neurologic exam (sensation, motor function) 3. Vascular (pulses, capillary refill)
What x-rays should be ordered with a fractured extremity?	Two views of the extremity Make sure to include the joint proximal and distal
How are fractures described?	Open versus closed Location (proximal, middle, or distal) Pattern of fracture (comminuted, transverse) Degree of angulation

Define the following types of fracture.

Comminuted	Fracture with > 2 fragments
Pathologic	Fracture through a bone weakened by tumor, osteoporosis, or other bony abnormalities
Torus	Cortex buckled, but not disrupted, because of impaction injury; seen in children
Greenstick	Incomplete fracture with disruption of the cortex on only one side; seen in children

FRACTURE EPONYMS

Smith's fracture	Volarly displaced distal radius fracture, usually from fall onto dorsum of hand
Jones' fracture	Fracture at the base of the 5th metatarsal diaphysis
Bennett's fracture	Fracture of the base of the 1st metacarpal with involvement of the carpometacarpal (CMC) joint
Monteggia's fracture	Fracture of the proximal third of the ulna with dislocation of radial head
Galeazzi's fracture	Fracture of the radial shaft with disruption of the distal radioulnar joint (DRUJ)
Pott's fracture	Fracture of the distal fibula

FRACTURE HEALING

What are the 3 stages of fracture healing?	1. Inflammation: Infiltration of hematopoietic cells and osteogenic precursors 2. Repair (2 weeks): Callus, cartilage, and woven bone formation 3. Remodeling: Lamellar bone formation, development of normal shape and configuration, and repopulation of marrow
What type of bone formation occurs in fractures treated with a cast?	Endochondral ossification
What is the usual appearance on x-ray?	Fracture callus
What type of bone formation occurs in fractures treated with open reduction and internal fixation?	Primary bone formation

What is the usual appearance on x-ray?	Blurring of fracture line; no callus

OPEN FRACTURES

What is an open fracture?	Fracture that communicates with the external environment
What is the primary complication associated with these fractures?	Infection
What is the Gustillo classification for open fractures?	Grade I: Wound < 1 cm; minimal contamination and soft tissue injury; simple or minimal comminuted fracture Grade II: Wound 1–10 cm; moderate contamination; soft tissue injury; fracture comminution Grade III: Wound > 10 cm; gross contamination; severe soft tissue injury; fracture comminution
What additional features classify an open fracture as grade III, regardless of the size of the cutaneous lesion?	1. Soil contamination 2. Vascular injury 3. Close-range shotgun injury
What are the subgroups of grade III lesions?	Grade IIIA: Soft tissue adequate for coverage of wound Grade IIIB: Soft tissue loss that mandates flap coverage of wound Grade IIIC: Concurrent vascular injury requiring repair
What is the incidence of infection for grades I, II, and III?	Grade I: 0–2% Grade II: 2–7% Grade III: 10–50%
What is the treatment of an open fracture?	1. Operative irrigation and débridement within 6 hours; repeat débridement or irrigation may be needed in 24–72 hours 2. IV antibiotics 3. Tetanus inoculation 4. Open reduction and stabilization of the fracture

What is the antibiotic regimen for each grade?	Grade I: First-generation cephalosporin (i.e., cefazolin) for 48 hours
	Grades II and III: Add gram-negative coverage (i.e., gentamicin) for at least 72 hours
	For soil contamination, penicillin is provided for clostridial coverage.

What are the options for stabilizing open fractures?

1. Internal fixation
2. External fixation
3. Casting, splinting, and traction generally are **not** used for open fractures.

What are the benefits of external fixation?

1. No need for additional dissection of injured soft tissue
2. Placement of fixator out of the region of injury
3. Easy access to wound for observation and wound care

When is wound closure performed?

At 3–7 days **if** there is no evidence of infection

TRAUMA

A patient comes to the emergency department after a motor vehicle accident. She has an obviously deformed leg. What is the first step in management?

Airway, breathing, and circulation: ABCs of the advanced trauma life support (ATLS) protocol

In a trauma patient, after the ABCs are established, how are the following elements of the musculoskeletal survey addressed?

    Observation

Cervical spine immobilization is maintained until cleared; the patient is examined for any obvious deformities, abrasions, or open wounds

    Palpation

All long bones, even uninjured, nontender segments

Function	Range of all joints is determined, ligaments are stressed, an obviously fractured pelvis is not stressed, and neurologic and vascular evaluation is performed
What x-rays are mandatory in a patient with trauma?	Anteroposterior (AP) and lateral x-rays of cervical spine, AP x-ray of chest, and AP x-ray of pelvis
For a traumatized extremity, what x-rays are obtained?	AP and lateral views of the affected long bone **plus** an evaluation of the joints proximal and distal to the long bone
What is the initial treatment of a traumatized extremity?	1. Splinting 2. Reduction of deformities (i.e., restoration of normal alignment of bone or joint) 3. Irrigation of any open wounds and application of a sterile dressing
What are the general indications for open (surgical) reduction?	1. Failed closed reduction 2. Intra-articular fractures 3. Extremity function requiring perfect reduction 4. Multiple trauma 5. Advanced age (i.e., long nonambulatory period increases morbidity rate)
How does orthopaedic surgery help to prevent pulmonary complications in patients with multisystem trauma?	1. Early mobilization of the patient with operative fixation of fractures allows upright posture. 2. Surgery reduces the incidence of adult respiratory distress syndrome secondary to fat embolism in patients with long bone fractures.
Which fractured bone is most commonly associated with a fat embolism?	Femur
How does a fat embolism present?	Shortness of breath and petechiae across the chest and in the axilla 48 hours after injury
In an extremity that is deformed because of fracture or dislocation, what assessments are performed before reduction is attempted?	1. Vascular status 2. Neurologic status 3. Identification of open wounds

What treatment is performed emergently on a deformed extremity with vascular compromise?	Correction of the deformity by gentle traction in-line of the injured bone; splinting
What procedure is performed on a pulseless extremity whose pulses do not return after reduction?	Immediate operative exploration with intraoperative arteriogram to identify the level of vascular injury
What areas are incorporated into a splint?	The joints proximal and distal to the injured bone are immobilized.
What is the treatment of an extremity whose neurologic function was compromised before reduction and remains compromised after reduction?	Observation
What is the treatment if the neurologic function is compromised only after reduction?	Surgical exploration

ORTHOPAEDIC EMERGENCIES

What are the classic orthopaedic emergencies?	1. Unstable pelvic fracture 2. Unstable spine fracture 3. Open fracture 4. Septic joint 5. Septic osteomyelitis 6. Displaced long bone fracture with neurovascular compromise 7. Compartment syndrome 8. Dislocation

COMPARTMENT SYNDROME

What injuries are particularly susceptible to compartment syndrome?	1. Tibial shaft fractures 2. Extremity vascular injuries 3. Burn injuries (thermal or electric) 4. Supracondylar elbow fractures in children
What are the most reliable symptoms of compartment syndrome?	Pain out of proportion to the expected injury

What physical findings strongly suggest compartment syndrome?

Tense or firm compartments with pain on passive stretching of the involved compartments

What is the normal pressure of a compartment?

0–5 mm Hg

What pressure suggests compartment syndrome?

> 30 mm Hg

What is the usual treatment of compartment syndrome?

Emergent open fasciotomy

Should the skin be opened for the length of the fascial incision?

Yes. Skin can cause a compartment syndrome alone!

What are the muscular and neurovascular contents of the four compartments of the leg?

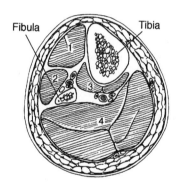

1. Anterior compartment

Muscles: Anterior tibialis, extensor hallucis longus, extensor digitorum longus, and peroneus tertius; **Nerve:** Deep peroneal; **Artery:** Anterior tibial

2. Lateral compartment

Muscles: Peroneus longus and peroneus brevis; **Nerve:** Superficial peroneal

3. Deep posterior compartment

Muscles: Posterior tibialis, flexor hallucis longus, and flexor digitorum longus; **Nerve:** Tibial; **Arteries:** Posterior tibial and peroneal

4. Superficial posterior compartment

Muscles: Gastrocnemius, soleus, and plantaris

What is the sequela of compartment syndrome that is not decompressed within 4–6 hours?	Muscle ischemia and necrosis resulting in contracture

CLAVICLE FRACTURES

What is the most common site of clavicular fracture?	Central one-third: 80% Distal one-third: 12–15% Proximal one-third: 5%
What is the usual treatment of this fracture?	Sling or figure-of-eight shoulder harness for 6–8 weeks
What clavicle fractures may require surgical fixation?	1. Concurrent vascular injury 2. Displaced distal clavicle fracture 3. Fracture end embedded in or piercing the trapezius muscle 4. Fracture end tenting the skin 5. Open fracture
What type of fixation is used for a clavicle fracture?	Plates and screws, not pins, because pins may migrate into the chest and erode into the chest cavities
What vascular structure is located directly beneath the clavicle?	Subclavian vein. Vascular injuries are rare.

SCAPULA FRACTURES

What is the significance of scapula fracture?	Indicates significant injury. The patient must be thoroughly evaluated for life-threatening lesions (i.e., pneumothorax, aortic injury, pelvic fracture).
What is the usual treatment?	Conservative management

SHOULDER TRAUMA

What is the most common direction of shoulder dislocation?	Anterior inferior
What is the usual presentation?	Pain and reduced shoulder mobility, with the injured arm held by the contralateral arm in slight abduction; prominent acromion

What x-ray views are included in a shoulder trauma series?	AP, lateral Y, and axillary views
What nerve is most commonly injured during shoulder dislocation?	Axillary nerve (almost always a neurapraxia)
What are the usual findings on physical exam if this nerve is injured?	Decreased sensation in region of lateral shoulder; decreased deltoid strength
What is the usual technique for reduction of anterior shoulder dislocation?	The patient lies prone with affected arm hanging over the side of the stretcher. A 5- to 10-lb weight is hung from the wrist. The patient is given muscle relaxant and medication for pain relief. After reduction, the arm is immobilized with a sling or swathe.
What step is important after reduction?	Reevaluation of neurovascular status of limb
What factor is most predictive of a recurrent shoulder dislocation?	Younger age at first dislocation increases risk of recurrence. Anterior shoulder reconstruction may be required.
What structure is at increased risk for injury during shoulder dislocation in the elderly?	Axillary artery
What is the usual presentation of posterior shoulder dislocation?	Arm is held adducted and internally rotated; the posterior shoulder is more prominent. Until proved otherwise, if the patient cannot externally rotate the shoulder beyond the neutral position or cannot supinate the hand, a posterior dislocation is present. These dislocations are frequently missed!
What are common mechanisms for posterior dislocation of the shoulder?	Seizure and electrocution
What is the usual treatment?	Closed reduction

HUMERUS FRACTURES

What are the 4 anatomic parts that can be displaced in a proximal humerus fracture?	1. Head 2. Shaft 3. Greater tuberosity 4. Lesser tuberosity

What muscle inserts on the:

Greater tuberosity?	Supraspinatus muscle
Lesser tuberosity?	Subscapularis muscle
What x-rays are mandatory for a proximal humerus fracture?	AP, Y, and axillary view
What nerve is at risk for injury in a humerus shaft fracture?	Radial nerve
What is the incidence of injury to this nerve?	5–10% of humerus shaft fractures
What muscles are innervated by the radial nerve distal to the shaft of the humerus?	Extensors of wrist and fingers
What is the usual treatment of nondisplaced fractures of the proximal humerus?	Sling for comfort. Begin gentle range of motion as soon as the proximal humerus can move as a unit.
What is the usual treatment of displaced proximal humerus fractures?	Open reduction, internal fixation, or hemiarthroplasty (replacement of proximal humerus only), with repair of rotator cuff tear
Should a humerus fracture with 30° angulation be corrected, and why?	No. The mobility of the shoulder joint allows the extremity to remain functional.
What is the usual treatment of humerus shaft fractures?	Coaptation or "U" splint and sling as long as there is bony opposition

What are the usual indications for surgical fixation of shaft fracture?	1. Segmental fracture 2. Distal fracture 3. Pathologic fracture 4. Concurrent forearm fracture (floating elbow) 5. Radial nerve injury during reduction

ELBOW DISLOCATIONS

What is the most common direction of an elbow dislocation?	Posterior (radius and ulna posterior to the humerus); others are rare.
What nerves are most commonly injured with an elbow dislocation?	Median and ulnar nerves
What muscles does the median nerve innervate distal to the elbow?	Radial wrist flexor (flexor carpi radialis) and deep flexor of thumb, index, and long finger, and all superficial flexors
What muscles does the ulnar nerve innervate distal to the elbow?	Ulnar wrist flexor (flexor carpi ulnaris), deep flexors to ring and small fingers, and intrinsic muscles to hand
What artery may be injured?	Brachial artery
What is the usual treatment of elbow dislocation?	Closed reduction with splinting. Splinting should last no more than 3 weeks to prevent joint contractures.
What are the indications for open reduction?	1. Irreducible dislocation 2. Incongruent reduction

ELBOW FRACTURES

What is a Monteggia fracture?	Proximal ulna fracture **plus** radial head dislocation
What nerve may be injured with this fracture?	Posterior interosseous nerve (PIN; distal radial nerve)
What muscles does the PIN innervate?	Extensor carpi ulnaris; finger and thumb extensors

What is a Galeazzi fracture?	Radial fracture at the junction of the middle and distal thirds **plus** subluxation of the radioulnar joint
What classic x-ray finding suggests occult elbow fracture?	"Sail sign": Fat anterior to distal humerus has a triangular appearance because of joint capsule distension.
What is the usual treatment of elbow fracture?	**Open** reduction and internal fixation. Precise alignment is needed for upper extremity function.

FOREARM FRACTURES

What is a Colles' fracture?	Fracture of the distal radius with **dorsal** carpal displacement
What is a Smith fracture?	Fracture of the distal radius with **volar** carpal displacement
What is the usual treatment of displaced midshaft radius fractures?	Open reduction with internal fixation
What is the usual treatment of displaced distal radius fractures?	Closed reduction with splinting
Why are distal radius fractures splinted initially?	Casts do not allow for swelling.
What joints are immobilized when a distal radius fracture is splinted?	Elbow and wrist
What postreduction parameters determine whether surgical intervention is warranted for a distal radius fracture?	1. Articular congruency 2. Radial length 3. Lack of volar tilt (in the AP plane)
What injury to the carpus is commonly missed with a distal radius fracture?	Scapholunate dissociation
What does "snuff-box" tenderness usually indicate?	Scaphoid (or navicular) bone fracture

PELVIC AND ACETABULAR TRAUMA

PELVIC FRACTURES

What bones are included in the pelvic ring?

Ilium, ischium, and pubis

What ligaments connect the:

    Sacrum to the ilium?

Anterior and posterior sacroiliac ligaments and interosseous ligaments

    Sacrum to the ischium?

Sacrotuberous ligament and sacrospinous ligament

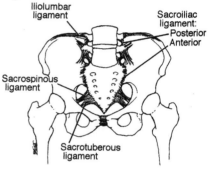

What ligament joins the ring anteriorly?

Pubic symphysis

What x-rays are necessary to evaluate a pelvic fracture or pelvic ring injury?

1. AP, inlet, and outlet
2. CT scan if the patient is hemodynamically stable

What aspect of a physical exam is mandatory before a Foley catheter is inserted?

Rectal exam (for high-riding prostate) and inspection for blood at the urethral meatus because of the risk of urethral disruption with pelvic fracture

What percentage of patients with a major pelvic fracture:

    Have concurrent intra-abdominal injury?

10–20%

    Require blood transfusion?

40%

    Have injury to a major pelvic arterial vessel?

2%

What are the usual applications for CT scan?	1. Evaluation of the posterior ligaments 2. Evaluation of the acetabulum 3. Identification of a pelvic hematoma or intraperitoneal injury
What is the quickest form of surgical treatment of a hemodynamically unstable patient with an unstable pelvic fracture?	External fixation, with pins placed through the skin and into the iliac wings and connected to a bar externally
What vessel is at risk for injury with a pelvic fracture through the greater sciatic notch?	Superior gluteal artery, a branch of the internal iliac artery

Describe a pelvis fracture classification by mechanism, including the feature that classifies each type as unstable.

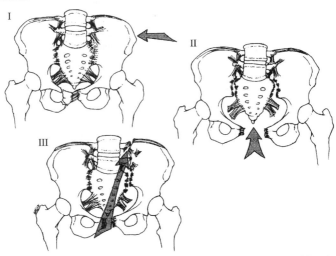

1. Type I	1. Lateral compression: Unstable when the posterior ligamentous or bony structure is disrupted
2. Type II	2. AP compression: Unstable when the pubic diastasis is > 2.5 cm, which indicates that the posterior ligamentous or bony structure is disrupted
3. Type III	3. Vertical shear: Unstable by definition

ACETABULAR FRACTURES

What is the basic anatomy of the acetabulum?	Rounded cavity whose walls contain anterior and posterior columns of bone that join at its dome
What x-rays are necessary to evaluate an acetabular fracture?	AP, Judet views CT scan if the patient is hemodynamically stable
Which fractures do not require surgical treatment?	< 2 mm displacement Satisfactory joint congruity
If surgery is necessary, when are these fractures usually repaired?	3–10 days after trauma, to reduce the risk of hemorrhage
What 3 complications are associated with acetabular fractures?	1. Sciatic nerve palsy 2. Post-traumatic arthritis 3. Heterotopic ossification that may limit hip motion

HIP TRAUMA

HIP DISLOCATION

What is the most common mechanism of injury?	Motor vehicle accident (75%)
What is the most common type of hip dislocation?	Posterior
What is the usual presentation of an anterior hip dislocation?	Externally rotated extremity with anterior hip fullness
What vascular structure can be injured with anterior dislocation?	Femoral artery
What is the usual presentation of posterior hip dislocation?	Internally rotated extremity with posterior fullness
What neurologic structure can be injured with posterior dislocation?	Sciatic nerve

What is the usual incidence of this injury?

10%

What is the usual treatment of hip dislocation?

Attempted closed reduction, followed by open reduction if dislocation is irreducible. Hip dislocation is an orthopaedic emergency!

How is the stability of reduction assessed?

Hip is flexed to 90° in neutral rotation. If the hip redislocates, it is considered unstable.

What are the usual indications for open reduction?

1. Failed closed reduction
2. Incongruent reduction
3. Intra-articular debris
4. Unstable reduction

What intervention is sometimes needed to prevent acute redislocation?

Traction

What follow-up study is necessary after reduction, and why?

X-ray (or, ideally, CT scan) to evaluate for:
1. Congruency of reduction
2. Presence of intra-articular bodies, which must be surgically removed

What are the usual late complications after hip dislocation?

1. Avascular necrosis (AVN; osteonecrosis) of the femoral head
2. Post-traumatic arthritis

What is the usual incidence of each complication?

1. AVN: 15–20% in posterior dislocation; 5–10% in anterior dislocation
2. Arthritis: 25–60% in both

HIP FRACTURE

Describe a hip fracture classification by location.

1. Femoral neck fracture
2. Intertrochanteric fracture—fracture traverses the metaphyseal region from greater to lesser trochanter
3. Subtrochanteric fracture—fracture extends in shaft of femur below lesser trochanter

What is the usual position of the lower extremity of a fractured hip?

Shortened and externally rotated

What is the usual treatment?	Closed reduction with internal fixation. In the elderly, traction is often the first line of therapy.

Describe a classification of femoral neck fractures.	Garden classification:
	    Type I: Incomplete; valgus impaction
	    Type II: Complete; undisplaced
	    Type III: Complete; partially
	        displaced
	    Type IV: Complete, totally displaced

What is the usual treatment of Garden type I and type II fractures?	Closed reduction with internal fixation
What is the usual treatment of Garden type III and type IV fractures?	Hip replacement (hemiarthroplasty vs. total hip replacement)
What is a common complication of femoral neck fractures?	AVN of the femoral head
Why is this a common complication?	Blood supply is disrupted as it travels distally to proximally.
What factors correlate most closely with the risk of AVN in femoral neck fractures?	Closeness of the fracture to the femoral head Degree of displacement at the time of injury
What is the usual mortality rate after hip fractures:	
In hospital?	10%
At 1 year?	35%

FEMORAL SHAFT FRACTURES

What fracture commonly occurs at the same time as a femoral shaft fracture?	Ipsilateral femoral neck fracture
What is the usual treatment of adult femoral shaft fractures?	Closed intramedullary nailing (with locking screws)

What is the usual treatment
of pediatric femoral shaft
fractures?

Hip spica cast

TRAUMATIC KNEE INJURIES

Name the labeled
structures (patella and
patella tendon removed).

1. Medial collateral ligament
2. Lateral collateral ligament
3. Anterior cruciate ligament
4. Posterior cruciate ligament
5. Medial meniscus
6. Lateral meniscus

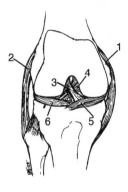

KNEE DISLOCATIONS

What neurovascular
structures are most
commonly injured during
knee dislocations?

1. Popliteal artery
2. Peroneal nerve

What is the usual incidence
of injury of each structure?

Popliteal artery: 20–40%
Peroneal nerve: 15%

What is the usual treatment?

Closed reduction is attempted; however,
open reduction may be necessary.

What study is performed
after reduction?

Arteriogram to evaluate the popliteal
artery

What may result from knee
dislocations?

Multi-ligament disruptions, which require
surgical reconstruction. If peroneal nerve
palsy exists, decompression of the nerve
should be performed urgently.

In which direction does the
patella most commonly
dislocate?

Laterally

What is the usual treatment?	Closed reduction by knee extension and manipulation. The dislocation often reduces spontaneously.
Why is a postreduction x-ray necessary?	To identify osteochondral fractures that require surgical repair

PATELLAR FRACTURES

What is a bipartite patella?	Patella with a well-defined superior-lateral secondary ossification center that is often mistaken for a fracture
What is the usual treatment of nondisplaced patellar fracture?	Cylinder cast
What is the usual indication for surgical repair of a patellar fracture?	> 3 mm of displacement or loss of the extensor mechanism

TIBIAL SHAFT FRACTURES

What complications often affect patients with tibial fractures?	1. Open fracture 2. Compartment syndrome
Why are tibial fractures prone to open wounds?	Subcutaneous location of the tibia
What flap can be used for coverage of an open fracture wound in the:	
Proximal one-third of the tibia?	Gastrocnemius muscle
Middle one-third of the tibia?	Soleus muscle
Distal one-third of the tibia?	Soleus muscle
What fracture configuration is most amenable to:	
Intramedullary rod fixation?	Transverse

External fixation?	Open, comminuted
Casting?	Spiral, nondisplaced

TRAUMATIC ANKLE AND FOOT INJURIES

What x-rays are mandatory in evaluating an ankle fracture?	AP, lateral, and mortise views
What does the mortise view evaluate?	Articular congruency (medially, superiorly, and laterally) and competency of the tibiofibular interosseous membrane
What ligament is most commonly injured in an ankle sprain?	Anterior talofibular ligament
What is the most common mechanism of ankle fracture?	Externally rotated leg on a supinated foot
What are the indications for surgery for ankle fractures?	1. Unstable ankle fractures (lateral and medial malleolus fracture or ligamentous disruption) 2. Incongruent joint after closed reduction 3. Syndesmotic rupture (disruption of distal tibiofibular ligamentous complex)
Where does the talus usually fracture?	Talar neck
What are the complications of talus fractures?	AVN of the body or dome; severe soft tissue injury
What is the usual mechanism of injury for calcaneus fractures?	Axial load (fall from a height)
What other fracture is common with a calcaneus fracture?	Lumbar spine fracture (10%)
What is the goal of treatment of a calcaneus fracture?	1. Prevent widened heel so that the foot can fit into a shoe 2. Maintain subtalar joint congruency to minimize risk of post-traumatic arthritis

What is a Lisfranc fracture or dislocation?	Fracture or dislocation of the base of the second metatarsal-cuneiform joint
What is the usual treatment?	Displaced injuries require anatomic reduction (open or closed) and fixation (percutaneous pin or screw).
What tendon is responsible for avulsion injuries to the base of the fifth metatarsal?	Peroneus brevis
What is the usual treatment?	Hard-soled shoe or cast for 2–3 weeks

PERIPHERAL NERVE INJURY

For each listed nerve, identify the contributing spinal levels and the motor test used to evaluate motor function.

Axillary nerve	C5 to C6; abduction of the shoulder
Musculocutaneous nerve	C5 to C6; flexion of the elbow
Radial nerve	C6 to C8; extension of the thumb
Median nerve	C6 to T1; flexion of the thumb interphalangeal joint
Ulnar nerve	C7 to T1; abduction of the index finger
Femoral nerve	L2 to L4; extension of the knee
Obturator nerve	L2 to L4; adduction of the hip
Superior gluteal nerve	L5; abduction of the hip
Inferior gluteal nerve	S1; extension of the hip
Tibial nerve (sciatic nerve)	L4 to S3; plantar flexion of the toe and ankle
Deep peroneal nerve (sciatic nerve)	L4 to S2; dorsiflexion of the toe

SPORTS MEDICINE

SPRAINS AND STRAINS

What is a sprain? Ligament tear

What is the usual presentation? Swelling and tenderness over the ligament; increased pain on stretching of the ligament

How are sprains graded? Grade I: Minor incomplete tear; no laxity compared with the contralateral ligament

Grade II: Significant incomplete tear; increased laxity; significant swelling and ecchymosis

Grade III: Complete tear; no end point felt when stress is applied to the ligament. Diagnosis may be missed because of muscle spasm and pain that prevent adequate examination of the ligament.

What is a strain? Partial tear of the musculotendinous unit

SHOULDER SEPARATION

What shoulder joint is most commonly sprained? Acromioclavicular (AC) joint

What ligaments stabilize the AC joint?
1. AC ligaments
2. Coracoclavicular (CC) ligaments (conoid and trapezoid)

What is the usual mechanism of ligament injury? Fall on the side of the shoulder

How are these injuries evaluated? AP x-ray taken with weight (10 lb) hanging from the arm, and compared with contralateral side

How are AC sprains graded? Grade I: Ligament continuity; no joint opening

Grade II: Ligament continuity; joint opening

Grade III: No ligament continuity; complete tear of AC and CC ligaments

What is the usual treatment?	Sling for comfort for all grades with early range of motion; orthopaedic referral in 3–5 days for grades I and II and immediately for grade III because surgery may be indicated

ROTATOR CUFF PATHOLOGY

How does rotator cuff tendinitis usually present?	Middle-aged man (40s) with gradually increasing pain in the shoulder and difficulty raising the arms above the head
What clinical findings support the diagnosis of rotator cuff tendinitis?	Passive internal rotation, flexion, and abduction of the shoulder cause severe pain.
What are the muscles of the rotator cuff?	**SITS:** 1. **S**upraspinatus muscle 2. **I**nfraspinatus muscle 3. **T**eres minor muscle 4. **S**ubscapularis muscle
Which muscle tendon is usually affected by tendinitis?	Supraspinatus muscle
What factors contribute to rotator cuff tendinitis?	1. Impingement from bone spur of the acromion or AC joint 2. Vascular watershed of the tendon 3. Repetitive trauma from overhead activities
What is the end-stage condition of rotator cuff impingement?	Rotator cuff tear with eventual proximal migration of the humerus; severe pain
What is the usual presentation of acute tear of the rotator cuff?	Acute onset of pain and inability to raise the arm over the head after a traumatic event
What radiographic studies are used to diagnose rotator cuff tears?	MRI or arthrogram
What is the usual medical treatment?	1. Physical therapy 2. Nonsteroidal anti-inflammatory drug (NSAID) 3. Steroid injection

What is the usual surgical treatment of severe impingement or rotator cuff tear?	1. Removal of bony spurs (acromioplasty) 2. Repair of rotator cuff

KNEE INJURIES

What is a common mechanism for rupturing the anterior cruciate ligament (ACL)?	Changing direction at high speed on a planted foot
What is the most common finding on knee aspiration after an ACL rupture?	Hemarthrosis (blood); 70% of patients with hemarthrosis and **stable** ligamentous findings actually have an ACL injury.
What physical findings are consistent with ACL injury?	1. Increased anterior translation of the tibia on the femur with the knee in 90° flexion (**anterior drawer** test) 2. Increased translation of the tibia on the femur with the knee in 20–30° flexion (**Lachman** test)
What study best evaluates intra-articular abnormalities of the knee?	MRI
What intra-articular structure is most commonly injured with a traumatic ACL rupture?	Lateral meniscus
What physical finding is consistent with a medial collateral ligament rupture?	Increased pain and medial joint opening with the knee in slight flexion and valgus stress applied
What physical finding is consistent with a lateral collateral ligament rupture?	Lateral joint opening with the knee in slight flexion and valgus stress applied
What is the most sensitive physical finding that suggests an acute posterior cruciate ligament rupture?	**Quadriceps active** test: Increased anterior translation of the tibia on the femur from a posteriorly displaced position when the knee is actively extended against gravity from a position of flexion

What is the usual conservative therapy?	Ice, elevation, compression, immobilization, non–weight-bearing with crutches, and physical therapy (**NICE: n**on–weight-bearing, **i**ce, **c**ompression, **e**levation)
What is the usual surgical therapy?	Reconstruction of the ligament with arthroscopic assistance, using the patella tendon or a hamstring autograft
What is the "unhappy triad"?	Knee injury that includes the ACL, medial collateral ligament (MCL), and the medial meniscus

FOOT AND ANKLE SPORTS INJURIES

What are the signs of an Achilles tendon rupture?	Calf pain, palpable disrupted tendon, unable to plantar flex ankle
What physical exam finding is indicative of an Achilles tendon tear?	Positive Thompson test: Squeezing the gastrocnemius muscle does not result in plantar flexion of the foot.
What is turf toe?	Hyperextension injury of the first metatarsophalangeal (MTP) joint resulting in a strain or avulsion of volar plate from the metatarsal head; often occurs on artificial turf

ORTHOPAEDIC INFECTIONS

SEPTIC ARTHRITIS

What is the most common route of infection that causes a septic joint?	Hematogenous
What is the usual presentation of bacterial septic arthritis?	Localized joint pain, erythema, warmth, swelling with pain on active and passive range of motion, inability to bear weight, ± fever
What are the components of the diagnostic evaluation?	X-ray (to rule out osteomyelitis), erythrocyte sedimentation rate, WBC count, blood cultures, and aspirate

What findings on aspirate are diagnostic of infection?	1. WBC $> 80{,}000$; $> 90\%$ neutrophils 2. Protein level > 4.4 gm/dL 3. Glucose level significantly $<$ blood glucose level 4. No crystals 5. Positive Gram stain results
What is the most common organism that causes septic arthritis?	*Staphylococcus aureus*
What other organism must be considered in a sexually active patient?	*Neisseria gonorrhoeae*
What is the usual treatment of septic arthritis?	1. Hip joint is emergently decompressed and drained surgically; other joints may be serially aspirated 2. IV antibiotics

OSTEOMYELITIS

What is the usual presentation of osteomyelitis?	Localized extremity pain, $\pm$ fever, 1–2 weeks after respiratory infection or infection at another nonbony site
What is the most common organism in the bacteriology of osteomyelitis?	*S. aureus*
Which patients are susceptible to gram-negative organisms?	Neonates and immunocompromised patients
Which additional organism is common in patients with sickle cell disease?	*Salmonella*
What classic radiographic findings are associated with osteomyelitis?	Lytic, eccentrically located serpiginous lesion involving the cortex
What other studies confirm the diagnosis?	Blood cultures, aspirate cultures, erythrocyte sedimentation rate, leukocytosis, and increased uptake on bone scan

What other organism must be considered when osteomyelitis occurs in a child < 5 years old?

Haemophilus influenzae

What organisms must be considered in the IV drug abuser?

Gram-negative organisms and *Pseudomonas aeruginosa*

What organism must be considered in the patient with sickle cell disease?

Salmonella typhi

What organism must be considered in patients with foot puncture wounds?

Pseudomonas

What is the usual treatment of osteomyelitis?

Surgical decortication and drainage; IV antibiotics

PEDIATRIC ORTHOPAEDIC SURGERY

Name and describe the classification used for pediatric fractures.

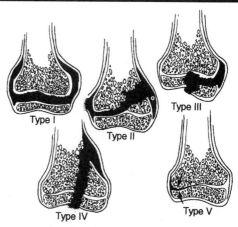

Salter classification of fractures involving the physis (growth plate):
  I.   Through the growth plate only
  II   Through the metaphysis and growth plate
  III. Through the epiphysis and growth plate
  IV. Through the epiphysis, growth plate, and metaphysis
  V.   Crushed growth plate
Most "ligamentous" injuries in children are actually fractures involving the physis.

What possibility should be investigated in children with spiral or oblique fractures?	Child abuse
What is the most commonly fractured bone in childhood?	Clavicle

LEG LENGTH DISCREPANCY

What leg length discrepancy goes unnoticed by patients?	1 cm
What leg length discrepancy can be treated with a shoe lift?	2.5 cm
What leg length discrepancy is generally treated by epiphysiodesis (i.e., limb shortening)?	2.5–5 cm (discrepancy > 5 cm is generally treated with limb lengthening)

HIP DISORDERS

How do hip abnormalities commonly present in children?	Knee pain referred from the hip
What nerve is responsible for this referred hip pain?	Obturator nerve
What is the differential diagnosis for a child with hip or knee pain and a waddling gait?	1. Late developmentally dysplastic hip 2. Perthes disease 3. Slipped capital femoral epiphysis
What is the usual presentation of developmentally dysplastic hips?	1. Hip "click" detected by newborn screening 2. Asymmetric skinfolds and thigh lengths in newborns. Most common in girls, firstborns, and infants presenting in breech position
What physical maneuver is used to screen a newborn's hips?	**Barlow test:** Hip is dislocated by adducting the leg while driving the hip posteriorly **Ortolani test:** Hip is reduced by abducting the leg while pulling the hip anteriorly

What is the usual treatment in a child 0–6 months old?	Pavlik harness (straps that hold the hips flexed and slightly abducted)
What is the usual treatment in a child > 6 months old?	Traction or surgery

LEGG-CALVÉ-PERTHES DISEASE

What is Legg-Calvé-Perthes disease?	Osteochondritis of the capital femoral epiphysis
What is the usual presentation?	Painless limp in a child 4–8 years old; knee pain
What is the differential diagnosis?	Hypothyroidism, infection, and epiphyseal dysplasia
What are the principles of treatment for Perthes disease?	1. Maintain hip range of motion. 2. Contain the softened revascularizing femoral head in the acetabulum during remodeling.
How are these goals achieved?	Bilateral walking long leg casts fixed together with transverse bars until x-rays show that mature bone has replaced the avascular epiphysis (usually 18 months)

SLIPPED CAPITAL FEMORAL EPIPHYSIS (SCFE)

What is the usual presentation of SCFE?	Painful, waddling gait in an adolescent; most common in African-American obese males
What is the classic physical finding?	Obligatory external rotation with hip flexion
How is SCFE quantified?	Degree or percentage of translation of the capital femoral epiphysis in relation to the femoral neck as seen on a lateral (frog leg) hip x-ray
What steps are mandatory in the evaluation of a patient diagnosed with SCFE?	1. Evaluation of the contralateral hip ($\approx 25\%$ are bilateral) 2. Endocrine evaluation to rule out hypothyroidism
What is the usual treatment?	Mandatory admission with strict non-weight-bearing until operative pinning is performed. Some deformities require an osteotomy.

What maneuver is avoided during the treatment of SCFE?	Forceful reduction of the hip

SCOLIOSIS

What is scoliosis?	Lateral curvature of a segment of the spine
What are the etiologies?	1. Idiopathic (most common) 2. Neuromuscular (neuropathic and myopathic) 3. Congenital defect in formation, segmentation, or both 4. Neurofibromatosis 5. Connective tissue disorders (Marfan's, Ehlers-Danlos) 6. Osteochondrodystrophy 7. Metabolic 8. Nonstructural (painful lesion) 9. Trauma (thoracic surgery)
What are the 2 general types?	1. Structural: Does not correct with positional changes 2. Nonstructural: Corrects with positional changes
What is the most common form of scoliosis?	Adolescent idiopathic scoliosis
What is the usual presentation?	Adolescent girl with painless curvature or asymmetric shoulders, pelvis, or rib hump (seen with forward bending)
What is the differential diagnosis?	Congenital vertebral malformation, neuromuscular disorders, tumors, or spinal dysraphism
What is the most common direction and location of adolescent idiopathic scoliosis?	Convexity to the right in the thoracic spine; look for chest rotation and rib hump
What findings require further evaluation with MRI or bone scan?	1. Pain 2. Left thoracic curve 3. Neurologic compromise

Which adolescent idiopathic scoliotic curves require treatment?

Curves that are likely to progress or those that show progression. Others need serial observation until the patient reaches maturity.

How is adolescent idiopathic scoliosis treated in skeletally immature patients?

1. Bracing for curves that are 25–30° and show progression of 5–10°
2. Bracing for any curve that is 30–40°
3. Surgical fusion for curves > 40°

What degree of scoliosis is likely to progress in skeletally mature patients?

> 50°

What degree of curvature is associated with cardiopulmonary compromise?

> 90°

CEREBRAL PALSY (CP)

What is CP?

Nonprogressive, neuromuscular disease secondary to injury of the immature brain

What types of movement characterize CP?

Spasticity, athetosis, ataxic, and mixed

What are the patterns of movement of the extremities?

Hemiplegic (upper and lower extremities on the same side), diplegic (both lower extremities), and totally involved

What is the most common type of CP?

Spastic and diplegic

Which type has the worst prognosis for ambulation?

Totally involved

Which type has the best prognosis for ambulation?

Hemiplegic

What is the usual treatment?

Physical therapy and orthotics. Surgery is not commonly used, but may be necessary for lengthening or transplantation of the tendons, arthrodesis of the joints, or correction of limb length inequality.

MYELODYSPLASIA (SPINAL DYSRAPHISM)

What is myelodysplasia?	Defect of spinal cord closure ranging from only the posterior vertebral arch (spina bifida occulta) to exposed neural elements (rachischisis)
Compare meningocele and myelomeningocele.	Meningocele: Exposed sac protruding into the defect **without** neural elements Myelomeningocele: Protruding sac containing neural elements
What factors determine the functional prognosis in myelodysplasia?	Level of defect and extent of neurologic injury
What is the highest level of myelodysplasia that allows ambulation?	Fourth lumbar
What muscle group is innervated by the fourth lumbar nerve roots?	Quadriceps by L2, L3, and L4
What are the usual orthopaedic manifestations of myelodysplasia?	Scoliosis, dislocated hips (from unopposed flexion and adduction at the level of L3 to L4), lower extremity contraction and fractures

DUCHENNE MUSCULAR DYSTROPHY (DMD)

What is DMD?	X-linked recessive, noninflammatory disorder of progressive muscle weakness affecting young males
What is the usual presentation?	Young male with clumsiness, lumbar lordosis, and calf pseudohypertrophy
What is the Gowers' sign?	Child stands from the recumbent position by walking his hands up his legs
What laboratory value supports the diagnosis of DMD?	Highly elevated creatinine phosphokinase level
What are the orthopaedic manifestations of DMD?	Flexion contractures of the joints and neuromuscular scoliosis

What is the usual prognosis?	Most patients die by 20 years of age as a result of cardiopulmonary complications.

TOEING-IN

What is the differential diagnosis for pigeon toe (toeing-in gait) in a child?	1. Metatarsus adductus 2. Tibial torsion 3. Excessive femoral anteversion
Which type is the most common?	Tibial torsion
What is metatarsus adductus?	Adducted forefoot
What is the most commonly affected age group?	First year of life
What is the usual treatment?	If flexible, stretching; if inflexible, osteotomy
What is tibial torsion?	Rotational deformity of the tibia proximally to distally
What is the most commonly affected age group?	2 years of age
What is the usual treatment?	None. Spontaneous resolution is the norm.
What is femoral anteversion?	Increased internal rotation of the femur in relation to the femoral neck and head
What is the most commonly affected age group?	3–6 years of age
What is the usual treatment?	Spontaneous resolution by 10 years of age is the norm.

NURSEMAID'S ELBOW

What is it?	Subluxation of the radial head because of a sudden tug on a child's pronated, extended arm
What is the usual presentation?	Local tenderness, limited use of the arm, but no swelling or x-ray abnormalities

What is the usual treatment?	Closed reduction by the supinating arm; no immobilization is necessary.

JOINT RECONSTRUCTION

What 3 forms of arthritis commonly require joint replacement?	1. Osteoarthritis 2. Rheumatoid arthritis 3. AVN
What are the radiographic hallmarks of osteoarthritis?	Loss of joint space, periarticular osteophytes, subchondral sclerosis, and subchondral cyst formation
What are the radiographic hallmarks of rheumatoid arthritis?	Periarticular erosions and osteopenia
What are the radiographic hallmarks of AVN of the femoral head?	Stage I: Normal x-ray findings; decreased signal by MRI Stage II: Femoral head that has subchondral radiodensity or radiolucency, but no collapse Stage III: Femoral head that has collapse, with a "crescent sign" and no acetabular involvement Stage IV: Femoral head involvement with acetabular involvement
Describe the ideal candidate for joint replacement surgery.	Elderly patient with debilitating pain localized to a joint and radiographic evidence of arthritis; failed nonoperative treatment
What are the classic nonoperative treatment modalities?	Unloading of joints through weight loss or a cane; support of joints through muscle strengthening or bracing; and relief of symptoms with an NSAID or joint injections with anesthetics and steroids
What are the contraindications to joint replacement surgery?	1. Active infection 2. Neurologic compromise 3. Young, active patient
What surgical options are available for the young patient with debilitating arthritis?	1. Osteotomy: Controlled fracture of the bone and fixation to correct the alignment 2. Arthrodesis: Joint fusion

What are the major complications after total hip arthroplasty (replacement) and the incidence of each?	1. DVT: 70% (by venogram) 2. Infection: 1% 3. Dislocation: 1%–5%
What structures are at risk because of screw penetration of the inner wall of the acetabulum during total hip arthroplasty?	1. External iliac artery and vein in the anterior superior quadrant 2. Obturator nerve artery and vein in the anterior inferior quadrant

FOOT AND ANKLE

DIABETIC FOOT

What 2 entities in patients with diabetes cause deformity and radiographic obliteration of the affected joints?	1. Infection 2. Neuropathic joint (Charcot's joint)
How do these 2 entities differ?	Charcot's joint presents with a swollen, warm, relatively painless deformed foot with no systemic fever and a low WBC count.
What is the usual treatment of Charcot's joint?	Immobilization in a cast until the inflammation resolves

FLATFOOT

What is the differential diagnosis for flatfoot in adulthood?	1. Posterior tibial tendon rupture 2. Talonavicular arthritis 3. Neuropathic arthritis
What is the differential diagnosis for rigid flatfoot in childhood?	1. Tarsal coalition 2. Congenital vertical talus
When is treatment of flatfoot indicated?	When it becomes painful
What is the usual treatment?	Flexible flatfoot is generally treated with orthotics (arch supports). Rigid flatfoot requires surgical correction.

TOE ABNORMALITIES

What is a claw toe?	Extended MTP joint and flexed proximal interphalangeal (PIP) and distal interphalangeal (DIP) joints
What is a hammer toe?	Flexed PIP joint ± extended MTP joint
What is a mallet toe?	Flexed DIP joint
What is the most common cause of deformed toes?	Narrow toe box of shoes

SPINE

LOW BACK PAIN

What is the most common cause of low back pain in children?	Spondylolysis
What are the common intrinsic spine disorders of children with back pain?	Congenital, developmental, and infectious disorders; tumors
What are the common intrinsic spine disorders of young adults with back pain?	Disc disease, spondylolisthesis, and acute fractures
What are the common intrinsic spine disorders of older adults with back pain?	Spinal stenosis, metastatic disease, and osteoporotic compression fractures
What percentage of the population shows evidence of herniated nucleus pulposus by MRI?	≈ 30%; most are asymptomatic

SPONDYLOLYSIS

What is spondylolysis?	Bony defect in the pars interarticularis, usually caused by a fatigue fracture
What x-ray views best show spondylolysis?	Oblique lumbar spine views, which show a break in the neck of the "Scottie dog"

What is the usual treatment of spondylolysis?	Asymptomatic spondylolysis is not treated. Symptomatic cases are treated with activity restrictions and, rarely, fusion.

SPONDYLOLISTHESIS

What is spondylolisthesis?	Slippage of one vertebra on another
What are the causes of spondylolisthesis?	Congenital, elongation of the pars interarticularis, degenerative, traumatic, pathologic, and postsurgical
What is the usual presentation of childhood spondylolisthesis?	Tight hamstrings, low back pain
At what level does childhood spondylolisthesis typically occur?	L5 to S1
At what level does adult degenerative spondylolisthesis usually occur?	L4 to L5
What is the usual treatment of spondylolisthesis?	Mild slips are treated with activity restriction until symptoms disappear. Severe slips are treated with fusion.

SPINAL INFECTIONS

What is Pott's disease?	Tuberculosis infection of the spine
What is the usual presentation?	Back pain, ± fever and weight loss, in an exposed or immunocompromised patient
What is the usual treatment?	Immobilization and IV antibiotics; if this treatment fails, then surgical débridement and stabilization
How is pyogenic vertebral osteomyelitis differentiated radiographically from tumor?	Infection often involves the disc space; tumor commonly spares the disc space

MUSCULOSKELETAL ONCOLOGY

What is the usual treatment for extremity tumors?	Wide excision or amputation; adjunctive chemotherapy or radiation therapy

SOFT TISSUE TUMORS

What is the most common soft tissue sarcoma of late adulthood?	Malignant fibrous histiocytoma
What is the most common soft tissue mesenchymal tumor?	Lipoma
What is the most common soft tissue sarcoma of childhood?	Rhabdomyosarcoma
What is the most common sarcoma of the hand?	Epithelioid sarcoma

BONE TUMORS

What is the most common malignancy of bone?	Metastatic disease
What is the most common tumor of the spine?	Metastatic disease
What primary malignancies commonly metastasize to bone in adults?	Breast, lung, prostate, kidney, and thyroid carcinoma
What primary malignancies commonly metastasize to bone in children?	Neuroblastoma and Wilms' tumor
What is the usual treatment of metastatic disease to the bone?	Radiation therapy and, in some cases, prophylactic fixation
What is the most common benign primary bone tumor?	Nonossifying fibroma

Primary Bone Malignancies

What is the most common primary bone malignancy in adults?	Multiple myeloma
What are the most common primary bone malignancies in children and adolescents?	1. Osteosarcoma 2. Ewing's sarcoma
What is the most common location for each type?	Both are usually found in the knee region (distal knee, proximal tibia).
What are the classic radiographic findings for each type?	1. Osteosarcoma: Sunburst pattern 2. Ewing's sarcoma: "Onion skinning" pattern
What is the usual treatment?	1. Osteosarcoma: Wide or radical excision with multiagent chemotherapy 2. Ewing's sarcoma: Chemotherapy with wide excision or radiation therapy

UNICAMERAL BONE CYST

What is it?	Benign fluid-filled cyst found in bone
What is the most common location?	Proximal humerus
What is the most common age group?	5–15 years
What is the usual presentation?	Pain or pathologic fracture
What is the usual treatment?	Steroid injections

71

Neurosurgery

ADVANCED NEUROANATOMY

What is the pterion?

The H-shaped junction of the frontal, parietal, temporal, and greater wing of the sphenoid bones. Its location is roughly 2.5 cm above the zygomatic arch and 1.5 cm behind the zygomatic process of the frontal bone.

Why is the pterion important?

Its position represents the central focus of one of the more common craniotomies in neurosurgery.

What is the largest foramen of the skull?

Foramen magnum

What does each foramen in the skull contain?

    Foramen magnum

Spinal cord and medulla, the anterior and posterior spinal arteries, the spinal accessory nerve (cranial nerve 11), and the vertebral arteries

    Foramen ovale

Mandibular branch of cranial nerve 5 and the motor branches to the jaw musculature

    Jugular foramen

Internal jugular vein and cranial nerves 9, 10, and 11

    Foramen lacerum

Although the foramen lacerum appears large when viewing the base of the skull, usually no structures enter or exit from this foramen.

What constitutes the base of the skull?

1. Orbital roofs of frontal bones
2. Cribriform plate of ethmoid bones
3. Sphenoid bone
4. Squamous and petrous portions of temporal bones
5. Occipital bones

What are the major anatomic divisions of the brain?

1. Two cerebral hemispheres
2. Brain stem
3. Cerebellum

What are the lobes of the cerebral hemispheres?

1. Frontal lobes
2. Parietal lobes
3. Temporal lobes
4. Occipital lobes

What are the 3 divisions of the brain stem?

1. Midbrain
2. Pons
3. Medulla

What are the functions of the frontal lobes?

Planning and sequencing of movement, voluntary eye movements, and emotional affect

What are the functions of the parietal lobes?

Subserve motor control and cortical sensation. The dominant parietal lobe governs motor programs, whereas the nondominant lobe governs spatial orientation.

What are the functions of the occipital lobes?

Visual perception and involuntary eye movements

What are the functions of the temporal lobes?

Subserve olfaction, memory, and certain components of auditory and visual perception

What region of the brain governs the comprehension of speech, and in which lobe is it located?

Wernicke's area; located in the dominant temporal lobe of the brain

What region of the brain governs the motor component of speech, and in which lobe is it located?

Broca's area; within the posterior portion of the dominant frontal lobe

What are the major vessels supplying blood to the brain and their branches?	1. The **anterior circulation** of the brain consists of the internal carotid arteries, which further divide into the anterior cerebral artery and the middle cerebral artery.
	2. The **posterior circulation** consists of the vertebral arteries, which join to form the basilar artery, which divides into the 2 posterior cerebral arteries. The vertebral arteries also give off the anterior spinal artery of the spinal cord and the posterior inferior cerebellar artery (PICA), whereas the basilar artery gives off the anterior inferior cerebellar artery (AICA) and the superior cerebellar artery (SCA).
What is the "circle of Willis"?	An arterial anastomosis of vessels that enables the entire brain to be reliably vascularized from 1 main feeding vessel. The anterior communicating artery between the 2 anterior cerebral arteries, and the 2 posterior communicating arteries between the internal carotid artery and the posterior cerebral arteries serve as the main conduits between the anterior and posterior circulatory systems as well as the right-and left-sided circulatory systems.

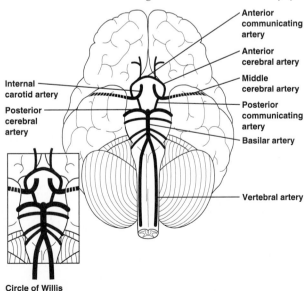

Circle of Willis

What are the main draining vessels of the brain?	The venous drainage systems of the brain are divided into superficial and deep systems:

1. In the superficial system, the superior sagittal sinus joins the straight sinus at the confluence of the sinuses, known as the torcular. Blood then drains from the cranial vault via the transverse and sigmoid sinuses to exit the skull via the internal jugular veins.
2. The deep system starts with the internal cerebral veins and inferior sagittal sinus draining into the straight sinus.

What is the cavernous sinus?	The cavernous sinus is a plexus of veins located on both sides of the bony sella turcica. A number of veins, including orbital and cortical vessels, contribute to its flow.
Which nerves travel within the lateral walls of the cavernous sinus?	Cranial nerves III, IV, and the ophthalmic and maxillary divisions of cranial nerve V
Which nerve and artery travel within the sinus itself?	Cranial nerve VI and the carotid artery
What is a carotid cavernous fistula?	Carotid cavernous fistulas are the general arterialization of the cavernous sinus. The fistulas are of 2 types: traumatic and spontaneous.
What symptoms are associated with carotid cavernous fistulas?	Headache, orbital pain, and diplopia
What signs are associated with carotid cavernous fistulas?	Ophthalmoplegia, arterialization of the conjunctiva (chemosis), and ocular or cranial **bruit**
What is the treatment of carotid cavernous fistulas?	Although some low-flow lesions may spontaneously thrombose, high-flow lesions often require balloon embolization.

Where is CSF produced?

The bulk of CSF is produced by the choroid plexus, which is located in the lateral and fourth ventricles. Small amounts are also produced in the interstitial spaces, the ependymal linings of the ventricles, and the dural root sleeves.

How much CSF is produced daily in the adult?

Typically, 500–750 mL (0.35 mL/min)

What is the pathway for CSF egress from the lateral ventricles to the surface of the brain?

CSF produced in the choroid plexus of the lateral ventricles travels first through the foramen of Monro of the lateral ventricles into the midline third ventricle. From the third ventricle, CSF travels through the narrow aqueduct of Sylvius to the fourth ventricle. CSF then exits the brain via the midline foramen of Magendie or the lateral foramina of Luschka. Once over the surface of the brain, CSF is primarily absorbed by the arachnoid granulations located in continuity with the superior sagittal sinus.

What are the principles of the Monro-Kellie doctrine?

For intracranial pressure to remain constant, the sum of the volumes of the intracranial contents (brain, blood, CSF) must remain constant.

What is the normal cerebral perfusion pressure (CPP) and how is it maintained?

The brain, through autoregulation, maintains CPP at ≥ 50 mm Hg.

What is normal cerebral blood flow (CBF)?

CBF in the normal resting brain is 50 mL/100 mg brain/min.

At what CBF does the electroencephalogram become flatline?

At 25 mL/100 mg brain/min

At what CBF does neuronal cell death ensue?

At 10 mL/100 mg brain/min

What is Kernohan's phenomenon?

Contralateral cerebral peduncle compression against the tentorial notch, resulting in contralateral dilated pupil and ipsilateral hemiparesis, is seen in 10–20% of epidural hematomas.

What is a subdural hygroma?	A subdural fluid collection due to a tear in the arachnoid membrane
What is the radiographic appearance of subdural hygroma?	A hypodense crescent of fluid displacing brain tissue

SPINAL INJURIES AND INTERVERTEBRAL DISC DISEASE

Are neurologic deficits more common with cervical or thoracolumbar vertebral fractures, and why?	Thoracolumbar fractures. Spinal canal is smaller at more caudal levels.
How is motor strength graded on physical examination?	Grade 0: No contraction Grade 1: Muscle contracts Grade 2: Movement without gravity Grade 3: Movement against gravity Grade 4: Movement against resistance Grade 5: Normal strength

Which sensory levels correspond to the following?

Shoulders	C4
Nipples	T4
Umbilicus	T10
Knees	L3
Perianal region?	S5

CERVICAL SPINE

What are the 3 functional columns of the cervical spine and the ligamentous complexes of each column?

Anterior column	1. Anterior half of vertebral body and disc 2. Anterior longitudinal ligament and anulus fibrosus
Middle column	1. Posterior half of vertebral body and disc 2. Posterior longitudinal ligament and anulus fibrosus

Posterior column

1. Lamina, pedicles, spinous processes, and facet joints
2. Interspinous ligaments and facet capsules

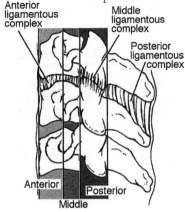

When is a cervical spine generally considered unstable? | When 2 or more of these functional columns are damaged

When is a cervical spine generally considered unstable?

When 2 or more of these functional columns are damaged

What are the names given to the first 2 cervical vertebrae (C1 and C2)?

C1: Atlas
C2: Axis (has an anterior protuberance called the odontoid)

What is the usual mechanism of C1 versus C2 fracture?

C1: Axial loading
C2 (including odontoid): Hyperextension

What is a Hangman's fracture?

Fracture through pedicles of C2 at the pars interarticularis

What is a Jefferson fracture?

A fracture of the ring of C1 at more than 1 site

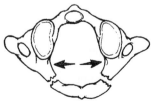

What is the radiographic criterion for a Jefferson fracture?

The "rule of Spence" provides that if the sum of the overhang of both lateral masses is ≥ 7 mm (on AP view), an abnormality exists at the level of C1.

Are neurologic deficits common with this injury, and why?

Given the large size of the spinal canal at this level, neurologic deficits are rare if this lesion occurs in isolation.

What is the treatment of a Jefferson fracture?

External fixation in a halo device

What are the 3 types of odontoid fractures?

Type I: Fracture of the apical portion of the dens
Type II: Fracture of the dens at its base
Type III: Fracture of the dens extending into the body of C2

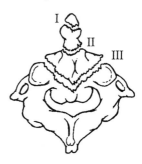

What is the treatment of odontoid fractures?

Type I: Stable fracture; treatment rarely necessary
Type II: Unstable fracture; surgical fusion
Type III: Stable fracture; immobilization with halo device

What surgical procedures are used for fixation of odontoid fracture?

1. Posterior approach: C1 can be plated or wired to C2.
2. Anterior approach: A screw can be placed into the body of C2 through the axis of the dens.

Which of these approaches preserves rotation of the head?

The anterior approach preserves rotation, which at C1 to C2 represents 50% of all rotation of the head at the neck. This technique is generally reserved for younger individuals.

How many cervical nerve roots are there?

There are 8 cervical nerve roots (C1 to C8), but only 7 cervical vertebrae.

What nerve root exits between vertebrae C3 and C4?

Nerve root C4

What are the clinical components of a radiculopathy?	Weakness, reflex changes, and dermatomal sensory changes ascribed to a particular nerve root
What is the most common cervical disc herniation and its associated radiculopathy?	Disc herniations at the C6 to C7 interval represent roughly two-thirds of all disc herniations. A C7 radiculopathy develops in these cases.
What are the clinical correlates of a C5 radiculopathy?	1. Deltoid weakness 2. Diminished sensation over the shoulder
What are the clinical correlates of a C5 radiculopathy?	1. Diminished biceps reflex 2. Biceps weakness 3. Decreased sensation over the upper arm, radial forearm, and thumb
What are the clinical correlates of a C7 radiculopathy?	1. Diminished triceps reflex 2. Triceps muscle weakness
What is the usual treatment of cervical disc herniation?	Over 95% of cervical disc herniation radiculopathies heal spontaneously.
What are the surgical approaches for those that fail to heal?	1. Anterior cervical discectomy (ACDF) with or without fusion 2. Posterior foraminotomy and disc excision
What is cervical spondylosis?	A degenerative disease of the spine associated with osteophytic spurs, hardening of the intervertebral discs, and hypertrophy of the vertebral ligaments, particularly the posterior longitudinal ligament
How does cervical spondylosis present?	Neck pain and the physical findings associated with cervical spondylitic myelopathy (CSM)
What is CSM?	A syndrome commonly associated with clinical findings including hyperreflexia, spasticity, weakness of the hands, proximal lower extremity weakness, and a paucity of sensory changes

What is the physiologic basis for CSM?

Repetitive trauma to the spinal cord by a narrowed canal and associated with normal movement, ischemia of the cord associated with vascular compression with a narrow canal, or direct cord compression

What is the treatment of CSM?

Physiologic decompression of the cord, which may be achieved by cervical laminectomy. Despite the sound theory, some patients have progression of disease and confinement to a wheelchair.

LUMBAR SPINE

How many lumbar nerve roots are there?

5 lumbar nerve roots (and 5 lumbar vertebrae)

What is the relationship of a nerve root to a vertebra of the same number?

The root exits between the vertebral bodies of its own number and the one below. Thus, the L4 root exits between L4 and L5.

A herniated disc between L4 and L5 generally affects which nerve root?

Counterintuitive: A herniated disc between vertebrae L4 and L5 impinges the L5 nerve root. Anatomically, the L4 nerve root has exited the spinal canal before the disc herniation. The shoulder of the L5 root, however, is readily impinged.

Can an L4 disc ever impinge on an L4 nerve root?

Yes. This is known as a far lateral disc herniation.

What is pain traveling down the lower extremity associated with nerve root impingement called?

Sciatica

What are the 3 main components of an L4 radiculopathy?

1. Diminished knee jerk
2. Weakness of knee extension
3. Decreased sensation over the medial malleolus

What are the 2 main components of an L5 radiculopathy?

1. Weakness in dorsiflexion of the great toe and foot
2. Decreased sensation at the web space of the great and second toes

What are the 3 main components of an S1 radiculopathy?

1. Diminished ankle jerk
2. Plantar flexion weakness at the foot
3. Decreased sensation over the lateral foot

What is the treatment for acute disc herniation?

More than 85% of patients with acute lumbar disc herniation improve without surgical intervention. Conservative care includes:

1. Not more than 1 or 2 weeks of bed rest (only a few days if axial back pain is the predominant pain)
2. A short course of analgesics (nonsteroidals and/or narcotics)
3. Education to protect the patient's back
4. After recovery is underway, physical therapy or a supervised exercise regimen may be beneficial for some patients.

What are the indications for emergent surgery in the setting of acute disc herniation?

1. Acute or progressive development of motor weakness
2. Cauda equina syndrome

NEURO-ONCOLOGY

Define benign versus malignant in the setting of CNS tumors.

Malignant tumors: highly aggressive/proliferative tumors of poorly differentiated cells. Benign: less aggressive, more differentiated cell line. A benign tumor can be as lethal as a malignant variety, however, because of the continued ability to grow within the confines of the skull.

What are the most common presentations of brain tumors?

1. Progressive neurologic deficit
2. Headache
3. Seizure

What is the difference between an intra-axial and an extra-axial mass?

An intra-axial mass is within the substance of the brain itself, whereas an extra-axial mass impinges on the brain.

What is the most common location of brain tumors in adults versus children?

Adults: Supratentorial (anterior or middle fossa) Children: Infratentorial (posterior fossa)

Which group has the higher incidence of seizures?	Supratentorial tumors (adults)
What is the most common intra-axial primary brain tumor in adults?	1. Astrocytoma (#1) 2. Meningioma
What is the most common intra-axial primary tumor in children?	1. Astrocytoma (#1) 2. Medulloblastoma

ASTROCYTOMA

How are astrocytomas graded?	There are several astrocytoma grading systems, but the most commonly used is a 3-tiered system with:
	    Grade 1: Low-grade astrocytoma
	    Grade 2: Anaplastic astrocytoma
	    Grade 3: Glioblastoma multiforme
	      (GBM)

Which grade of primary brain tumor is most common in adults versus children?	Grade 3 (GBM) is by far the most common in adults. Grade 1 is most common in children.
What MRI findings are typical in low-grade glioma?	Low-grade gliomas typically do not enhance with contrast. High signal on the T2 or proton density images is always present. High-grade gliomas typically enhance on T1-weighted images. GBMs often have cysts or obvious areas of necrosis.
How do primary gliomas spread?	Primarily through the white matter tracts of the brain and through the CSF pathways
What is the cure rate for GBM?	There is no cure.
What is the treatment of GBM?	Chemotherapy and external beam radiation
What are the 1- and 2-year survival rates?	The 1-year survival rate is approximately 33%, whereas the 2-year survival rate is approximately 10%.

MENINGIOMA

What are the most common locations for a meningioma?	Parasagittal region and sphenoid bone
Is this tumor usually benign or malignant?	Benign
How does it cause focal neurologic deficits?	Compression (rather than invasion) of adjacent neural structures (an extra-axial tumor). Examples include unilateral exophthalmos and optic nerve compression.
What is the peak age of incidence for meningioma?	Age 45
What is the treatment of meningioma?	Surgical removal
What anesthetic decreases the seizure threshold?	Enflurane, so **isoflurane** is preferred in neurosurgical cases
What is the 5-year survival rate?	90%. However, recurrences are common and often necessitate additional surgical interventions.

ACOUSTIC NEUROMA

What histologic type are the cells of an acoustic neuroma?	The term acoustic neuroma is actually a misnomer. The tumor cells are actually Schwann cells that typically arise from the vestibular portion, not the cochlear portion of cranial nerve 8.
What are the most common symptoms associated with acoustic neuroma?	1. Hearing loss (virtually all patients) 2. Tinnitus 3. Dysequilibrium
Other than hearing loss, what is the most common physical finding?	Roughly one-third of patients lose the corneal reflex.
What is the treatment of acoustic neuroma?	Surgical removal (via craniotomy and/or translabyrinthine approach)

PITUITARY TUMORS

What are the 2 general presentations of pituitary tumors?	1. Endocrine disturbance (excess adrenocorticotropic hormone [ACTH], growth hormone, or prolactin) 2. Neurologic deficits due to mass effect
Do pituitary tumors most commonly arise in the anterior or posterior pituitary?	Anterior pituitary
Pituitary tumors are associated with what endocrine syndrome?	Multiple endocrine neoplasia I (MEN I).
What are the 3 components of this syndrome?	1. Pancreatic islet-cell tumors 2. Nonsecretory pituitary adenomas 3. Parathyroid tumors
What is the common visual field defect associated with pituitary adenomas?	Bitemporal hemianopsia (due to compression of the medial retinal fibers at the chiasm)
What is the difference between Cushing's syndrome and Cushing's disease?	1. Cushing's syndrome is the result of hypercortisolism. 2. Cushing's disease is caused by overproduction of ACTH by a pituitary adenoma.
What are the treatments for pituitary tumors?	1. For tumors that secrete prolactin, medical treatment with bromocriptine (dopamine agonist) is often helpful. 2. Otherwise, transsphenoidal surgery or open craniotomy, with or without adjuvant external beam irradiation

NEUROCUTANEOUS DISORDERS

What are the 4 principal neurocutaneous disorders?	1. Neurofibromatosis (NF) 2. Tuberous sclerosis 3. Von Hippel-Lindau disease 4. Sturge-Weber syndrome
Which of these disorders usually initially present with seizures?	Tuberous sclerosis, von Hippel-Lindau disease, and Sturge-Weber syndrome

Which is the most common NF?	NF-1, also called von Recklinghausen's disease, represents 90% of cases of NF.
What is the inheritance pattern of this syndrome?	NF-1 has an autosomal dominant inheritance with nearly 100% penetrance.
What are the clinical features of this syndrome?	Café au lait spots, optic gliomas, cutaneous neurofibromas, and Schwann-cell tumors on any nerve
What is the hallmark of NF-2?	Bilateral acoustic neuromas, which are virtually never seen in NF-1 patients
What is the most common cutaneous lesion in tuberous sclerosis?	Adenoma sebaceum (reddened nodules on face)

Where are the vascular malformations located in von Hippel-Lindau disease?

1. Retina (results in progressive vision loss)
2. Cerebellum (results in progressive ataxia)

What are the clinical features of Sturge-Weber syndrome?

1. Unilateral, cutaneous capillary angioma (nevus flammeus or port-wine stain of upper face)
2. Leptomeningeal venous hemangiomas with intracranial calcification (classic "railroad track" appearance on x-ray)

ASSORTED NEURO-ONCOLOGY TOPICS

Where do chordomas commonly arise?

Chordomas are tumors of the notochord remnant. They typically arise at either end of the notochord (i.e., at the clivus and at the sacrum/coccyx).

What is a PNET, and what is the most common type?

PNET stands for **p**rimitive **n**euroectodermal **t**umor. The most common type is the medulloblastoma, which accounts for about 20% of all intracranial tumors in children.

What are the most common metastases to the brain?

In descending order of frequency:
1. Lung
2. Breast
3. Renal
4. Gastrointestinal
5. Melanoma

Which primary brain tumors have potential to spread systemically?	Although brain tumors rarely spread systemically, medulloblastoma, meningioma, pineoblastomas, and choroid plexus tumors have the potential for systemic spread.
Which tumor generally arises from the roof of the fourth ventricle?	Medulloblastoma
Which tumor arises from the remnants of Rathke's pouch above the sella?	Craniopharyngioma (results in bitemporal field defects)
What are false lateralizing signs?	Clinical findings that are due to tumors but are not due to direct infiltration or compression of tumor. This situation may result in false localization of the primary tumor.
What are 2 examples of false lateralizing signs?	1. CN III or CN VI palsy secondary to herniation syndromes 2. Ipsilateral hemiparesis secondary to compression of the contralateral cerebral peduncle against the tentorial ridge

NEUROVASCULAR MALFORMATIONS

What are the basic types of vascular malformations?	1. Venous angioma 2. Capillary telangiectasias 3. Cavernous angioma 4. Arteriovenous malformations (AVM)
What is the histological appearance of AVMs?	A tangle of abnormal vessels that do not have normal brain tissue between the vessels
What is the common presentation of AVMs?	Hemorrhage (peak age 15–20) and seizure are the most common features. Headache is rare.
What are the treatment options for AVMs?	1. Surgical excision 2. Intra-arterial embolization for AVMs that are not surgically accessible 3. Gamma knife

HYDROCEPHALUS

What is hydrocephalus?	Enlargement of CSF compartments of the brain; generally results from obstruction of CSF reabsorption
What are examples of congenital and acquired etiologies of hydrocephalus?	Congenital: Aqueductal stenosis, myelomeningocele, and Dandy-Walker malformation Acquired: Meningitis, intraventricular hemorrhage, and obstruction of CSF passage by tumor
How often is hydrocephalus due to overproduction of CSF?	Very rarely (e.g., choroid plexus papilloma)
What are the signs and symptoms of hydrocephalus?	Presentation of increasing ICP with headache, nausea, vomiting, and papilledema. Late signs of impending herniation include lethargy and diplopia.
What is the level of obstruction in communicating versus noncommunicating hydrocephalus?	Communicating: At the level of the arachnoid granulations Noncommunicating: Proximal to the level of the arachnoid granulations
Why is it important to distinguish communicating from noncommunicating hydrocephalus?	Pressure engendered by an obstruction can be relieved by lumbar puncture in the case of communicating hydrocephalus, whereas noncommunicating hydrocephalus generally requires ventricular drainage.
How is persistent hydrocephalus treated?	Ventriculoperitoneal shunting (or, alternatively, ventriculopleural, ventriculoatrial, or ventriculoureteral shunting)

CONGENITAL NEUROMALFORMATIONS

What is the most common congenital neuromalformation?	Spina bifida occulta
What is the most common form of neural tube defect?	Myelomeningocele (due to failure of closure of posterior neuropore)

What is spina bifida?	Congenital absence of posterior elements of spinal vertebra (e.g., spinous processes and lamina)
What differentiates spina bifida occulta from spina bifida aperta?	Occulta form has skin overlying the spinous defect.
What is an encephalocele?	Protrusion of neural tissue through a cranial defect (due to failure of closure of anterior neuropore)
What is the most common site of encephalocele?	Occipital region
What is a meningocele?	A membrane- or skin-covered, cystic, posterior midline mass containing CSF and meninges (no neural elements)
What is the most common site of meningocele?	Lumbosacral region

INFECTIONS

BRAIN ABSCESS

What are the 5 predisposing factors for brain abscess?	1. Systemic infection 2. Immunosuppression (e.g., AIDS) 3. Localized sinus infection 4. Cranial trauma 5. Pulmonary arteriovenous fistulae
What is the most common systemic source?	Pulmonary infections; but in 25% of cases, no source is identified.
What is the most common bacterial organism?	1. In adults, *Streptococcus* species predominate, but in 80% of cases, multiple organisms (often anaerobes like *Bacteroides*) are cultured. 2. In trauma, *Staphylococcus* is the most common pathogen. 3. In infants, gram-negative organisms predominate.
What is the most common organism in patients with AIDS?	Toxoplasmosis

What is the usual treatment of brain abscess?	Medical management with a 6- to 8-week course of intravenous antibiotics is effective in many cases.
When is surgical intervention for abscess indicated?	1. If abscess exhibits significant mass effect (evidence of increased ICP or neurologic deficit) 2. If abscess approaches the ventricles (ventricular rupture carries high mortality)

SUBDURAL EMPYEMA

What are the most common sources?	1. Paranasal sinus infection 2. Otitis infection
With what dangerous vascular complication is subdural empyema associated?	Thrombophlebitis of the cerebral veins
What is the treatment?	Intravenous antibiotics and emergent surgical evacuation

PAIN SYNDROMES

What are the symptoms associated with trigeminal neuralgia (TN)?	The symptoms of TN (tic douloureux) are episodes of severe lancinating pain lasting only a few minutes. It is often triggered by facial or oral sensory stimuli.
Which divisions of the trigeminal nerve (CN V) are most commonly involved in TN?	V2 and V3 combined are most commonly involved, followed by V2 alone and V3 alone.
What are the major treatment modalities of TN?	1. Lesioning of trigeminal nerves with radio frequency, glycerol, or balloon inflation has proved reliable. 2. Posterior microvascular decompression of the nerve from associated arteries and veins has also proved reliable.
What is a cordotomy?	Interruption of the lateral spinothalamic tracts. It may be performed as an open procedure anywhere along the spinal cord or percutaneously at the level of C1–C2.

When is cordotomy most useful?	For unilateral pain below the nipple
What nerve is trapped in carpal tunnel syndrome?	The median nerve
Under what structure is the nerve trapped?	The transverse carpal ligament
Which fingers typically experience decreased pinprick sensation in carpal tunnel syndrome?	The thumb and first and second fingers
What is Tinel's sign?	Production of pain or paresthesia in the thumb and first and second fingers by gentle tapping over the transverse carpal ligament
What is meralgia paresthetica?	Pain over the anterior lateral aspect of the thigh associated with entrapment of the lateral femoral cutaneous sensory nerve
Which patients are at risk of meralgia paresthetica?	1. Obese patients 2. Patients undergoing iliac bone graft harvesting or abdominal surgery near the iliac crest

EPILEPSY SURGERY

What are the indications for surgery?	Poorly controlled severe epilepsy lasting > 1 year
What is the goal of surgery?	Resect seizure focus
How is seizure focus located?	CT, MRI, with or without surface electrodes (subdural grids)

SYRINGOMYELIA

What is syringomyelia?	Central pathologic cavitation of the spinal cord
What is the etiology?	Unknown, but associated with cranial base malformations, intramedullary tumors, or traumatic necrosis of the cord

What is the anatomic location?	Most are in the cervical/upper thoracic region; they can extend either way (syringobulbia = extension into medulla).
What are the signs/ symptoms?	First, bilateral loss of pain and temperature sensation in "cape-like" distribution (lateral spinothalamic tract involvement); enlargement of syrinx will cause further motor and sensory loss
How is the diagnosis made?	MRI will show defect in cord
What is the treatment?	Surgical (syringosubarachnoid shunt)

72

Urology

SCROTUM AND SPERMATIC CORD

ANATOMY

What are the 6 major layers of the scrotal sac and the corresponding layers of the abdominal wall?	1. Skin 2. Dartos muscle 3. External spermatic fascia: Derived from external oblique 4. Cremaster muscle: Derived from internal oblique and transversus abdominis 5. Internal spermatic fascia: Derived from transversalis fascia 6. Tunica vaginalis: Derived from peritoneum
Which nerves receive sensory information from the scrotum?	Anterior scrotum Ilioinguinal nerve Genitofemoral nerve Posterior scrotum Perineal division of the pudendal nerve Posterior femoral cutaneous nerve
What common surgical procedure can result in anesthesia of the scrotum, and why?	Inguinal hernia repair complicated by injury to the ilioinguinal nerve

INFECTIOUS DISORDERS

Fournier's Gangrene

What is Fournier's gangrene	Rapidly progressive gangrenous infection that usually involves scrotum, penis, and perineum (may extend up the abdominal wall)

What is the bacteriology?	Usually mixed infection of gram negatives and anaerobes
What is the most common origin of the infection?	Urinary tract (usually the urethra)
What are other origins?	Perianal, external genitalia, intra-abdominal process, and retroperitoneum
What is the clinical presentation?	Abrupt onset of severe pain and erythema of scrotum, penis, and perineum. The patient often declines rapidly into florid sepsis.
What are the classic physical findings?	Erythema, induration, necrosis and crepitance of involved regions; grayish discharge with foul odor
What is the mortality rate?	50%
What are the predisposing conditions?	1. Diabetes mellitus 2. Corticosteroid usage 3. Immune compromise 4. Alcohol abuse 5. Obesity 6. Trauma or surgery
What is the treatment?	IVF, IV antibiotics (triples), immediate surgical débridement

TUMORS OF THE SPERMATIC CORD

What is the most common benign tumor of the spermatic cord?	Lipoma
What is the most common malignant tumor of the spermatic cord?	Rhabdomyosarcoma
What is the usual pathologic cell type of paratesticular rhabdomyosarcoma?	Embryonal
What is a common site of early metastasis?	Retroperitoneal lymph node (LN)

What is the treatment for paratesticular rhabdomyosarcoma?

Inguinal orchiectomy and radiologic evaluation of retroperitoneal LN status:
1. If LN negative: Chemotherapy only (with vincristine and dactinomycin); no radiation
2. If LN positive: Unilateral retroperitoneal lymph node dissection (RPLND); chemotherapy with vincristine, dactinomycin, and cyclophosphamide. Radiation therapy depends on the amount of residual local or nodal disease.

PENIS AND MALE URETHRA

ANATOMY

What are the 3 erectile bodies of the penis and where does each originate?

1. Paired (2) corpora cavernosa: Just anterior to the ischial tuberosities
2. Corpora spongiosum: At the urogenital diaphragm, and expands distally to form the glans penis

Within which corporal body does the urethra run?

Corpora spongiosum

What are the covering layers of the penis?

1. Tunica albuginea: Surrounds each corpora
2. Buck's fascia: Envelops all 3 corpora
3. Colles' fascia: Lies beneath the skin of the penis from the base of the glans to the urogenital diaphragm; continuous with Scarpa's fascia of the abdominal wall
4. Skin

What are the labeled structures or layers in the cross-section of the penis?

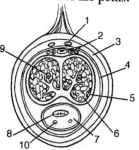

1. Cutaneous dorsal vein
2. Deep dorsal vein, artery, and nerve
3. Colles' fascia
4. Buck's fascia
5. Tunica albuginea
6. Corpora cavernosa
7. Corpus spongiosum
8. Urethra
9. Cavernosal artery and vein
10. Bulbourethral artery and vein

What are the 3 regional segments of the male urethra?	1. Prostatic urethra: Begins at bladder neck, traverses prostate, and ends at urogenital (UG) diaphragm; approximately 3 cm long 2. Membranous urethra: Traverses UG diaphragm; these encircling muscles function as the external (voluntary) urethral sphincter; approximately 2–2.5 cm long 3. Penile urethra: Begins after UG diaphragm and extends to external meatus; often subdivided into bulbous and pendulous portions; approximately 15 cm long
Which branch of the hypogastric artery supplies the majority of blood to the penis?	Internal pudendal artery
What are the 4 main branches of the previously mentioned artery that supply the penis?	1. Deep cavernosal artery of the penis 2. Deep dorsal artery of the penis 3. Bulbar artery 4. Urethral artery

INFECTIOUS DISORDERS

Urethritis

What is the classic presentation of gonococcal urethritis?	Thick, yellow urethral discharge with dysuria
How long is the incubation period?	Usually 1–5 days
What is the causative organism?	*Neisseria gonorrhoeae*
How is gonorrhea diagnosed?	1. Positive Gram stain (urethral swab showing gram-negative diplococci within PMNs), and/or 2. Positive culture growth on a modified Thayer-Martin culture plate
What are the treatment options for gonococcal urethritis?	1. Ceftriaxone 250 mg IM, plus 2. Doxycycline 100 mg PO bid for treatment of chlamydia

What is the classic presentation of nongonococcal urethritis?

Thin, white, mucoid discharge with or without dysuria

How long is the incubation period?

1–3 weeks

What is the causative organism?

1. *Chlamydia trachomatis* (most common)
2. *Ureaplasma urealyticum*
3. *Mycoplasma hominis*
4. *Trichomonas vaginalis*

How is nongonococcal urethritis diagnosed?

1. More than 4 PMNs per high-power field (hpf) in a urethral swab, and
2. Exclusion of gonococcal urethritis by Gram stain and culture

How can the presence of chlamydia be confirmed?

Conjugated monoclonal antibody test (sensitivity 93%; specificity 96%)

What are the complications of urethritis?

1. Urethral stricture
2. Epididymitis
3. Prostatitis
4. Impaired fertility

GENITAL HERPES

What is the classic presentation?

1. Primary infection: Grouped vesicles followed by painful shallow erosion lasting 4 days to 2 weeks; often associated fever, myalgias, and/or lymphadenopathy. Urinary retention can occur because of local pain.
2. Secondary infection: Usually constitutional, and local symptoms less severe; reappearance of classic painful vesicles and ulcerations

What is the causative organism?

Herpes simplex virus (HSV) type I or II

What is the regional predilection of each type?

In general, type II infects the genital region and type I infects the oral mucosal surface, but either organism can infect the external genitalia.

Where does the virus establish its latent infection?	Dorsal root ganglion
When does viral shedding occur?	When vesicles rupture. It can also occur when the patient is asymptomatic.
Which diagnostic test is used?	1. Tzanck prep of a skin lesion often reveals the virus. 2. If Tzanck is negative, obtain a viral culture.
What is the treatment?	7-day course of acyclovir can be used to decrease severity and duration of primary and secondary infections.

SYPHILIS

What is the causative organism?	The spirochete *Treponema pallidum*
What is the incubation period?	Usually 2–4 weeks
What is the classic presentation?	1. Primary syphilis: Shallow painless ulcer with rolled borders (chancre) lasting 1–5 weeks; nontender unilateral or bilateral inguinal adenopathy 2. Secondary syphilis: Copper-colored maculopapular lesions on palms, soles, oral and anogenital region; generalized lymphadenopathy 3. Tertiary (latent) syphilis: No outward signs of disease; all organs of body now infected; late manifestations in CNS, peripheral nerves (tabes dorsalis), and/or aortic arch (aortitis)
How is syphilis diagnosed?	1. Demonstration of spirochetes on dark-field exam of chancre scrapings 2. Rapid plasma reagin (RPR) serology test for syphilis may be negative for up to 3 weeks after appearance of chancre. 3. Fluorescent treponema antibody-absorption (FTA-ABS) test
What is the treatment of primary syphilis?	Benzathine penicillin G 2.4×106 U IM (1 dose)

CHANCROID

What is the clinical presentation?	Deep, ragged, painful ulcer or ulcers; foul smelling with unilateral or bilateral adenopathy
What is the causative organism?	*Haemophilus ducreyi*
How long is the incubation period?	1–5 days following exposure (usually intercourse)
How is chancroid diagnosed?	Usually clinical. Occasionally the organism grows from cultures of the ulcer.
What is the treatment?	Ceftriaxone 250 mg IM x 1 dose

LYMPHOGRANULOMA VENEREUM

What is the classic presentation?	Painless primary papule or vesicles that ulcerate, then heal. Fixed matted unilateral adenopathy develops and can form multiple draining fistulae.
What is the causative agent?	*Chlamydia trachomatis* (an obligate intracellular organism)
How long is the incubation period?	From 1 week to 3 months following exposure (usually intercourse)
How is lymphogranuloma venereum diagnosed?	Immunofluorescent serologic testing
What is the treatment?	Doxycycline 100 mg PO bid × 7 days

CONGENITAL AND ACQUIRED DISORDERS

Paraphimosis

What is paraphimosis?	A foreskin with a narrowed opening that forms a tight band behind the coronal ridge when retracted, leading to inflammation and inability to pull the foreskin back over the glans
What is the primary sequela?	Further painful swelling of the glans and foreskin, which can lead to decreased arterial flow and necrosis of the glans

| What is the treatment? | 1. Manual compression of the glans for 5–10 minutes after a penile block with 1% lidocaine may reduce its size enough to allow the foreskin to be pulled back into place. |
| | 2. If this fails, a dorsal slit is made in the constricting foreskin, followed by a formal circumcision when inflammation has resolved. Antibiotics should also be administered. |

PRIAPISM

| What is priapism? | Prolonged, often painful, erection not associated with sexual desire and lasting 4 or more hours |

What are the etiologic classifications?	1. Primary (idiopathic)
	2. Secondary
	Intracavernous injections for impotence (PGE, phentolamine, papaverine)
	Hematologic (sickle-cell disease, leukemia, hypercoagulable states)
	Oral agents (alcohol, psychotropics, antihypertensives)
	Neurogenic (anesthesia and spinal cord injury)
	Traumatic injury of cavernosal artery within corporal tissue causing traumatic arteriovenous (A-V) fistula (pelvic fracture or laceration from injection therapy)
	Malignant metastasis to the corpora

| What are the 2 most common causes? | 1. Primary ($> 50\%$) |
| | 2. Intracavernous injections for impotence |

| What are the differences between classic low-flow priapism and the high-flow priapism associated with pelvic trauma? | |

Low-flow priapism	1. Usually painful
	2. Dark, poorly oxygenated blood obtained on corporal aspiration
	3. Associated with sludging, thrombosis, and fibrosis if not treated within 24 hours

High-flow priapism	1. Usually painless 2. Red, well-oxygenated blood obtained on corporal aspiration 3. An A-V fistula exists between the injured cavernosal artery and the corpora, resulting in a persistent erection without associated sludging and thrombosis
What are the classic treatment approaches to priapism associated with sickle cell disease?	1. Oxygenation 2. Hydration 3. Alkalinization 4. Needle corporal aspiration followed by intracavernous injection of a dilute α-adrenergic compound (e.g., phenylephrine or epinephrine)
What are the general treatment approaches to the other types of low-flow priapism?	1. Aspiration of 10–20 mL of corporal blood followed by injection of dilute α-adrenergic compound every 5 minutes up to 10 doses (Note: Monitor blood pressure and heart rate; use caution in patients with cardiac or cerebrovascular disease.) 2. Surgical shunting (Multiple procedures have been described to shunt blood from the corpora cavernosa to the spongiosum or directly to the venous system.)
What is a simple, effective shunting procedure?	Winter's shunt: Shunt generated by passing a 16-gauge IV or Tru-Cut needle several times through the glans into the cavernosal bodies

PEYRONIE'S DISEASE

What is Peyronie's disease?	Fibrosis and plaque formation in the tunica albuginea of the corpora cavernosa, often associated with pain and a bending deformity with erection
What are the common etiologic theories?	1. Vasculitic immune-mediated process 2. Repeated microtrauma to the tunica during intercourse
What percentage of these conditions will resolve spontaneously?	Approximately 50%

What is the medical treatment if no resolution?	1. Vitamin E 2. Potassium para-aminobenzoate (Potaba) 3. Dimethyl sulfoxide (DMSO) 4. Intralesional steroids (triamcinolone 40 mg)
What is the surgical treatment?	Excision of plaque and placement of a dermal patch graft with or without a penile prosthesis (Note: This treatment is usually reserved for patients with angulation too severe for successful intercourse.)

TUMORS

Urethral Cancer

What is the most common histologic type?	Squamous cell carcinoma
What are the risk factors?	1. Stricture disease 2. Chronic irritation and infection
What is included in the evaluation?	1. Urethroscopy with transurethral biopsy or brushings 2. Pelvic CT to evaluate lymph node status 3. CXR
What is the difference in pattern of nodal drainage between anterior and posterior tumors?	Anterior (distal) tumors: Drain to the inguinal chain Posterior tumors: Drain to the pelvic nodes (e.g., external iliac, obturator, and hypogastric)
What are the treatment options?	1. Transurethral resection: For superficial, low-grade lesions of the proximal penile or prostatic urethra 2. Segmental urethrectomy and reanastomosis: For superficial, low-grade cancers of the penile urethra 3. Partial penectomy: For invasive lesions of the distal urethra 4. Extended en bloc cystectomy including proximal urethrectomy with excision of the pubic symphysis and subsymphyseal soft tissue: For proximal invasive bulbous or membranous urethral lesions

Is therapeutic lymph node dissection effective?	Occasional long-term survivors with inguinal or pelvic lymph node metastases have been reported following lymphadenectomy.

PENILE CANCER

What is the incidence of penile cancer in United States males?	< 1% of all malignancies
What is another name for squamous cell carcinoma in situ?	Bowen's disease
What is its appearance?	Red plaque with encrustations
What is the incidence of visceral malignancy in association with this condition?	Approximately 25%
What is the most common location of invasive penile squamous cell carcinoma?	Glans
What is the primary route of dissemination?	Lymphatic
How does location of the primary tumor affect its pattern of spread?	1. Prepuce and shaft: Superficial inguinal nodes 2. Glans and corporal bodies: Superficial and deep inguinal nodes (Note: Due to extensive cross-communications, penile lymphatic drainage is bilateral.)
What percentage of patients present with palpable nodes?	> 50%
What percentage of this enlargement is secondary to inflammation?	Approximately 50%
What is the classic Jackson staging system for penile cancer?	Stage I: Tumor involving glans or prepuce only Stage II: Tumor involving penile shaft Stage III: Operable nodal involvement Stage IV: Inoperable local, nodal, or distant metastasis

What does the metastatic workup include?	1. CXR 2. Bone scan 3. Abdominal pelvic CT scan

What is the treatment of:

Carcinoma in situ (CIS)?	Conservative treatment with fluorouracil cream or neodymium/YAG laser
Carcinoma of prepuce?	Circumcision only, provided the margin is adequate
Carcinoma of glans or distal penile shaft?	Distal penectomy with 2-cm margin
Proximal lesions?	If unable to maintain enough length for direction of urinary stream or sexual function, then total penectomy with perineal urethrostomy

TESTIS AND EPIDIDYMIS

ANATOMY

From the epithelial lining of what structures within the testis do spermatozoa develop?	Seminiferous tubules
What is the arterial blood supply to the testis?	1. Internal spermatic artery 2. Cremasteric artery 3. Artery of the vas
What is the clinical significance of this collateral blood supply?	Blood flow via the collaterals is often sufficient to allow ligation and division of the internal spermatic artery to gain extra length during orchiopexy (Fowler-Stephens orchiopexy)

What are the primary lymphatic drainage sites of the:

Right testicle?	Interaortocaval LNs followed by precaval, pre-aortic, and paracaval LNs
Left testicle?	Left para-aortic LNs followed by the preaortic LNs

| **Where is the epididymis located in relation to the normal testicle?** | Along the posterolateral surface of the testis |

ACQUIRED AND CONGENITAL DISORDERS

Ectopic Testis

| **What is the difference between an ectopic testis and a cryptorchid testis?** | An ectopic testis has descended along an abnormal path, whereas a cryptorchid testis has descended along the normal course but has not made it out of the inguinal canal. |

| **What are some observed ectopic positions and which is most common?** | 1. Superficial inguinal (most common): Migrates cephalad and lateral to the external ring
2. Femoral: Lies in the superficial femoral triangle
3. Perineal: Lies in the perineum anterior and lateral to the anus
4. Penile: Lies subcutaneously at the base of the penis
5. Crossed descent: Both testicles descending through the same inguinal canal |

CRYPTORCHID TESTIS

| **What are the etiologic theories?** | 1. Deficient maternal gonadotropin stimulation
2. Intrinsic gonadal defect, making the testicle nonresponsive to gonadotropin stimulation
3. Abnormal gubernaculum formation |

| **Why is it important for the testicles to descend?** | The scrotal location is 1–2 degrees cooler than the rest of the body, a condition that is necessary for normal spermatogenesis. |

What is the incidence of cryptorchidism in:

Preterm infant?	30%
Full-term infant?	3.5%
1 year?	0.8%
Adulthood?	0.8%

What is the single most common factor that causes a misdiagnosis of a cryptorchid testis?

A retractile testis from cremasteric contraction

If a testis is not retractile or ectopic and it cannot be palpated, what are the possible locations?

1. Canalicular: Located between the internal and external rings
2. Intra-abdominal: Located proximal to the internal ring
3. Absent

How is bilateral cryptorchidism distinguished from bilateral anorchia?

Baseline testosterone levels are obtained. Then human chorionic gonadotropin (hCG) is given for 3 days; if testicular tissue is present, an elevation in serum testosterone will be seen.

By what age should intervention for a cryptorchid testis be initiated, and why?

By 1 year of age; after this:
1. Spontaneous descent is extremely unlikely.
2. Significant histologic changes (fibrosis) occur, greatly increasing the risk of diminished fertility of the involved testis.

What is the incidence of neoplasm formation in a cryptorchid testis versus a normally descended testis?

35–50 times greater in a cryptorchid testis

Does the timing of orchiopexy affect the risk of neoplasm formation in a cryptorchid testis?

No (However, it improves the ability to examine the testis.)

Due to its abnormal position and lie, what other complication can be seen in association with an undescended testis?

Torsion (especially in the enlarged postpubertal testis)

What is the medical treatment of cryptorchid testes?

1. hCG stimulation: Increasing testicular testosterone production (Success rate 15–50%)
2. Gonadotropin-releasing hormone (Gn-RH) [specifically luteinizing hormone-releasing hormone (LH-RH)]

What are the surgical treatment options for cryptorchid testes?	Standard orchiopexy, Fowler-Stephens orchiopexy, laparoscopic orchiopexy, and testicular autotransplantation
What is a standard orchiopexy?	Incision is made in the groin, the external oblique muscle is split, and the testicle is delivered to the base of the scrotum through a separate skin incision.
What is the Prentiss maneuver?	A Prentiss maneuver may be performed by opening the floor of the inguinal canal and dividing the inferior epigastric vessels to gain additional length.
What is a Fowler-Stephens orchiopexy?	In cases with insufficient length to bring the testicle into the scrotum, the internal spermatic artery is clamped, and if adequate testicular collateral blood supply is demonstrated, the artery is divided and the testis is brought into the scrotum.
What is testicular autotransplantation?	The testicular artery is anastomosed to the inferior epigastric artery and the testicle is transplanted into the scrotum. (Note: This technically difficult procedure has relatively poor success rates.)

TUMORS

Epididymal Adenomatoid Tumors

At what age do these tumors usually present?	Third and fourth decades
What is the classic presentation?	Round, discrete, usually painless mass that can be found in any region of the epididymis
In what other regions are these lesions found?	1. Tunica albuginea of the testicle 2. Spermatic cord
What is the histologic appearance?	Acidophilic epithelial-like cells in a collagenized stroma
What are the theories of etiology?	1. Reaction to injury 2. Some ultrastructural similarities to mesotheliomas

KIDNEYS

ANATOMY

What are the dimensions of a normal adult kidney?

Vertical: 10–12 cm
Transverse: 5–7 cm
Anteroposterior: 3–4 cm

Which intra-abdominal organs are in contact with the labeled regions of anterior surface of the kidneys?

1. Adrenal gland
2. Liver
3. Colon
4. Ileum
5. Adrenal gland
6. Stomach
7. Pancreas
8. Ileum
9. Spleen
10. Colon

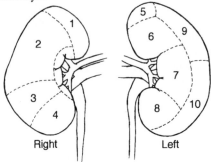

Right   Left

What is the normal location of the upper pole of each kidney relative to the:

Vertebral bodies?

Left: T12; Right: Top of L1

Ribs?

Left: To 11th rib; Right: To 11th interspace

What is the clinical significance of the location of the upper pole with regard to:

Penetrating chest trauma?

Stab wounds to the lower chest may injure the kidneys.

Surgical incision?

Inadvertent entry into the pleural space can occur during a standard flank incision (obtain a postoperative CXR).
Access to large renal tumors can be facilitated by a thoracoabdominal incision that enters the chest and splits the diaphragm to expose the upper pole.

Which structures are contained within Gerota's fascia?

1. Perirenal fat
2. Kidney
3. Adrenal gland
4. Ureter
5. Gonadal vessels

What is the order of structures in the renal hilum (anterior to posterior)?

Renal vein > Renal artery > Renal pelvis

The main renal artery:

    Arises at which vertebral level?

L2, below the superior mesenteric artery (SMA)

    Divides into what 5 segmental branches?

Anterior division: Apical, upper, middle, and lower
Posterior division: Posterior
(Segmental divisions are named after the region of parenchyma they supply.)

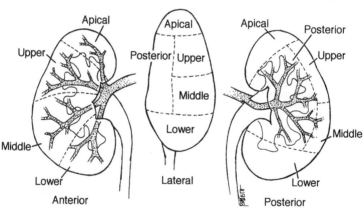

Which segmental branch is the first and most constant branch?

Posterior

What collateral drainage exists to the left renal vein?

1. Left inferior phrenic vein
2. Left adrenal vein
3. Left ascending lumbar vein
4. Left gonadal vein

What is the clinical significance of collaterals?

Surgical ligation or occlusion of the left renal vein is tolerated in most cases.

What are the components of the intrarenal collecting system?

1. Minor (tertiary) calyx: 7–9 cup-shaped structures surrounding the papilla of each renal pyramid
2. Infundibula: Narrowing of each minor calyx, which coalesces to form a major calyx
3. Major calyx: Coalescence of several infundibula to form these 2 or 3 larger drainage channels
4. Renal pelvis: Main collection chamber, which can be completely contained within the substance of the kidney or can be a large saccular extrarenal structure

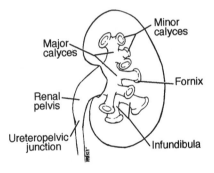

What is the fornix?

The delicate rim of each calyx or "edge of the wineglass"

RENAL PHYSIOLOGY

What are the 4 major functions of the kidney?

1. Excretion of metabolic waste products
2. Reabsorption of necessary solutes
3. Secretion of unnecessary solutes
4. Endocrine function (e.g., erythropoietin, renin, and vitamin D)

What percentage of normal cardiac output do the kidneys receive?

20–25%

What is renal clearance?

Rate at which the kidney excretes a substance in relation to its plasma concentration (mL/min)

What does clearance indirectly measure?

Glomerular filtration

How is clearance calculated?	$C = (U \times V)/P$ C = clearance (mL/min) U = urine concentration of creatinine (Cr) P = plasma concentration of Cr V = volume of urine flow in 1 minute (Note: To compare values for persons of different size, glomerular filtration rate is standardized per unit of body surface [1.73 m^2].)
Which formula allows a quick calculation of Cr clearance based on serum Cr (SCr)?	$[(140 - \text{age}) \times (\text{weight})]/(72 \times \text{SCr})$
How is the calculation altered for women?	Multiply by 0.85
What is the normal adult value for Cr clearance?	75–120 mL/min
Where is most filtered sodium reabsorbed in the nephron?	Proximal tubule (70–80% of the filtered load)
Is this an active or passive process?	Active. The energy for the function of the Na$^-$ K$^+$-pump comes from aerobic metabolism.
Where is renin produced, and what stimulates its release?	The myoepithelial (juxtaglomerular) cells of the afferent arteriole. Release is stimulated by: 1. Decreased renal perfusion 2. β-adrenergic stimulation 3. Decreased salt delivery to the distal tubule
What is the major effect of renin?	Renin converts angiotensinogen to angiotensin I, which is then converted to angiotensin II in the lung. Angiotensin II is a potent vasoconstrictor and also stimulates the release of aldosterone.
Where is aldosterone produced, and what are its major effects?	Zona glomerulosa of the adrenal cortex; it acts upon the collecting tubule, causing: 1. Increased Na$^+$ reabsorption 2. Increased H$^+$ secretion 3. Increased K$^+$ secretion

How much acid must the kidney excrete per day to maintain acid-base balance?	0.3–1.0 mEq/kg/day

How does the kidney accomplish this task, and in what part of the nephron do these mechanisms occur?

1. Reclamation of filtered HCO_3^-: Primarily in the proximal tubule
2. Generation of new HCO_3^-: Via net acid excretion (collecting tubule secretes H^+ ions, which are then bound to titratable buffers, e.g., PO_4 and NH_4^+)

INFECTIOUS DISEASES

Pyonephrosis

What is pyonephrosis?

An obstructed, infected, hydronephrotic kidney filled with purulent debris

What is the clinical presentation?

Flank pain, fever, and chills. Patients are often floridly septic.

What is the treatment?

1. Emergent drainage via percutaneous nephrostomy
2. Triple IV antibiotic coverage (e.g., ampicillin, aminoglycoside, and Flagyl)

XANTHOGRANULOMATOUS PYELONEPHRITIS

What is xanthogranulomatous pyelonephritis?

A chronic bacterial infection of the kidney associated with calculi and often partial obstruction/dilation of the collecting system

What is the classic histology?

Localized yellow nodules composed of inflammatory infiltrate and foamy macrophages

What is the target population?

Middle-aged or older women

What is the usual presentation?

Fever, flank tenderness, anorexia, or malaise

What are the common laboratory findings?

1. Anemia: 65%
2. Leukocytosis: 50%
3. Pyuria
4. Microhematuria
5. Positive urine culture (*Proteus mirabilis* and *Escherichia coli* are the most often isolated organisms)

CONGENITAL AND ACQUIRED DISORDERS

Renal Tubular Acidosis (RTA)

From what defect does type I RTA result?

Distal tubule is unable to secrete H^+ ions across a large gradient.
(Note: Proximal tubule's ability to absorb HCO_3^- is not affected.)

What are the clinical features?

1. Systemic acidosis
2. Inappropriately alkaline urine
3. Hypokalemia/hyperchloremia
4. Calcium phosphate stone formation (70%) due to hypercalciuria in the setting of low urinary citrate levels

What is the treatment?

1. Increased fluid intake
2. Sodium bicarbonate or potassium citrate to alkalinize the urine (Note: Effect can be monitored by measuring urinary citrate.)

From what defect does type II RTA result?

Proximal tubule decreased HCO_3^- reabsorptive ability, which causes extracellular fluid contraction, Cl^- reabsorption, and acidosis

What is the treatment of type II RTA?

Sodium bicarbonate or potassium citrate to correct HCO_3^- loss

PELVIC KIDNEY

What is the incidence of pelvic kidney?

1:500 to 1:1000 (the most common location of ectopic kidney)

In which sex and on which side is this condition found most commonly?

Boys; left side

Are these kidneys normal?

Approximately 50% are pathologic with poor function. Reflux is common.

What is the treatment?

Correction of reflux, if possible. Most remain asymptomatic.

ADULT POLYCYSTIC KIDNEY DISEASE

What is the pattern of inheritance?

Autosomal dominant—100% penetrance

What are the classic clinical findings?	1. Bilateral flank masses: Large cystic enlargement of both kidneys 2. Hypertension (65%) 3. Renal failure 4. Lumbar pain 5. Recurrent pyelonephritis: Infection of cysts is also common.
What are 2 associated nonrenal lesions, and what is the incidence of each?	1. Hepatic cysts (33%) 2. Aneurysm of the circle of Willis (10 to 40%)
What is the treatment?	1. General conservative measures (e.g., low protein diet, 0.5–0.75 g/kg/day) 2. Cyst decompression or drainage: Indicated for infection, obstruction, or severe distension and compression of the diaphragm 3. Nephrectomy: Indicated in a few patients with severe hemorrhage, complicated infections, or obstruction 4. Dialysis versus renal transplant (progression to renal failure common)

MULTICYSTIC DYSPLASTIC KIDNEY DISEASE (MCKD)

What is the typical renal appearance in this disorder?	Grape-like cystic structures replace the kidney, which has little true stroma and no calyceal system.
What are the etiologic theories?	1. Severe hydronephrosis secondary to atresia of the ureter or pelvis 2. Failure of union between the ureteric bud and metanephric blastema
On which side is this disorder more typically seen?	Left
What is the presentation of MCKD?	Diagnosis may be via prenatal ultrasound, or later in life on evaluation of abdominal pain, hematuria, or hypertension
What abnormalities of the contralateral kidney are associated with MCKD?	1. Ureteropelvic junction obstruction 2. Obstructive megaureter
What name is given to the syndrome of bilateral MCKD?	Potter's syndrome

What are the clinical features of this syndrome?	1. Classic facial appearance (blunted nose, prominent skinfold beneath each eye, depression between lower lip and chin, and broad ear lobes) 2. Bilateral multicystic dysplastic kidneys 3. Oligohydramnios
What is the prognosis of this syndrome?	Incompatible with life
What test is most useful in differentiating MCKD from severe hydronephrosis?	Dimercaptosuccinic acid (DMSA) renal scan: Function (i.e., radioisotope clearance) is usually present with hydronephrosis and not with MCKD.
What is the treatment?	Controversial. Most advocate conservative management unless severe flank pain is present. Then, the best management is with simple nephrectomy.

TUMORS

Oncocytoma

What is the distinguishing histologic feature?	Uniform cells with eosinophilic granular cytoplasm due to increased number of mitochondria
Are the cells benign or malignant?	Benign
Which characteristic angiographic feature is often noted?	"Spoke wheel" configuration of arterioles (Note: This appearance can also be seen in renal cell cancers.)
What is the treatment?	Due to the similar radiographic and clinical appearance with renal cell cancer, these lesions are usually treated with nephrectomy.

PROSTATE

ANATOMY

What percentage of the prostate gland is:	
Fibromuscular stroma?	40%
Glandular epithelial tissue?	60%

From what embryonic structures does the prostate originate?

Urogenital sinus (with the exception of the central zone and ejaculatory ducts, which are of wolffian origin)

What are the major zones of the prostate?

1. Peripheral zone: Together with the central zone, it makes up 95% of the gland.
2. Central zone: Surrounds the ejaculatory ducts and is found in the posterior portion of the gland
3. Transition zone: Surrounds the urethra and verumontanum
4. Anterior fibromuscular area: Forms a cap over the anterior surface of the prostate and has some sphincteric action

In which zone does benign hyperplasia arise?

Transition zone

In which zones do adenocarcinomas arise?

Peripheral (60–70%), transition (10–20%), and central (5–10%) zones

Which vessel supplies the majority of blood to the prostate?

Inferior vesical artery. Branches supply the seminal vesicle, and then the artery divides into the urethral group (supplying bladder neck and periurethral gland) and the capsular group (supplying the outer prostate).

Which nerve roots contribute autonomic innervation to the prostate and seminal vesicles?

Parasympathetic visceral efferents from S2 to S4 and sympathetics from T11 through L2

Which structures mark the macroscopic location of the nerves supplying innervation to the cavernosal bodies?

The lateral pedicle of the inferior vesical artery marks the location of the "neurovascular bundle," which runs dorsolaterally (outside Denonvilliers fascia) in the lateral pelvic fascia.

INFECTIOUS DISORDERS

Acute Bacterial Prostatitis

What are the causative organisms?

1. *E. coli*
2. *Pseudomonas* species
3. *Streptococcus faecalis*

What are the routes of infectious spread?	1. Retrograde ascent up the urethra 2. Reflux of infected urine into the prostatic ducts 3. Direct lymphatic spread from the rectum 4. Blood-borne infection
What are the usual presenting symptoms?	Perineal or low sacral pain, fever, chills, irritative voiding symptoms, and varying degrees of obstruction
What is found on digital rectal exam?	Swollen, firm, indurated, and extremely tender prostate
Should a prostatic massage be performed to express the infecting pathogen, and why?	No. Vigorous prostatic manipulation can result in significant bacteremia, and urine cultures alone are often positive.
If the patient cannot empty his bladder completely, should a Foley catheter be inserted?	No, for the reason mentioned previously. If significant residual urine exists, a percutaneous suprapubic tube should be placed.
What are the complications of prostatitis?	1. Septic shock 2. Pyelonephritis 3. Epididymitis 4. Prostatic abscess
What is the treatment for *acute* prostatitis in an uncompromised patient?	Trimethoprim-sulfamethoxazole (TMP/SMX) PO for 14 days
What is the treatment for *chronic* prostatitis?	TMP/SMX for 3 months or quinolones × 1 month
What is the treatment of prostatitis in a septic or otherwise compromised patient?	1. Gentamicin IV or IM and ampicillin IV for 1 week 2. Thereafter, oral agents for 30 days

PROSTATIC ABSCESS

What is the difference between causative organisms seen today and those seen prior to widespread antibiotic use?	The primary causative agent is now *E. coli*, whereas *N. gonococcus* predominated in the pre-antibiotic era.

What is the etiology?	Usually a complication of acute bacterial prostatitis
What are the clinical symptoms?	Identical to those of acute prostatitis
What are the findings on digital rectal exam?	Tender, fluctuant prostate with asymmetric enlargement
What is the best imaging modality for confirming the diagnosis?	Transrectal ultrasound
Which patient group has a much higher incidence of abscess formation?	AIDS patients
What is the treatment of prostatic abscess?	1. Surgical drainage via transurethral unroofing or transperineal drainage 2. Antibiotic coverage: Similar to that for acute prostatitis

BLADDER

ANATOMY

What is the capacity of the normal adult bladder?	350–450 mL
What is the urachus?	The fibrous remnant of the allantois, which joins the dome of the bladder with the umbilicus
What is the clinical significance?	1. Varying degrees of patency can result in urachal cysts, diverticula, or sinuses. 2. Often the site of origin of bladder adenocarcinoma
What is the main muscle of the bladder, and how are its fibers arranged?	Detrusor muscle: 1. Inner: Longitudinal 2. Middle: Circular 3. Outer: Longitudinal
In the male bladder, from what vessels does the major arterial blood supply come?	The superior, middle, and inferior vesical arteries, which arise from the anterior division of the hypogastric artery (Minor branches arise from the obturator and inferior gluteal artery.)

Where is the major lymphatic drainage of the bladder?	External iliac, common iliac, and hypogastric LNs
Which nerve fibers supply the contractile innervation of the detrusor muscle?	Parasympathetic fibers via S2 to S4
What supplies the motor innervation of the trigone and bladder neck sphincter?	Sympathetic fibers from T11 to T12 and L1 to L2

INFECTIOUS DISORDERS

Acute Cystitis

What are the most common causative organisms?	1. Coliform bacteria (*E. coli* most common) 2. Gram-positive organisms are also occasionally found (e.g., *Enterococci* and *Staphylococcus saprophyticus*)
How do these organisms gain access to the bladder?	Ascending infections from the urethra
What viral infection is reported to cause hemorrhagic cystitis in children?	Adenoviral infection
Are men or women more commonly affected?	Women
What is the clinical presentation?	1. Irritative voiding symptoms (e.g., frequency, urgency, and dysuria) 2. Suprapubic discomfort 3. Hematuria or foul-smelling urine
What are the laboratory findings?	1. CBC may show mild WBC elevation with a left shift. 2. UA shows WBCs, RBCs, and bacteria.
What are the complications?	1. Ascending pyelonephritis 2. Epididymitis 3. Prostatitis

What is the treatment?	1. Hydration 2. In uncomplicated patients, oral antibiotic therapy for 1–3 days is usually adequate (e.g., ampicillin, nitrofurantoin, or TMP/SMX). 3. In complicated patients (e.g., associated calculi, diabetes, or immunocompromise), intravenous therapy may be necessary.

CONGENITAL AND ACQUIRED DISORDERS

Interstitial Cystitis

What is interstitial cystitis?	Chronic irritative process of the bladder wall leads to fibrosis, pelvic pain, and irritative voiding symptoms.
Which group of patients does it tend to affect?	Middle-aged women
What are the etiologic theories?	1. Autoimmune collagen disease 2. Hypersensitivity response to food allergens 3. Obstruction of the pelvic lymphatics secondary to surgery causing fibrosis 4. Fibrosis secondary to thrombophlebitis from recurrent bladder infections 5. Arteriolar spasm secondary to vasculitic or psychogenic impulses
What is the clinical presentation?	1. Worsening irritative voiding symptoms (e.g., frequency, urgency, and nocturia) 2. Suprapubic pain made worse by bladder distension and relieved with voiding 3. Microscopic hematuria, which may progress to gross hematuria with bladder overdistension
What are the classic cystoscopic findings?	Areas of punctate hemorrhage (i.e., glomerulations), stellate splitting of the dome, and occasional areas of ulceration (i.e., Hunner's ulcer)

What is the treatment?	No definitive treatment; the goal is symptomatic pain relief. The following methods have been tried with varying degrees of success: 1. Hydraulic distension under anesthesia 2. Instillations of dimethyl sulfoxide (DMSO) every 2 weeks 3. Irrigations with 0.4% oxychlorosene sodium (Clorpactin) 4. Corticosteroids (unpredictable results) 5. Surgical therapies such as augmentation and loop diversion (unpredictable results)

Hemorrhagic Cystitis

What chemotherapeutic agent is most often associated with this condition?	Cyclophosphamide (the urotoxic metabolite acrolein is the etiologic agent)

TUMORS

Adenocarcinoma of the Bladder

What percentage of bladder cancer does adenocarcinoma represent?	< 2%
What are the 3 possible sites of origin?	1. Primary bladder adenocarcinoma arising from the base of the bladder 2. Urachal remnant 3. Metastatic adenocarcinoma from the gastrointestinal or the female gynecologic tract
What developmental abnormality is associated with increased risk of this condition?	Classic bladder extrophy
What is the treatment?	Preoperative radiotherapy with 3000 cGy followed by radical cystectomy

SQUAMOUS CELL CARCINOMA (SCCa) OF THE BLADDER

What percentage of bladder lesions does SCCa represent?	< 8%

What are the risk factors?	1. Chronic indwelling catheter or other foreign body irritation
	2. Vesical calculi
	3. Stricture disease
	4. Infection with *Schistosoma haematobium*
What is the treatment?	1. Superficial well-differentiated tumors can be treated with transurethral resection or partial cystectomy.
	2. Locally invasive lesions should receive preoperative radiotherapy with 3000 cGy and radical cystectomy.
	3. There is no effective chemotherapy for metastatic squamous cancers.

Transitional Cell Carcinoma (TCCa) of the Bladder

What are the classic demographics in terms of age, sex, and race?	1. Mean age 65 years
	2. Male-to-female ratio of 2.7:1
	3. White to African American ratio of 4:1
What are the known occupational risk factors?	Exposure to the aromatic amines:
	1. Benzidine
	2. β-naphthylamine
	3. 4-aminobiphenyl (Note: These substances are most commonly encountered in the manufacturing of dyes, rubber, textiles, and plastics.)
What are the known nonoccupational risk factors?	1. Cigarette smoking: This risk factor is present in 50% of men and 30% of women.
	2. Dietary nitrosamines
	3. Cytoxan exposure
What are the TMN stage groupings of TCCa of the bladder?	T0—Papillary lesion confined to the mucosa
	TIS—Carcinoma in situ (CIS)
	T1—Tumor invading submucosa or lamina propria
	T2—Tumor invading superficial muscle
	T3—Tumor invading deep muscle or perivesical fat; LN negative
	T4—Tumor extending into adjacent organs, LN involvement, or distant metastasis

Which histologic features determine the grade of a lesion, and how does this correlate with tumor invasiveness?	Grade is determined by:
	1. Cellular atypia
	2. Nuclear abnormalities
	3. Number of mitotic figures
	    Grade 1: Well differentiated (10% are invasive)
	    Grade 2: Moderately differentiated (50% are invasive)
	    Grade 3: Poorly differentiated (> 80% are invasive)

What is the most common presenting sign of bladder cancer?	Hematuria, either gross or microscopic (present in 85–90%)
What is another common presenting complaint more often seen in association with diffuse CIS?	Irritative voiding symptoms such as dysuria, frequency, and urgency
What is the evaluation?	1. UA, culture, and bladder washings for cytology 2. Bimanual exam (usually performed under anesthesia at the time of cystoscopy and deep bladder biopsy) 3. Intravenous pyelogram to rule out concomitant upper tract disease 4. Cystoscopy with directed deep biopsy of any suspicious lesions and random cold-cup biopsies of the 4 walls, trigone, and prostatic urethra 5. CT scan to determine presence of intra-abdominal metastases and nodal involvement > 1.5 cm
What is the treatment of CIS?	1. Due to the high risk of progression to invasive disease (50–75%), these lesions are treated with intravesical bacillus Calmette-Guérin (BCG; an attenuated strain of *Mycobacterium bovis*) 2. Recurrences can be treated by a repeat course of BCG or radical cystectomy.
What is the treatment of stage T0 and T1?	1. Transurethral resection of the bladder tumor (TURBt) 2. Recurrences can be treated with repeat TURBt with or without intravesical chemotherapy.

What are the indications for intravesical chemotherapy in superficial bladder TCCa?	1. CIS 2. Multicentricity 3. Rapid recurrence 4. Progression to higher grade
What are the most common intravesical agents?	1. Thiotepa 2. Mitomycin C 3. Doxorubicin 4. BCG
How often should superficial lesions be followed with repeat cystoscopy and cytology?	Every 3 months
What is the treatment of stage T2 and T3 (muscle-invasive) TCCa?	1. Radical cystectomy with bilateral pelvic LN dissection and urinary diversion 2. Preoperative radiotherapy (3000 cGy) is controversial; some studies have shown a decrease in the incidence of recurrence in patients with full-thickness muscle invasion. 3. Partial cystectomy may be performed for isolated lesions of the posterior wall, lateral wall, dome, or within a diverticulum in the absence of CIS.
What is the treatment of stage T4?	1. Combination methotrexate, vinblastine, adriamycin, and cisplatin (MVAC) 2. A cystectomy may be performed for uncontrolled bleeding, but does not improve overall survival rate.

COLLECTING SYSTEM AND URETERS

ANATOMY

From what major vessels does the ureter receive its arterial blood supply?	1. Upper and middle ureter: Renal, gonadal, aorta, and common iliac arteries 2. Distal ureter: Internal iliac, superior vesical, uterine and vaginal (in females), middle rectal, and inferior vesical arteries
What are the 3 anatomic narrowings of the ureter and their usual calibers?	1. Ureteropelvic junction: 2 mm 2. Iliac vessel crossing: 4 mm 3. Ureterovesical junction: 3–4 mm

What is the significance of these narrowings?	They are the most common sites of stone obstruction.

CONGENITAL AND ACQUIRED DISORDERS

Ureteropelvic Junction Obstruction

What are the etiologies?	1. Intrinsic circular smooth muscle disorder 2. Compression due to a crossing vessel from the lower pole of the kidney 3. High insertion of the ureter on the renal pelvis 4. Valvular fold of mucosa (rare)
What is the male to female ratio?	2.5:1
What are the usual presenting symptoms?	1. Infants usually present with an asymptomatic flank mass, evaluation of hydronephrosis detected on prenatal U/S, or urosepsis. 2. Children and adults usually present with episodic flank pain with or without associated vomiting.
What percentage present during the first year of life?	25%
Which studies are included in the evaluation?	1. Intravenous pyelogram (IVP) can usually establish the diagnosis. 2. Diuretic DTPA renogram is useful in equivocal cases. 3. Retrograde pyelogram is often attempted to further define the region of obstruction.
What are the treatment options?	1. Open pyeloplasty (gold standard therapy) 2. Laparoscopic pyeloplasty 3. Antegrade or retrograde pyelotomy

VESICOURETERAL REFLUX (VUR)

What is VUR?	Abnormal backward flow of urine from the bladder up the ureter (and possibly into the intrarenal collecting system)
What are the complications?	1. Recurrent infections 2. Renal parenchymal scarring 3. Renal damage (reflux nephropathy)

Which factors contribute to the occurrence of reflux?

1. Shortened intramural segment of ureter (less than a 4:1 ratio of intramural segment to ureteral diameter)
2. Abnormal ureteral orifice due to varying degrees of diminished supporting musculature (i.e., stadium orifice or golf hole)
3. Ectopic lateral displacement of the ureter
4. Edema secondary to infection or inflammation
5. Displacement from a diverticulum or from the ureterocele of a duplicated ureter

What is the gold standard diagnostic test for VUR?

Voiding cystourethrogram

What is the radiographic grading system for VUR?

Grade I: Ureter only
Grade II: Into the intrarenal collecting system without dilation
Grade III: Reflux into the calyceal system with loss of the fornices
Grade IV: Moderate dilation of renal pelvis, calyces, and ureter with or without ureteral tortuosity
Grade V: Severe dilation of the ureter, renal pelvis, and calyces with a markedly tortuous ureter

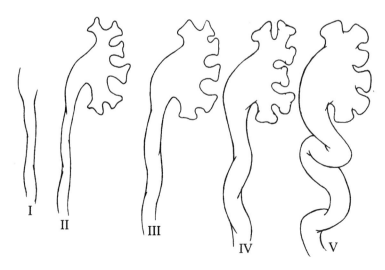

What is a "Boari Flap"?

Provides length to a shortened ureter

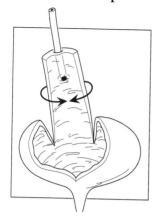

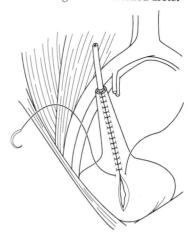

What is a "Psoas Hitch"?

Provides length to a shortened ureter

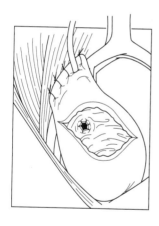

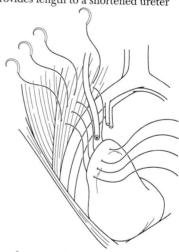

What is the medical treatment of VUR?

Low-dose suppressive antibiotics, frequent urine culture, yearly nuclear or voiding cystourethrogram, and an IVP every 2 years

What are the indications for medical treatment?

Young patients without evidence of progressive renal damage and a normal appearing ureteral orifice

What is the surgical treatment of VUR?

Ureteral reimplantation (Of the many techniques, the primary principle of each is to increase the length of the intravesical ureter.)

What are the indications for surgical treatment?

1. Progressive scarring or pyelonephritis despite medical therapy
2. Poor compliance with medical therapy
3. Reflux in association with a significant anatomic abnormality such as a diverticulum, duplication, ureterocele, or ectopic location

What is its claim to fame?

Most common anomaly of the urinary tract

What is the female-to-male ratio?

2:1

What is the Meyer-Weigert rule?

In a duplicated system, the ureteral orifice draining the upper pole is located inferiorly and medial to the lower pole ureter.

Which of the duplicated ureteral orifices most commonly refluxes?

The lower pole ureter

ECTOPIC URETER

What is ectopic ureter?

The ureteral orifice opens into the urinary tract in a position other than its normal location on the trigone

With what other condition is this anomaly often associated?

Ureteral duplication

What are the most common extravesical ectopic sites in men?

1. Posterior urethra
2. Seminal vesicle

What are the most common extravesical ectopic sites in women?

1. Urethra
2. Vestibule
3. Vagina

What is the treatment?

1. Partial nephroureterectomy if the ectopic ureter drains a nonfunctioning renal segment
2. Pyeloplasty and distal ureterectomy if the renal moiety is functioning
3. A primary reimplantation if a single ureter is ectopic

IDIOPATHIC RETROPERITONEAL FIBROSIS

What is idiopathic retroperitoneal fibrosis?

A chronic inflammatory process in the retroperitoneum, which can encompass the ureters

What is the primary complication?

Ureteral obstruction and hydroureteronephrosis

What are the etiologies?

1. Primary: Idiopathic
2. Secondary:
   Cancer (e.g., breast, ovarian, prostate)
   Several drugs/medications (e.g., methysergide, hydralazine, β-blocker)
   Infections (e.g., tuberculosis, syphilis)
   Radiation exposure
   Inflammatory processes (e.g., leaking aortic aneurysm, inflammatory bowel disease)

What is the usual presentation?

Flank or abdominal pain

What is the most useful diagnostic modality for evaluating this condition?

Abdominal and pelvic CT scan with contrast to define extent of involvement and to evaluate for underlying malignancy

What is the treatment?

Diagnostic biopsy of the retroperitoneal process followed by intraperitonealization of the ureters (Note: Some surgeons advocate wrapping the ureters with segments of omentum to keep them from becoming reincorporated in the process.)

TUMORS

Transitional Cell Carcinoma (TCCa) of the Renal Pelvis or Ureter

What percentage of TCCa tumors are located in either the renal pelvis or ureter?

Approximately 4%

What percentage of patients with an upper tract tumor will develop a lesion in the lower tract?

33%

What are the most common presenting complaints?	1. Hematuria: Most common (70–80%) 2. Flank pain: Due to obstruction from clot or tumor
What studies and procedures are included in the evaluation?	1. UA with cytology 2. IVP: Often the initial study; also to evaluate the contralateral collecting system 3. Cystoscopy with retrograde pyelogram and selective ureteral washings: To further define the lesion and to gain a pathologic diagnosis. Cystoscopy is necessary to rule out concomitant disease in the bladder. 4. Ureteropyeloscopy with brush biopsies (occasionally necessary) 5. Abdominal and pelvic CT scan: To evaluate for obvious metastases 6. Chest x-ray
What is the staging system?	Stage 0: CIS or superficial papillary cancer Stage I: Invasion of the lamina propria Stage II: Invasion of the underlying smooth muscle Stage III: Invasion of the peripelvic fat, periureteral fat, or renal parenchyma Stage IV: Invasion through the renal capsule, into adjacent organs or metastases to LN or distant organs
What is the treatment of:	
Low-stage, low-grade distal ureteral tumor?	Distal ureterectomy, excision of a cuff of bladder and ureteral reimplantation
Stage I to III tumors?	Nephroureterectomy (Note: In patients with a solitary renal unit, more conservative therapy such as segmental ureteral resection or endoscopic pelvic resections followed by chemotherapeutic instillations have all been tried, with variable results.)
Stage IV tumors?	Combination chemotherapy using MVAC

MISCELLANEOUS

On what side is testicular cancer more common?	Right
What is a "Goldblatt kidney"?	A small shrunken kidney due to renal artery stenosis
What is a varicocele?	Dilation of spermatic cord veins (no valves), pampiniform plexus, and spermatic veins

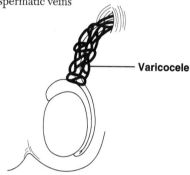

Varicocele

On what side is a varicocele more common?	Left
What is the "BCG" intravesical agent, and how does it work?	**B**acillus **C**almette-**G**uérin (BCG) tuberculin agent: Works by increasing patient's own immune response against the tumor
What is the recurrence rate of TURB (transurethral resection of the bladder)?	Increased risk because of "field effect" (i.e., the uniform exposure of the urothelium as it is bathed in urinary carcinogens). Therefore, surveillance with repeat cystoscopy and urinary cytology every 3–4 months is required.
What is the most likely outcome with TURP (transurethral resection of the prostate)?	More than two-thirds of patients have improvement in urinary symptoms.
What is a complication from forceful digital rectal exam with patient with severe prostatitis?	Bacteremia and septic shock

ANATOMY

What are the labeled ocular structures?

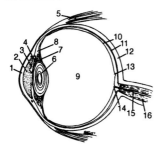

1. Cornea
2. Anterior chamber
3. Iris
4. Posterior chamber
5. Conjunctiva
6. Lens
7. Zonular fibers
8. Ciliary body
9. Vitreous humor
10. Retina
11. Choroid
12. Sclera
13. Macula
14. Optic disk
15. Retinal artery and vein
16. Optic nerve

What are the labeled structures in this anterior view of the dissected orbital cavity?

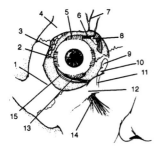

1. Zygomatic bone
2. Lateral rectus muscle
3. Lacrimal gland
4. Frontal bone
5. Superior rectus muscle
6. Superior oblique tendon
7. Supraorbital muscle
8. Trochlea of superior oblique muscle
9. Lacrimal canaliculi (duct)
10. Lacrimal sac
11. Nasolacrimal duct
12. Maxilla
13. Inferior rectus muscle
14. Infraorbital nerve
15. Inferior oblique muscle

OPHTHALMOLOGIC EXAMINATION

What are the basic components of the bedside ophthalmologic examination?

Systematically evaluate structures from anterior to posterior:

Orbital rim—Palpate for crepitus, step-off deformities; test for periorbital hypesthesia

Eyelid—Inspect lid for lacerations/foreign bodies (examination should include careful lid eversion)

Visual acuity—Test with counting of fingers (or reading of card eye chart)

Globe—Test extraocular muscles; inspect for laceration or rupture

Conjunctiva—Inspect for subconjunctival hemorrhage, laceration, emphysema, or foreign body

Anterior chamber—Inspect for hyphema and chamber depth (tangential lighting)

Iris—Inspect for shape and reactiveness

Lens—Inspect for transparency and position (dislocated?); red reflex?

Vitreous humor—Inspect for transparency

Retina—Inspect for hemorrhage and detachment

What may absence of red reflex suggest?

Cataract, vitreous hemorrhage, or retinal detachment

What may lid ptosis suggest?

Injury to levator palpebrae or its innervation (CN III)

NONTRAUMATIC OCULAR EMERGENCIES

ORBITAL CELLULITIS

What are the most common microbial etiologies?

Gram-positive cocci (*Streptococcus, Staphylococcus*); *Haemophilus influenzae* (in children < 5 years of age)

What are the routes to orbit?

Direct extension via paranasal sinuses, vascular drainage from periorbital soft tissue, and occasionally hematogenous spread from distant site

What is the usual presentation?	Acute onset of severe orbital pain, reduced mobility of eye, conjunctival chemosis (edema), reduced vision, malaise, fever, and in some cases, marked periorbital erythema and edema
What are the sequelae?	Cavernous sinus thrombosis due to thrombophlebitis of the orbital veins, blindness due to optic neuritis, spread of infection to brain or meninges
What is the treatment?	Hospitalization, systemic antibiotics, warm packs, bed rest; occasionally, surgical drainage indicated (Note: Most experts recommend CT scan of orbit to exclude abscess.)

GLAUCOMA

What is it?	An ocular disease complex primarily characterized by an **increased intraocular pressure.**
What are the 3 different types?	1. **Chronic open angle:** Bilateral, insidious, slowly progressive; most common type (90%) 2. **Narrow angle:** Acute obstruction of aqueous outflow; painful, acute visual loss, cloudy cornea 3. **Congenital:** Genetically transmitted; often appearing in first year of life
What is the pathophysiology?	Increased ocular pressure related to increased intraocular aqueous humor production, decreased outflow of aqueous humor from the eye, or both, leading to optic nerve degeneration
How is the diagnosis made?	1. Increased intraocular pressure 2. Retinoscopy (optic disc cupping) 3. Peripheral visual field testing
What is the treatment?	Decrease intraocular pressure through topical eyedrops, surgery, or both
What are the surgical treatment options?	Laser iridotomy (Note: The contralateral eye is also prophylactically treated.)

HYPHEMA

What is hyphema?	Hemorrhage into anterior chamber of the eye; seen as meniscus or layering of blood anterior to iris
What percentage of patients rebleed?	Between 10% and 30% rebleed in the first week post-trauma.
What is the medical management of hyphema?	Controversial. The most conservative treatment involves elevation of head for 5 to 7 days ($\pm$ admission to hospital), bed rest, daily examination, and tonometry (to ensure absorption of blood without development of glaucoma).
What are the indications for surgical washout of hyphema?	Blood staining of cornea, secondary glaucoma

CONJUNCTIVAL EMPHYSEMA

What is the usual etiology of conjunctival emphysema?	Fracture of sinus (often the lamina papyracea of the ethmoid bone) permitting air to dissect under the conjunctiva
What special instructions should be given to the patient?	Patient should not blow nose, because acute increases in sinus pressure result in further dissection.

LENS DISLOCATION

What is the mechanism of lens dislocation?	Disruption of > 25% of zonular fibers (anchored to ciliary body), which hold lens to posterior surface of iris
What is the usual presentation?	Blurred vision (often subtle)
Which general type of lens dislocation is a surgical emergency, and why?	Anterior; can cause acute glaucoma (Note: Posterior dislocation into vitreous humor is treated electively after resolution of inflammation.)
What is the classic LATE complication of blunt trauma?	Retinal detachment (due to retinal tear)

What is the usual presentation?	Decreased visual acuity (due to slowly progressive and painless dissection of retina from choroid)
What is the treatment?	Cryosurgery and/or scleral buckling (performed emergently if the macula is threatened because it can prevent permanent loss of central vision)

CORNEA

What is keratitis?	Inflammation of the **cornea** secondary to an infectious or mechanical etiology
What infectious agents are frequently involved?	*Staphylococcus, Streptococcus, Pseudomonas,* herpes, *Chlamydia*
What predisposes the cornea to infection?	Exposure, trauma
What is the treatment of corneal opacities secondary to scarring?	Corneal transplant

MISCELLANEOUS

What are the terms used to describe the constriction and dilatation of the iris?	Miosis-parasympathetic-mediated constriction Mydriasis-sympathetic-mediated dilatation
What type of ophthalmologic medication should not be given to the patient for outpatient use, and why?	Local anesthetics. Patient may further injure eye without realizing it, and these agents often delay healing.
What drugs are used to reduce the spasm of the ciliary muscle frequently seen with ocular injuries?	Cycloplegic-anticholinergic agents (e.g., atropine drops)
What are the untoward sequelae of topical corticosteroids?	Herpes simplex keratitis, cataract formation, fungal infection, and acute-angle glaucoma

Which injuries to the eye classically first present with symptoms 4 to 12 hours after injury?

Ultraviolet burns of cornea (e.g., welding arc, "snow blindness")

What is the associated finding on examination?

Diffuse punctate fluorescein staining of corneas

What is the treatment?

Topical corticosteroids, oral analgesia (Note: Resolution of symptoms in 1–2 days without sequela)

Which lacerations to the eyelid should be repaired by an ophthalmologist or plastic surgeon?

Lacerations involving:
1. Medial canthal region
2. Deep or through-and-through laceration involving the tarsal plate
3. Edge of lid (risk of obvious lid notching)

What is a cataract?

Opacification of the lens

What is dacrocystitis?

Infection of the lacrimal sac

What is the usual etiology?

Obstruction of nasolacrimal duct with resultant *Streptococcus pneumoniae* infection (In infants, *Haemophilus influenzae* is the responsible organism.)

THE RED EYE

What are the 8 signs of serious ocular pathology in a red eye?

1. Visual loss
2. Pain
3. Opacities
4. Pupil irregularities
5. Perilimbal erythema
6. Increased pressure
7. History of eye disease
8. Refractory to treatment

Index

Page numbers followed by t indicate table. Page numbers in *italics* indicate figure.